Study Guide for

Brunner and Suddarth's Textbook of Medical-Surgical Nursing

TWELFTH EDITION

Mary Jo Boyer, R.N., M.S.N., Ph.D.
Vice Provost and Adjutant Nursing Faculty
Former Dean and Professor of Allied Health and Nursing
Delaware County Community College
Media, Pennsylvania

Wolters Kluwer | Lippincott Williams & Wilkins
Health
Philadelphia · Baltimore · New York · London
Buenos Aires · Hong Kong · Sydney · Tokyo

Acquisitions Editor: Hilarie Surrena
Product Manager: Mary Kinsella
Editorial Assistant: Victoria White
Design Coordinator: Joan Wendt
Manufacturing Coordinator: Karin Duffield
Prepress Vendor: Aptara, Inc.

12th edition

9 8 7 6 5 4

Printed in China

ISBN: 978-0-7817-8594-5

Care has been taken to confirm the accuracy of the information presented and to describe generally accepted practices. However, the author(s), editors, and publisher are not responsible for errors or omissions or for any consequences from application of the information in this book and make no warranty, expressed or implied, with respect to the currency, completeness, or accuracy of the contents of the publication. Application of this information in a particular situation remains the professional responsibility of the practitioner; the clinical treatments described and recommended may not be considered absolute and universal recommendations.

The author(s), editors, and publisher have exerted every effort to ensure that drug selection and dosage set forth in this text are in accordance with the current recommendations and practice at the time of publication. However, in view of ongoing research, changes in government regulations, and the constant flow of information relating to drug therapy and drug reactions, the reader is urged to check the package insert for each drug for any change in indications and dosage and for added warnings and precautions. This is particularly important when the recommended agent is a new or infrequently employed drug.

Some drugs and medical devices presented in this publication have Food and Drug Administration (FDA) clearance for limited use in restricted research settings. It is the responsibility of the health care provider to ascertain the FDA status of each drug or device planned for use in his or her clinical practice.

This book is dedicated to

. . . my son, Brian, and my daughter, Susan, whose career choices reflect their commitment and appreciation of lifelong learning and teaching

. . . my students whose energy, motivation, and dedication to learning challenges and enriches my professional life

Preface

The *Study Guide for Brunner and Suddarth's Textbook of Medical-Surgical Nursing, Twelfth Edition*, was developed as a learning tool to help you, a nursing student, focus on content areas considered essential for understanding the concepts, techniques, and disease processes presented in the textbook. A Critical Thinking approach was used to present facts from a knowledge-based level (using multiple choice, matching and fill in) to the highest levels of analysis and syntheses (using comparison analysis, pattern identification, contradiction recognition, supportive argumentation, and critical analysis and discussion). The application of theory to practice is tested by having you complete nursing care plans, outline detailed patient teaching guides, and complete decision-making trees and critical clinical pathways. Case studies are offered at the end of most sections.

The answer to every question is presented in the Answer Key at the end of the book. Critical thinking, the nursing process, and a community-based focus to nursing care are incorporated throughout; information is tested from the viewpoint of nursing intervention. Some answers are derived from analysis and are implied. They may not be found specifically in the chapter. Pathophysiologic processes are included only if relevant to specific nursing actions.

It was my intent to present information in a manner that will stimulate critical thinking and promote learning. It is my hope that knowledge gained and reinforced will be used to provide competent nursing care to those in need.

Mary Jo Boyer, R.N., M.S.N., Ph.D.

Contents

CHAPTER 1

Health Care Delivery and Nursing Practice

I. Interpretation, Completion, and Comparison

MULTIPLE CHOICE

Read each question carefully. Circle your answer.

1. The definition of nursing has evolved over time. According to the Social Policy Statement (2003) of the American Nurses Association (ANA), registered nurses can and should:
   a. diagnose human responses to illness.
   b. promote optimum levels of wellness.
   c. prevent illness and maintain health.
   d. do all of the above.

2. An underlying focus in any definition of nursing is the registered nurse's responsibility to:
   a. appraise and enhance an individual's health-seeking perspective.
   b. coordinate a patient's total health management with all disciplines.
   c. diagnose acute pathology.
   d. treat acute clinical reactions to chronic illness.

3. A Jewish patient who adheres to the dietary laws of his faith is in traction and confined to bed. He needs assistance with his evening meal of chicken, rice, beans, a roll, and a carton of milk. Choose the nursing approach that is most representative of promoting wellness.
   a. Nurse "A" removes items from the overbed table to make room for the dinner tray.
   b. Nurse "B" pushes the overbed table toward the bed so that it will be within the patient's reach when the dinner tray arrives.
   c. Nurse "C" asks a family member to assist the patient with the tray and the overbed table while the nurse straightens the area in an attempt to provide a pleasant atmosphere for eating.
   d. Nurse "D" prepares the environment and the overbed table and inspects the contents of the dinner tray. The nurse asks the patient whether he would like to make any substitutions in the foods and fluids he has received.

4. Using the concept of the wellness–illness continuum, a nursing care plan for a chronically ill patient would outline steps to:
   a. educate the patient about every possible complication associated with the specific illness.
   b. encourage positive health characteristics within the limits of the specific illness.
   c. limit all activities because of the progressive deterioration associated with all chronic illnesses.
   d. recommend activity beyond the scope of tolerance to prevent early deterioration.

5. To be responsive to the changing health care needs of our society, registered nurses will need to:

    a. focus their care on the traditional disease-oriented approach to patient care, because hospitalized patients today are more acutely ill than they were 10 years ago.

    b. learn how to delegate discharge planning to ancillary personnel so that registered nurses can spend their time managing the "high tech" equipment needed for patient care.

    c. place increasing emphasis on wellness, health promotion, and self-care, because the majority of Americans today suffer from chronic debilitative illness.

    d. stress the curative aspects of illness, especially the acute, infectious disease processes.

6. Continuous quality improvement (CQI) was mandated in health care organizations in 1992. This system focuses on all of the following processes *except*:

    a. analyzing similar clinical situations.

    b. assessing the impact of financial decisions on patient care delivery.

    c. examining processes that affect patient care.

    d. reviewing medication errors for individual patients.

7. Quality assurance programs created in the 1980s required that hospitals be accountable for all of the following *except*:

    a. appropriateness of care related to established standards.

    b. cost of services.

    c. staff–patient ratios for nursing care.

    d. quality delivery of services.

8. The primary focus of the nurse advocacy role in managing a clinical pathway is:

    a. continuity of care.

    b. cost-containment practices.

    c. effective utilization of services.

    d. a patient's progress toward desired outcomes.

9. Nursing practice in the home and community requires competence and experience in the techniques of:

    a. decision making.

    b. health teaching.

    c. physical assessment.

    d. all of the above.

10. Common features that characterize managed care include all of the following *except*:

    a. fixed-price reimbursement.

    b. mandatory precertification.

    c. preferred provider choice.

    d. prenegotiated payment rates.

SHORT ANSWER

Read each statement carefully. Write your response in the space provided.

1. List four phenomena frequently identified by the American Nurses Association (ANA) in 2003 as the focus of nursing care and research. An example is given:

    Pain and discomfort (Example)

    _____, _____, _____, and _____.

2. List six significant changes (socioeconomic, political, scientific, and technological) that have evolved over the last hundred years that have influenced where nurses practice.

    _____, and _____

    _____, and _____

    _____, and _____

3. List four major health care concerns that practitioners are facing today with the shift from acute to chronic illnesses: _____, _____, _____, and _____.

4. Choose four health and illness problems and write a human response to each that would require nursing intervention. An example is provided.

Health and Illness Problems	Human Response Requiring Nursing Intervention
Fractured right arm (Example)	Self-care limitations (Example)
1. _____	_____
2. _____	_____
3. _____	_____
4. _____	_____

5. According to Hood and Leddy (2007), wellness involves proactively working toward physical, psychological, and spiritual well-being. Four major concepts supporting wellness are: _____, _____, _____, and _____.

6. List Maslow's hierarchy of needs, and give an example for each need. The first need is provided as an example.

Need	Example
Physiologic (Example)	Food and water (Example)
_____	_____
_____	_____
_____	_____
_____	_____
_____	_____
_____	_____

7. Health promotion efforts today target negative lifestyle behaviors. List six examples.

_____ _____
_____ _____
_____ _____

8. Three infectious diseases that presently seem to be on the rise are: _____, _____, and _____.

9. List four comorbidities that are associated with the major health concern of obesity: _____, _____, _____, and _____.

10. Define the term *evidence-based practice* (EBP).

_____

11. Define the term *clinical pathway* as it relates to the concept of managed care.

_____

12. In addition to clinical pathways, there are four other EBP tools a nurse can use. They are:

_____, _____, _____, and _____.

13. Explain when "care mapping" may be more beneficial than "clinical pathways" for managing care.

_____

_____

14. List five common features of managed care: _____, _____,

_____, _____, and _____.

15. List the purpose and goals of case management.

_____

_____

16. List four categories of advanced practice nurses: _____, _____, _____,

and _____.

II. Critical Thinking Questions and Exercises

DISCUSSION AND ANALYSIS

Discuss the following topics with your classmates.

1. Review the clinical pathway for acute ischemic stroke that is presented in Appendix B. Discuss the range of assessments, expected outcomes, nursing diagnoses, and treatment modalities listed in the chart.
2. Discuss the primary differences between community-based nursing and community-oriented/public health nursing.
3. Discuss the current and future role of the *advanced practice nurse* (APN).

SUPPORTING ARGUMENTS

Read the paragraph below. Fill in the space provided with the best response.

Many recent changes in health care have significantly affected nursing care delivery and nursing education, including the aging population, increased cultural diversity, changing patterns of disease, the rising cost of health care, and federally legislated health care reform. Choose one factor that you believe has had *the most impact* on nursing care in the last 5 years, and support your argument with data.

The most important factor is:

_____

Supporting argument:

_____

RECOGNIZING CONTRADICTIONS

Rewrite each statement correctly. Underline the key concepts.

1. The majority of health problems in the United States today are of an infectious and acute nature.

   _____

2. A person with a chronic illness can never attain a high level of wellness, because part of his or her health potential will never be reached.

   _____.

3. It is predicted that by the year 2030, people older than 65 years of age in the United States will constitute about 35% of the total population; racial and minority groups could approach 60% of the population.

   _____

4. Those individuals with infectious diseases are the largest group of health care consumers in the United States.

   _____

5. The largest group of health care consumers in the United States is children and the middle-aged.

   _____

6. Home health care nursing is a major component of public health nursing.

   _____

EXAMINING ASSOCIATIONS

Answer the following.

1. Examine the progression of Maslow's hierarchy of needs in Figure 1-1. Consider one or more recent clinical situations where the patient's physical symptoms prevented him or her from attending to higher level needs.

   _____

   _____

2. Using Figure 1-2 in the text, examine and explain the expected behaviors among the physician, patient, nurse, and ancillary personnel in the collaborative practice model.

   _____

3. Compare the two most common models of nursing care delivery in practice today: primary nursing and patient-focused or patient-centered care.

   _____

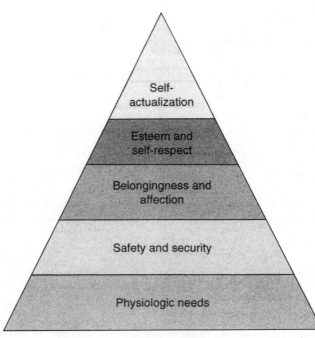

FIGURE 1-1. This scheme of Maslow's hierarchy of human needs shows how a person moves from fulfillment of basic needs to higher levels of needs, with the ultimate goal being integrated human functioning and health.

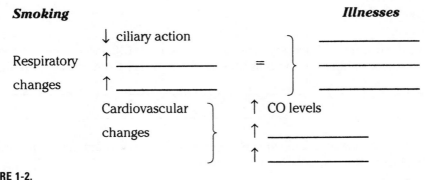

FIGURE 1-2.

CLINICAL SITUATIONS

Complete the following flow charts.

1. Continuous quality improvement (CQI) mandates the standardization of processes that are implemented and improved on a continuous basis. Complete the blank lines on the flow chart for the process of radial pulse assessment.

Radial Pulse Assessment

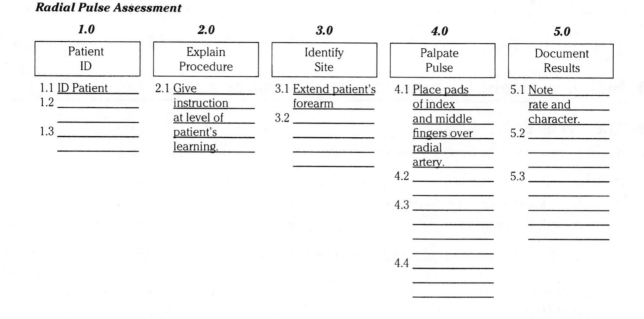

1.0	2.0	3.0	4.0	5.0
Patient ID	Explain Procedure	Identify Site	Palpate Pulse	Document Results

1.1 ID Patient
1.2 _____
    _____
1.3 _____
    _____

2.1 Give _____
    instruction _____
    at level of _____
    patient's _____
    learning. _____

3.1 Extend patient's forearm
3.2 _____
    _____
    _____
    _____

4.1 Place pads of index and middle fingers over radial artery.
4.2 _____
4.3 _____
    _____
    _____
    _____
4.4 _____
    _____
    _____

5.1 Note rate and character.
5.2 _____
    _____
    _____
5.3 _____
    _____
    _____

2. The Joint Commission on Accreditation of Healthcare Organizations (JCAHO) mandated in 1992 that health care organizations move toward implementation of CQI. A cause-and-effect diagram can illustrate potential causes of a process so that the cause can be examined and corrected and patient care improved. Complete the following diagram.

CQI Cause and Effect Diagram: Delayed Medication

Possible Causes

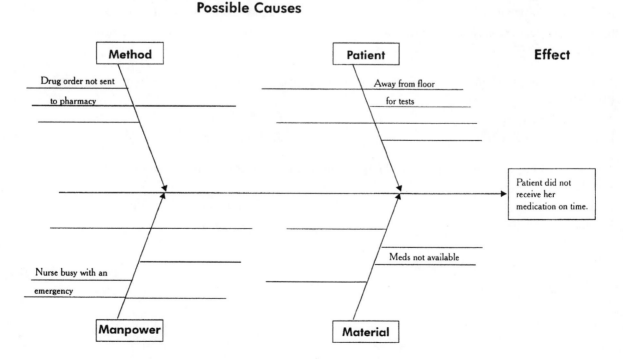

Method
Drug order not sent
to pharmacy

Patient
Away from floor
for tests

Effect

Patient did not receive her medication on time.

Nurse busy with an
emergency

Meds not available

Manpower

Material

CHAPTER 2

Community-Based Nursing Practice

I. Interpretation, Completion, and Comparison

MULTIPLE CHOICE

Read each question carefully. Circle your answer.

1. The shift in health care delivery from acute care to community-based care is primarily the result of:
   a. alternative health care delivery systems.
   b. changes in federal legislation.
   c. tighter insurance regulations.
   d. the interfacing of all three conditions.

2. Choose an alternative health care delivery system that has dramatically reduced patient-care days in acute care settings.
   a. Health Maintenance Organizations.
   b. Managed Health Care Systems.
   c. Preferred Provider Organizations.
   d. Each of the three is equally significant.

3. The most frequent users of home health services are:
   a. children with chronic, debilitating disorders.
   b. newborns who are sent home with apnea monitors.
   c. the frail and elderly who need skilled care.
   d. young adults on prolonged intravenous therapy.

4. Discharge planning from the hospital to home care begins when the:
   a. discharge order is written.
   b. nurse receives the physician's order for discharge.
   c. physician notifies the insurance company.
   d. patient is admitted to the hospital.

5. Nurses working in elementary schools are trained to deal with one of the most frequent health care problems:
   a. eating disorders.
   b. emotional problems.
   c. infections.
   d. drug abuse.

6. Nurses working with high school students are prepared to deal with the common health care problem of:
   a. influenza.
   b. cancer.
   c. alcohol and drug abuse.
   d. pneumonia.

SHORT ANSWER

Read each statement carefully. Write your response in the space provided.

1. Name three chronic conditions that are increasing in prevalence and causing an increased need for community health services: _____, _____, and _____.

2. List four factors that have affected the shift of health care delivery from inpatient to outpatient settings: _____, _____, _____, and _____.

3. List specific skills a nurse will need to function in community-based care.

   _____

4. Community-based nursing practice focuses on three primary goals: _____, _____, and _____.

5. List the four primary concepts supporting community-based nursing care: _____, _____, _____, and _____.

6. List several examples of "skilled" nursing services provided by home care.

   _____

7. The first step in preparing for a home visit is for the nurse to:

   _____

8. Explain the purpose of the initial home visit.

   _____

   _____

9. List the range of nursing responsibilities within ambulatory health care settings.

   _____

   _____

10. The homeless have high rates of health care problems such as:

    _____

II. Critical Thinking Questions and Exercises

DISCUSSION AND ANALYSIS

Discuss the following topics with your classmates.

1. Distinguish among primary, secondary, and tertiary levels of preventive care and cite a clinical case example for each level.
2. Discuss one of the major financial incentives for discharging patients from acute care facilities prior to full recovery.

3. Explain the concept of "telehealth" and its implications for nursing care. Refer to the book, *Community and Public Health Nursing*, by M. Stanhope and S. Lancaster, 2008, St. Louis, Mosby.

CLINICAL SITUATIONS

CASE STUDY: Assessing the Need for a Home Visit

Read the following case study and assess the patients' need for a home visit.

Mrs. Flynn is an 85-year-old lady who suffered a stroke on December 28. She was admitted to the emergency department and suffered another stroke on December 30. The left occipital area and the cerebellum were affected resulting in the loss of 50% of vision (right half of each eye) and loss of balance. After 2 weeks in the hospital and 10 days in a rehabilitation treatment center, Mrs. Flynn will be discharged to her one-floor home where she lives alone. Her son and daughter both live an hour away. She is capable of walking with a walker. Before the stroke, Mrs. Flynn was independent, an active member of several citizen groups, and participated in water walking at the YMCA three times a week. Her driver's license was revoked. Using Chart 2-2 in the text, complete the outline to assess Mrs. Flynn's need for a home visit. Create your own answers to several of the questions so you can complete the assessment.

Current Health Status

1. How well is the patient progressing?
2. How serious are the present signs and symptoms?
3. Has the patient shown signs of progressing as expected, or does it seem that recovery will be delayed?

Home Environment

1. Are worrisome safety factors apparent?
2. Are family or friends available to provide care, or is the patient alone?

Level of Self-Care Ability

1. Is the patient capable of self-care?
2. What is the patient's level of independence?
3. Is the patient ambulatory or bedridden?
4. Does the patient have sufficient energy or is she frail and easily fatigued?

Level of Nursing Care Needed

1. What level of nursing care does the patient require?
2. Does the care require basic skills or more complex interventions?

Prognosis

1. What is the expectation for recovery in this particular instance?
2. What are the chances that complications may develop if nursing care is not provided?

Educational Needs

1. How well has the patient or family grasped the teaching points made?
2. Is there a need for further follow-up and retraining?
3. What level of proficiency does the patient or family show in carrying out the necessary care?

Mental Status

1. How alert is the patient?
2. Are there signs of confusion or thinking difficulties?

Level of Adherence

1. Is the patient following the instructions provided?
2. Does the patient seem capable of following the instructions?
3. Are the family members helpful, or are they unwilling or unable to assist in caring for the patient as expected?

CHAPTER 3

Critical Thinking, Ethical Decision Making, and the Nursing Process

I. Interpretation, Completion, and Comparison

MULTIPLE CHOICE

Read each question carefully. Circle your answer.

1. The least effective decision-making process used in critical thinking is:
   a. analyzing data.
   b. establishing assumptions.
   c. formulating conclusions.
   d. synthesizing information.

2. The term *metacognition* refers to the critical-thinking skill of:
   a. consultation.
   b. data analysis.
   c. self-reasoning.
   d. validation.

3. *Morality* is defined as:
   a. adherence to specific codes of conduct.
   b. commitment to informal, personal values.
   c. dependence on specified principles of behavior.
   d. an understanding of defined rules of behavior.

4. When an ethical decision is made based on the reasoning of the "greatest good for the greatest number," the nurse is following the:
   a. deontological theory.
   b. formalist theory.
   c. moral-justification theory.
   d. utilitarian theory.

5. Individual patient rights regarding the freedom of choice and the right to privacy are subsumed under the ethical principle of:
   a. autonomy.
   b. beneficence.
   c. fidelity.
   d. paternalism.

6. Consider the ethical situation in which a nurse moves a confused, disruptive patient to a private room at the end of the hall so that other patients can rest, even though the confused patient becomes more agitated. The nurse's judgment is consistent with reasoning based on:
   a. "consequentialism," by which good consequences for the greatest number are maximized.
   b. "duty of obligation," by which an action, regardless of its results, is justified if the decision making was based on moral principles.
   c. "prima facie" duty, by which an action is justified if it does not conflict with a stronger duty.
   d. the "categorical imperative," by which the results of an action are deemed less important than the means to the end.

7. A hospital board of directors decided to close a pediatric burn treatment center (BTC) that annually admits 50 patients and to open a treatment center for terminally ill AIDS patients (with an expected annual admission of 200). This decision meant that the nearest BTC for children was 300 miles away. The board's decision was an example of ethical reasoning consistent with:
   a. a formalist approach.
   b. obligation or duty.
   c. "the means justifies the end."
   d. utilitarianism.

8. A terminally ill patient asks the nurse whether she is dying. The nurse's response is influenced by the moral obligation to:
   a. communicate the patient's wishes to the family.
   b. consult with the physician.
   c. provide correct information to the patient.
   d. consider all of the above measures before disclosing specific information.

9. A patient with a "Do Not Resuscitate" order requires large doses of a narcotic (which may significantly reduce respiratory function) for excruciating pain. After the patient requests pain medication, the nurse assesses a respiratory rate of 12 breaths per minute. The nurse's ethical decision should be to:
   a. ask the patient to wait 20 minutes and reassess.
   b. give half of the prescribed dose.
   c. give the pain medication without fear of respiratory depression.
   d. withhold the pain medication and contact the physician.

10. Choose the situation that most accurately represents a moral problem in contrast to a moral dilemma.
   a. Three days after surgery, a patient requests narcotic pain medication every 3 hours. The nurse administers a placebo that reduces pain.
   b. A 32-year-old father of three with advanced cancer of the lungs asks that everything be done to prolong his life, even though his chemotherapy treatments are no longer effective.
   c. A confused 80-year-old needs restraints for protection from injury, even though the restraints increase agitation.
   d. A young patient with AIDS has asked not to receive tube feedings to prolong life because of intense pain.

11. Assessment, the first of five steps in the nursing process, begins with initial patient contact. Nursing activities during this component of the nursing process include:
   a. interviewing and obtaining a nursing history.
   b. observing for altered symptomatology.
   c. collecting and analyzing data.
   d. all of the above.

12. The end result of data analysis during the assessment process is:
   a. actualization of the plan of care.
   b. determination of the patient's responses to care.
   c. collection and analysis of data.
   d. identification of actual or potential health problems.

13. A therapeutic communication technique that validates what the nurse believes to be the main idea of an interaction is known as:
   a. acknowledgment.
   b. focusing.
   c. restating.
   d. summarizing.

14. An example of a medical diagnosis, in contrast to a nursing diagnosis, is:
   a. fever of unknown origin.
   b. fluid volume excess.
   c. risk for falls.
   d. sleep-pattern disturbances.

15. In choosing the nursing action that illustrates planned nursing care prioritized according to Maslow's hierarchy of needs, a nurse would:

a. administer pain medication to an orthopedic patient 30 minutes before transportation to physical therapy for crutch-walking exercises.

b. discourage a terminally ill patient from participating in a plan of care, to minimize fears about death.

c. help a patient walk to the shower while the breakfast tray waits on the overbed table, because the shower area is vacant at this time.

d. interrupt a family's visit with a depressed patient to assess blood pressure measurement, because it is time to take the scheduled vital signs.

16. Consider the following nursing diagnosis: "Imbalanced nutrition, less than body requirements, related to inability to feed self." An example of an immediate nursing goal is that the patient will:

a. acquire competence in managing cookware designed for handicapped people.

b. assume independent responsibility for meeting self-nutrition needs.

c. learn about food products that require minimal preparation yet meet individual needs for a balanced diet.

d. master the use of special eating utensils to feed self.

17. Registered nurses are responsible for delegating patient care responsibilities to licensed practical nurses (LPNs) and ancillary personnel. The most appropriate task to delegate to a nurse aide is:

a. assessing the degree of lower leg edema in a patient on bed rest.

b. making the bed of an ambulatory patient.

c. measuring the circumference of a patient's calf for edema.

d. recording the size and appearance of a bed sore.

SHORT ANSWER

Read each statement carefully. Write your response in the space provided.

1. There are three consistent themes threaded through all definitions of critical thinking. These themes are: _____, _____, and _____.

2. List 10 characteristics of critical thinkers as identified by Alfaro-LeFevre (2008).

_____
_____
_____
_____
_____
_____
_____
_____
_____
_____

3. List six skills that are needed for nurses to be critical thinkers.

_____

_____

_____

_____

_____

_____

4. Explain this statement: How a nurse perceives a situation and employs critical thinking skills depends on the "lens" through which she sees the situation.

_____

5. Compare and contrast the meaning of the following terms: moral dilemma, moral problem, moral uncertainty, and moral distress.

_____

_____

6. Write the definition of nursing as proposed in Nursing's Social Policy Statement (ANA, 2003).

_____

_____

7. List five of the most common ethical issues that nurses face today: _____, _____,

_____, _____, and _____.

8. List two types of "advance directives" that specify a patient's wishes before hospitalization: _____ and _____.

9. Explain the concept of a "durable power of attorney."

_____

_____

10. Suggest an opening statement that a nurse can use during the interview process.

_____

11. Discuss how formulation of a nursing diagnosis and identification of collaborative problems differs from making a medical diagnosis.

_____

_____

12. Discuss the significance of establishing expected outcomes during the evaluation phase of the nursing process.

_____

_____

NURSING OR COLLABORATIVE PROBLEM

Read each statement below. Put "N" in front of every nursing diagnosis and "C" in front of every collaborative problem.

1. _____ Anxiety related to impending surgery.

2. _____ Constipation related to altered nutrition.

3. _____ Potential complication: paralytic ileus secondary to postoperative inactivity.

4. _____ Potential complication: sacral decubiti secondary to bed rest.

5. _____ Risk for impaired skin integrity related to prolonged bed rest.

6. _____ Ineffective breastfeeding related to fear of discomfort.

7. _____ Potential complication: hypoglycemia related to inadequate food intake.

8. _____ Potential complication: phlebitis related to intravenous therapy.

9. _____ Risk for posttraumatic syndrome related to an accident.

10. _____ Potential complication: oral lesions related to chemotherapy.

MATCHING

Match the critical-thinking strategy in column II with the nursing process skill listed in column I.

Column I

1. _____ Categorize information

2. _____ Design a plan of care

3. _____ Determine assessment processes

4. _____ Evaluate outcomes

5. _____ Implement a standard plan

6. _____ Make a nursing diagnosis

7. _____ Manage collaborative problems

Column II

a. Assert a practice role

b. Formulate a relationship

c. Generate a hypothesis

d. Provide an explanation

e. Recognize a pattern

f. Search for information

g. Set priorities

Match the definitions of ethical principles listed in column II with their associated terms listed in column I.

Column I

1. _____ Autonomy

2. _____ Beneficence

3. _____ Justice

4. _____ Nonmaleficence

5. _____ Paternalism

6. _____ Veracity

Column II

a. Limiting one's autonomy based on the welfare of another

b. Similar cases should be treated the same

c. The commitment to not deceive

d. Freedom of choice

e. The duty to do good and not inflict harm

f. The expectation that harm will not be done

II. Critical Thinking Questions and Exercises

DISCUSSION AND ANALYSIS

Discuss the following topics with your classmates.

Planning nursing care involves setting priorities and distinguishing problems that need urgent attention from those that can be deferred to a later time or referred to a physician. For each of the following patient care problems, circle the *initial priority of nursing care* from among the choices provided and write a rationale for your choice. For standardized interventions from the Nursing Interventions Classification (NIC), see Chart 3-7 in the text.

1. Activity intolerance, related to inadequate oxygenation:
   a. dyspnea
   b. fatigue
   c. hypotension

   Rationale for choice:

   _____

   _____

2. Alterations in bowel elimination: constipation, related to prolonged bed rest:
   a. abdominal pressure and bloating
   b. palpable impaction
   c. straining at stool

   Rationale for choice:

   _____

   _____

3. Altered oral mucous membrane, related to stomatitis:
   a. erythema of oral mucosa
   b. intolerance to hot foods
   c. oral pain

   Rationale for choice:

   _____

   _____

RECOGNIZING CONTRADICTIONS

Rewrite each statement correctly. Underline the key concepts.

1. Nursing ethics is considered an applied form of medical ethics because nurses work only under the direction of a physician.

   _____

2. A nurse experiences moral uncertainty when he or she is prevented from doing what he or she believes is the correct action.

   _____

3. A nurse should always honor a terminally ill patient's request to withhold food and hydration if the patient is competent.

_____

4. By design, living wills are very prescriptive and are always honored as legally binding documents.

_____

SUPPORTING ARGUMENTS

Read each paragraph. Offer logical supporting rationales for each answer.

1. In vitro fertilization, based on sophisticated technology, has resulted in women in their 50s and 60s giving birth. Physicians argue that this is ethically sound if the woman meets the criteria that she is healthy and could live another 25 years. List three rationales to support this argument.

_____

_____

_____

2. You are asked to defend the statement that "life support measures should never be used for anyone with a terminal illness." Develop three supporting arguments.

_____

_____

_____

3. List two rationales to support the argument that age should be used as a criterion for determining the allocation of health care resources.

_____

_____

CLINICAL SITUATIONS

Read each nursing diagnosis. Write a specific outcome.

The planning phase of the nursing process incorporates documented expected patient outcomes for specific nursing diagnoses (ND). Resources include the Nursing-Sensitive Outcomes Classification (NOC) (see Chart 3-6 in the text). Write one outcome that indicates an improvement for each diagnosis.

1. ND: Activity intolerance, related to dyspnea

   Outcome: _____

2. ND: Impaired physical mobility, related to total hip replacement

   Outcome: _____

3. ND: Fluid volume excess, related to compromised cardiac output

   Outcome: _____

4. ND: Imbalanced nutrition: less than body requirements, related to anorexia

   Outcome: _____

5. ND: Disturbed sleep-pattern disturbance, related to pain

   Outcome: _____

CASE STUDY: Ethical Analysis

Read the following case study. Fill in the blanks below.

You are a registered nurse and a board member of American Red Cross Disaster Relief Services. When a smallpox epidemic erupted among thousands in Washington, DC, as a result of terrorist activity, the board was asked by the Office of Homeland Security to allocate limited resources. The board decided that those with the greatest chance of survival and those working for the government would be treated. Those individuals with preexisting or terminal conditions would not be treated. The decision resulted in multiple deaths while preserving the lives of those most likely to survive. The framework for decision making followed the utilitarian approach.

Assessment

Write your response in the space provided.

1. List two possible conflicts between ethical principles and professional obligations.

   a. _____   b. _____

2. People involved in the decision:

   a. _____   c. _____

   b. _____

3. Those affected by the decision:

   a. _____   c. _____

   b. _____

Planning

1. Treatment options:

   a. _____   b. _____

2. Medical facts:

   a. _____   b. _____

3. Influencing information:

   a. _____   b. _____

4. Ethical/moral issues:

   a. _____   b. _____

5. Competing claims:

   a. _____   b. _____

Implementation

Compare the Utilitarian and the Deontological approaches.

Utilitarian	*Deontological or Formalist*

1. Basis of ethical principles:

    a. _____   a. _____

    b. _____   b. _____

2. Predict consequences of actions:

    a. _____   a. _____

    b. _____   b. _____

3. Assign a positive or negative value to each consequence.

    a. _____   a. _____

    b. _____   b. _____

4. Choose the consequence, decision, or action that predicts the highest positive value:

    a. _____   a. _____

    b. _____   b. _____

Evaluation

Finish the following statements.

1. The best, morally correct action is to:

    _____

    _____

2. This decision is based on the ethical reasoning that:

    _____

    _____

3. The decision can be defended based on the following arguments:

    a. _____

    b. _____

    c. _____

CHAPTER 4

Health Education and Health Promotion

I. Interpretation, Completion, and Comparison

MULTIPLE CHOICE

Read each question carefully. Circle your answer.

1. Health education is:
   a. a primary nursing responsibility.
   b. an essential component of nursing care.
   c. an independent nursing function.
   d. consistent with all of the above.

2. Nursing responsibilities associated with patient teaching include:
   a. determining individual needs for teaching.
   b. motivating each person to learn.
   c. presenting information at the level of the learner.
   d. all of the above.

3. A nurse assesses that a patient is emotionally ready to learn when the patient:
   a. has accepted the therapeutic regimen.
   b. is motivated.
   c. recognizes the need to learn.
   d. demonstrates all of the above.

4. Nursing actions that can be used to motivate a patient to learn include all of the following *except*:
   a. feedback in the form of constructive encouragement when a person has been unsuccessful in the learning process.
   b. negative criticism when the patient is unsuccessful, so that inappropriate behavior patterns will not be learned.
   c. the creation of a positive atmosphere in which the patient is encouraged to express anxiety.
   d. the establishment of realistic learning goals based on individual needs.

5. Normal aging results in changes in cognition. Therefore, when teaching an elderly patient how to administer insulin, the nurse should:
   a. repeat the information frequently for reinforcement.
   b. present all the information at one time so that the patient is not confused by pieces of information.
   c. speed up the demonstration because the patient will tire easily.
   d. do all of the above.

6. The nurse reviews a medication administration calendar with an elderly patient. Being aware of sensory changes associated with aging, the nurse should:
   a. print directions in large, bold type, preferably using black ink.
   b. highlight or shade important dates and times with contrasting colors.
   c. use several different colors to emphasize special dates.
   d. do all of the above.

Study Guide for Brunner and Suddarth's Textbook of Medical-Surgical Nursing, 12th edition.

7. A nursing action that involves modifying a teaching program because a learner is not experientially ready is:
   a. changing the wording in a teaching pamphlet so that a patient with a fourth-grade reading level can understand it.
   b. contacting family members to assist in goal development to help stimulate motivation.
   c. postponing a teaching session with a patient until pain has subsided.
   d. all of the above.

8. A nurse identifies a patient's inability to pour a liquid medication into a measuring spoon. This diagnosis is part of the nursing process known as:
   a. assessment.
   b. planning.
   c. implementation.
   d. evaluation.

9. A nurse develops a program of increased ambulation for a patient with an orthopedic disorder. This goal setting is a component of the nursing process known as:
   a. assessment.
   b. planning.
   c. implementation.
   d. evaluation.

10. Outcome criteria are expressed as expected outcomes of patient behavior resulting from teaching strategies. An example is:
    a. ability to climb a flight of stairs without experiencing difficulty in breathing.
    b. altered lifestyle resulting from inadequate lung expansion.
    c. inadequate ventilation associated with pulmonary congestion.
    d. potential oxygenation deficit related to ventilatory insufficiency.

11. Select the health promotion model that identifies why some people choose actions to foster health and others refuse to participate:
    a. Health Belief Model
    b. Resource Model of Preventive Health
    c. Achieving Health for All Model
    d. Social Learning Theory Model

12. The single, most important factor in determining health status and longevity is:
    a. adherence to a plan.
    b. good nutrition.
    c. motivation to change.
    d. stress reduction.

SHORT ANSWER

Read each statement carefully. Write your response in the space provided.

1. List three significant factors for a nurse to consider when planning patient education:

   _____, _____, and _____.

2. Explain why health education is so essential for those with a chronic illness.

   _____

3. List five common examples of specific activities that promote and maintain health: _____,

   _____, _____, _____, and _____.

4. Define the term *adherence* as it relates to a person's therapeutic regimen.

   _____

5. Name four classifications of variables (factors) that influence a person's ability to adhere to a program of care: _____, _____, _____, and _____.

6. There is a positive correlation between patient motivation and adherence to a teaching plan. Three significant variables affecting motivation and learning are: _____, _____, and _____.

7. List the six stages of personal change that an individual experiences as he or she moves toward a healthy behavior.

   _____   _____
   _____   _____
   _____   _____

8. Describe the nature of the teaching–learning process.

   _____

9. List at least six variables that make adherence to a therapeutic regimen difficult for the elderly.

   _____   _____
   _____   _____
   _____   _____

10. Increased age affects cognition by decreasing: _____, _____, and _____.

11. Discuss how learner readiness affects a learner and the learning situation.

   _____

12. Identify six teaching techniques the nurses frequently use:

   _____   _____
   _____   _____
   _____   _____

13. Two major goals from the Healthy People 2010 report are: _____ and _____.

14. Health promotion activities are grounded in four active processes:

   _____, _____, _____, and _____.

II. Critical Thinking Questions and Exercises

DISCUSSION AND ANALYSIS

Discuss the following topics with your classmates.

1. Using Table 4-1 in the text, design two teaching plans: one for a teenage diabetic patient who has an emotional disability and another for a 70-year-old individual with a visual impairment who had a stroke.
2. Discuss the positive relationship between health and physical fitness. Explain at least five ways that exercise can promote health.

RECOGNIZING CONTRADICTIONS

Rewrite each statement correctly. Underline the key concepts.

1. Health education is a dependent function of nursing practice that requires physician approval.

   _____

   _____

2. The largest groups of people in need of health education today are children and those with infectious diseases.

   _____

3. Patients are encouraged to evidence compliance with their therapeutic regimen.

   _____

4. Evaluation, the final step in the teaching process, should be summative (done at the end of the teaching process).

   _____

5. Elderly persons rarely experience significant improvement from health promotion activities.

   _____

6. About 50% of elderly persons have one or more chronic illnesses.

   _____

EXAMINING ASSOCIATIONS

The health status of residents of the United States is a serious concern to individuals, health care practitioners, and health-promotion groups. A nation's health status can be measured by evaluating certain indicators. (Refer to Chart 4-3 in the text.) After reading *Healthy People 2010* (U.S. Department of Health and Human Services, 2000), complete the following chart. For each indicator listed, assign a rating score (1 = not relevant, 2 = important, and 3 = very significant) reflecting the degree to which the indicator affects an individual's health, the rationale for the score, and an activity to improve the score. The first row has been filled in as an example.

Indicator	Rating Score	Rationale	Improvement Strategy
Physical activity	3	Research has shown an increased percentage of inactivity among young adults over the last 10 years.	Increase time for physical activity in K–12 schools. Limit TV, video games, and computer time in the home.
Obesity			
Tobacco use			
Substance abuse			
Sexual behavior			
Mental illness			
Violent behavior			
Environmental pollution			
Lack of access to health care			

CHAPTER 5

Adult Health and Nutritional Assessment

I. Interpretation, Completion, and Comparison

MULTIPLE CHOICE

Read each question carefully. Circle your answer.

1. The health history obtained by the nurse should focus on nursing's concern about:
   a. a comprehensive body systems review.
   b. current and past health problems.
   c. the family history.
   d. all of the above.

2. A patient has certain rights concerning data collection, such as the right to know:
   a. how information will be used.
   b. that selected information will be held confidential.
   c. why information is sought.
   d. all of the above.

3. Open-ended questions help persons describe their chief complaint. Choose the sentence that is *not* an open-ended question.
   a. "Describe the pain."
   b. "Tell me more about your feelings."
   c. "How did the accident happen?"
   d. "Is the pain sharp and piercing?"

4. The single most important factor in helping the nurse and physician arrive at a diagnosis is the:
   a. family history.
   b. history of the present illness.
   c. past health history.
   d. results of the systems review.

5. Choose the best question an interviewer would use to obtain educational or occupational information.
   a. "Are you a blue-collar worker?"
   b. "Do you have difficulty meeting your financial commitments?"
   c. "Is your income more than $20,000 per year?"
   d. "What college did you attend?"

6. Which of the following is an *inappropriate* interviewer response to the patient statement, "I will not take pain medication when I am in pain"?
   a. "Is there another way you have learned to lessen pain when you experience it?"
   b. "Let a nurse know when you are in pain so you can be helped to decrease stimuli that may exaggerate your pain experience."
   c. "Refusing medication can only hurt you by increasing your awareness of the pain experience."
   d. "You have the right to make that decision. How can the nurses help you cope with your pain?"

7. All of the following are questions that will provide information about a person's lifestyle *except*:
   a. "Do you have any food preferences?"
   b. "Have you always lived in this geographic area?"
   c. "How many hours of sleep do you require each day?"
   d. "What type of exercise do you prefer?"

8. When obtaining a health history from an older adult patient, the nurse must remember to:
   a. ask questions slowly, directly, and in a voice loud enough to be heard by those who are hearing-impaired.
   b. clarify the frequency, severity, and history of signs and symptoms of the present illness.
   c. conduct the interview in a calm, unrushed manner using eye-to-eye contact.
   d. do all of the above.

9. On initial impression, the nurse assesses a patient's posture, stature, and body movements. This assessment is part of the physical examination process known as:
   a. auscultation.
   b. inspection.
   c. palpation.
   d. percussion.

10. An examiner needs to determine the upper border of a patient's liver. With the patient in the recumbent position, the examiner would percuss for a:
   a. dull sound.
   b. flat sound.
   c. resonant sound.
   d. tympanic sound.

11. During a physical examination, the nurse noted hyperresonance over inflated lung tissue in a patient with emphysema. The process used for this assessment was:
   a. auscultation.
   b. inspection.
   c. palpation.
   d. percussion.

12. A heart murmur was detected during a physical examination. The process used to obtain this information was:
   a. auscultation.
   b. inspection.
   c. palpation.
   d. percussion.

13. A waist circumference measurement can be useful in assessing excess abdominal fat. Women should try to maintain a waist circumference of _____ to remain healthy.
   a. 30 to 34 in
   b. 35 in
   c. 36 to 38 in
   d. 39 to 41 in

14. A serum albumin level of 2.50 g/dL indicates:
   a. a severe protein deficiency.
   b. low levels of serum protein.
   c. an acceptable amount of protein.
   d. an extremely high measurement of protein.

15. Several factors contribute to the altered nutritional status of the elderly. A *primary nutritional nursing consideration* during physical assessment is:
   a. altered metabolism and nutrient use secondary to an acute or chronic illness.
   b. decreased appetite related to loneliness.
   c. limited financial resources.
   d. the patient's ability to shop for and prepare food.

SHORT ANSWER

Read each statement carefully. Write your response in the space provided.

1. The role of the nurse in assessment includes two primary responsibilities: _____ and _____.

2. Describe five basic guidelines that a nurse should use while conducting a health assessment: _____, _____, _____, _____, and _____.

3. Explain how mutual trust and confidence between the interviewer and the patient facilitate the communication process.

   _____

4. Define the term *chief complaint*.

   _____

5. A number of diseases of first- or second-order relatives are significant when a nurse takes a patient's family history. List six diseases that are considered significant.

   _____ _____

   _____ _____

   _____ _____

6. When questioning a patient about lifestyle and health-related behaviors, the nurse should ask about: _____, _____, _____, _____, and _____.

7. The *three leading causes of death* in the United States that are related in part to poor nutrition are: _____, _____, and _____.

8. A nurse used the Department of Agriculture's Food Guide Pyramid (Figure 5-6) to evaluate a patient's dietary information. The nurse knows that the minimum recommendations for five groups are:

   Grains: _____ Milk: _____

   Vegetables: _____ Meat and Beans: _____

   Fruits: _____

9. The body mass index (BMI), a number based on a weight-to-height ratio, provides a quick reference to a person's nutritional status. A person with a score of _____ is considered overweight, a score of _____ is considered obese, and a score greater than _____ is considered extremely obese. Those with a score of _____ are at risk for poor nutritional status.

10. In addition to BMI, waist circumference is an indication of weight problems. Men are at risk for obesity with a waist circumference of _____ in; women at _____ in.

11. Explain the concept of *negative nitrogen balance*.

    _____

    _____

12. Adolescent girls are particularly at risk for nutritional deficits in minerals, such as:

_____, _____, and _____.

13. Which of the following assessments was most likely used to obtain the data. Write the word on the line provided.

Inspection

Palpation

Percussion

Auscultation

a. _____ Asymmetry of movement is associated with a central nervous system disorder.

b. _____ Clubbing of the fingers is a diagnostic symptom of chronic pulmonary disorders.

c. _____ Tenderness is present in the area of the thyroid isthmus.

d. _____ Tactile fremitus is diagnostic of lung consolidation.

e. _____ Tympanic or drumlike sounds are produced by pneumothorax.

f. _____ The first heart sound is created by the simultaneous closure of the mitral and tricuspid valves.

g. _____ A friction rub is present with pericarditis.

h. _____ Nodules present with gout lie adjacent to the joint capsule.

MATCHING

Match the body area listed in column II with the descriptive sign of poor nutrition listed in column I.

Column I

1. _____ Atrophic papillae
2. _____ Brittle, dull, depigmented
3. _____ Cheilosis
4. _____ Flaccid, underdeveloped
5. _____ Fluorosis
6. _____ Xerophthalmia

Column II

a. Abdomen
b. Eyes
c. Hair
d. Lips
e. Muscles
f. Skeleton
g. Teeth
h. Tongue

II. Critical Thinking Questions and Exercises

DISCUSSION AND ANALYSIS

Discuss the following topics with your classmates.

1. Create a list of six questions that a nurse could incorporate into a genetic health assessment.
2. Review Figures 5-3 and 5-4 in the text. Discuss and then demonstrate the proper techniques to be used for abdominal palpation and percussion.

CLINICAL SITUATIONS

Read the following case study. Fill in the blanks below.

CASE STUDY: Calculating a Healthy Diet

Mrs. Allred is a 40-year-old Hispanic woman, 5 ft 5 in tall, with three children younger than 5 years of age. She weighs 175 lb. She had no known history of any physical illness before experiencing fatigue and irritability that she believed was the result of her parenting responsibilities. Mrs. Allred does not exercise regularly, eats snack foods while watching television with her children, and is too tired to prepare balanced meals for her family. She orders fast food or pizza for dinner at least three times a week.

Part I: Estimate ideal body weight

1. Calculate Mrs. Allred's frame size based on a wrist circumference of 16 cm.
   a. Small frame.
   b. Medium frame.
   c. Large frame.

2. Mrs. Allred's ideal body weight (IBW) is _____ lb. Therefore, she needs to _____ (gain/lose) approximately _____ lb.

3. Her body mass index (BMI) is _____, which is considered (ideal, overweight, obese) _____.

Part II: Calculate a balanced diet for Mrs. Allred's ideal body weight, as determined in Part I. Use Chart 5-5 from the text as a guide.

1. Convert IBW in pounds to kilograms. _____.

2. Determine basal energy needs (1 kcal/kg/hr): _____ calories.

3. Increase activity by 40% (moderate activity): _____ calories.

4. Divide calories into carbohydrates (50%) _____, fats (30%) _____, and proteins (20%) _____.

5. Estimate grams for each: carbohydrates _____, fats _____, and proteins _____.

Part III: Using the USDA's Food Pyramid Guide (Figure 5-6) design a 2000-calorie diet for Mrs. Allred.

1. The majority of foods from fat sources should come from _____, _____, and _____.

2. The majority of grains should be composed of: _____

3. Mrs. Allred should be advised to eat about _____ of vegetables daily.

4. The least amount of calories should come from two food groups: _____ and _____.

5. Milk products should always be: _____.

6. Mrs. Allred should eat about _____ servings of fruit daily.

CHAPTER 6

Homeostasis, Stress, and Adaptation

I. Interpretation, Completion, and Comparison

MULTIPLE CHOICE

Read each question carefully. Circle your answer.

1. Stress is a change in the environment that is perceived as:
   a. challenging.
   b. damaging.
   c. threatening.
   d. having all of the above characteristics.

2. An individual's adaptation to stress is influenced by the stressors:
   a. frequency and duration.
   b. number of occurrences and magnitude.
   c. sequencing (intermittent or enduring).
   d. combined characteristics as listed above.

3. An example of a functional, yet maladaptive, response of the body to a threat is:
   a. collateral circulation subsequent to diminished tissue perfusion.
   b. decreased cardiac output subsequent to cardiomegaly.
   c. increased pulmonary ventilation subsequent to increased levels of carbon dioxide.
   d. muscle atrophy subsequent to disuse.

4. Health promotion should be initiated before compensatory processes become maladaptive. Preventive nursing measures include all of the following *except*:
   a. demonstrating wound cleansing to a patient who has a necrotic leg ulcer resulting from vascular disease.
   b. showing a patient with a casted extremity how to perform isometric exercises.
   c. suggesting stress-reducing measures for a patient with a diagnosis of angina pectoris.
   d. teaching weight management to a patient who has a family history of obesity and a blood pressure reading of 125/90 mm Hg.

5. Maladaptive compensatory mechanisms result in disease processes in which cells may be:
   a. dead.
   b. diseased.
   c. injured.
   d. affected in all of the above ways.

6. Adaptation to a stressor is positively correlated with:
   a. previous coping mechanisms.
   b. the duration of the stressor.
   c. the severity of the stressor.
   d. all of the above.

7. During the initial stress response, primary appraisal refers to:
   a. evaluating the effectiveness of several coping mechanisms.
   b. organizing all available resources to deal with the stressor.
   c. identifying support services needed for coping.
   d. weighing the significance of the stressful event.

8. Helen, age 48, is diagnosed with pneumonia. She has been paralyzed from the chest down for 7 years. The nurse realizes that Helen needs additional support to cope with her infection because:
   a. coping measures become less effective with advancing age.
   b. the patient's available coping resources are already being used to manage the problems of immobility.
   c. an acute infectious process requires more adaptive mechanisms than a chronic stressor does.
   d. this additional physical stressor places unmanageable demands on the patient's internal and external resources.

9. Helen cooperates and willingly follows the treatment regimen. The nurse wonders how Helen can project such a positive outlook and cope with additional stress. Helen's ability to cope is probably due to all of the following *except*:
   a. acceptance that "life is not fair" and that people have limited control over their health.
   b. adoption of the problem-focused method of coping.
   c. her ability to draw on past coping behaviors and apply them to new situations.
   d. the support of family and friends who call and visit frequently.

10. The neural and hormonal activities that respond to stress and maintain homeostasis are located in the:
    a. cerebral cortex.
    b. hypothalamus.
    c. medulla oblongata.
    d. pituitary gland.

11. Elizabeth is newly admitted to the medical unit. She has periodic episodes of shortness of breath and tightness in her throat. She is crying. To evaluate the impact of physiologic and psychological components on her illness, the nurse should:
    a. perform a thorough physical examination and include subjective patient statements as well as objective laboratory data.
    b. focus primary attention on the respiratory system, because this is the patient's chief complaint.
    c. determine that the patient is not in acute distress, and then perform a complete physical examination and include data about the patient's lifestyle and social relationships.
    d. attempt to discover the reasons behind the patient's anxieties, because stress can cause breathing difficulties.

12. During the nursing interview, a patient with shortness of breath reveals that she is in the process of getting a divorce. This information alerts the nurse to initially:
    a. try to determine whether there is a psychological basis for the patient's physical symptoms.
    b. restrict family members from visiting, because their presence may aggravate the patient's symptoms.
    c. teach the patient specific breathing exercises that can be used to manage symptoms.
    d. request that the physician recommend counseling services.

13. A patient is admitted to the emergency department for observation after a minor automobile accident. On the basis of an understanding of the sympathetic nervous system's response to stress, the nurse would expect to find all of the following during assessment *except*:
    a. cold, clammy skin.
    b. decreased heart rate.
    c. rapid respirations.
    d. skeletal muscle tension.

14. Physiologically, the sympathetic-adrenal-medullary response results in all of the following *except*:
    a. decreased blood flow to the abdominal viscera.
    b. decreased peripheral vasoconstriction.
    c. increased myocardial contractility.
    d. increased secretion of serum glucose.

15. The hypothalamic-pituitary response is a long-acting physiologic response to stress that involves:
    a. stimulation of the anterior pituitary to produce adrenocorticotropic hormone (ACTH).
    b. the production of cortisol from the adrenal cortex.
    c. protein catabolism and gluconeogenesis.
    d. all of the above mechanisms.

16. An example of a negative feedback process is increased:
    a. aldosterone secretion in burn trauma, resulting in excess sodium retention.
    b. cardiac output in hemorrhage, resulting in increased blood loss.
    c. secretion of antidiuretic hormone (ADH) in congestive heart failure, causing increased fluid retention.
    d. secretion of thyroid-stimulating factor (TSF), which stops when circulating thyroxin levels reach normal.

17. A patient experiences lower leg pain associated with lactic acid accumulation (an example of a local response involving a feedback loop). The nurse expects the pain to lessen when:
    a. aerobic metabolism is reinstated.
    b. anaerobic metabolism becomes the major pathway for energy release.
    c. muscle use and subsequent glucose catabolism increase.
    d. vasoconstriction diminishes blood flow, thereby slowing the removal of waste products.

18. A patient has a diagnosis of hypertrophy of the heart muscle (an example of cellular adaptation to injury). The nurse expects all of the following *except*:
    a. compromised cardiac output.
    b. muscle mass changes evident on radiologic examinations.
    c. cellular alteration compensatory to some stimulus.
    d. decreased cell size, leading to more effective ventricular contractions.

19. Breast changes in a pregnant woman are an example of cellular adaptation to stress known as:
    a. dysplasia.
    b. hyperplasia.
    c. hypertrophy.
    d. metaplasia.

20. Cell injury results when stressors interfere with the body's optimal balance by altering cellular ability to:
    a. grow and reproduce.
    b. synthesize enzymes.
    c. transform energy.
    d. do all of the above.

21. An adult patient's hemoglobin level is 7 g/dL. This should alert the nurse to assess for signs and symptoms associated with:
    a. hyperemia.
    b. hypertension.
    c. hypoglycemia.
    d. hypoxia.

22. A diabetic patient is admitted to the hospital with a blood sugar level of 320 mg/dL. The nurse decides to monitor fluid intake and output because:
    a. decreased blood osmolarity causes fluid to shift into the interstitial spaces, resulting in polydipsia.
    b. polydipsia occurs when glucose catabolism is accelerated, thereby increasing the body's need for fluids.
    c. polyuria results from osmotic diuresis, which is compensatory to hyperglycemia.
    d. the blood's hypotonicity will result in tissue fluid retention and weight gain.

Study Guide for Brunner and Suddarth's Textbook of Medical-Surgical Nursing, 12th edition.

23. Nursing care for a patient with a fever is based on all of the following body responses *except*:
   a. diaphoresis, which is a compensatory mechanism that cools the body.
   b. increased heart rate, which helps to meet increased metabolic demands.
   c. increased nutrient catabolism, which influences the body's caloric needs.
   d. vasodilation of surface blood vessels, which prevents excessive heat loss.

24. Anti-infective drugs are not useful against biologic agents known as:
   a. bacteria.
   b. fungi.
   c. mycoplasmas.
   d. viruses.

25. Viruses are infectious agents that:
   a. burst out of invaded cells to enter other cells.
   b. infect specific cells.
   c. replicate within invaded cells.
   d. do all of the above.

26. Genetic disorders arising from inherited traits include all of the following *except*:
   a. hemophilia.
   b. meningitis.
   c. phenylketonuria
   d. sickle cell anemia.

27. A nurse who is caring for a patient with a localized response to a bee sting expects symptoms to include all of the following *except*:
   a. blanching due to compensatory vasoconstriction.
   b. hyperemia due to increased blood flow.
   c. pain due to pressure on the nerve endings.
   d. swelling due to increased vascular permeability.

28. While caring for a patient with an infected surgical incision, the nurse observes for signs of a systemic response. These include all of the following *except*:
   a. leukopenia owing to increased white blood cell production.
   b. a febrile state caused by the release of pyrogens.
   c. anorexia, malaise, and weakness.
   d. loss of appetite and complaints of aching.

29. Research has shown that the single most important factor influencing an individual's health is:
   a. health insurance coverage.
   b. income.
   c. level of education.
   d. social relationships.

30. Nursing assessment to determine individual social support systems includes obtaining information about the person's:
   a. belief that he or she belongs to a group that is mutually dependent and communicative.
   b. concept of being cared for and loved.
   c. impression of being esteemed and valued.
   d. perception of all of the above.

31. Mrs. Talbot is scheduled for a breast biopsy in the morning. There is a history of breast malignancy in her family. While caring for her the evening before surgery, the most appropriate nursing action would be to:
   a. administer a soothing back massage to promote relaxation and decrease stress.
   b. make sure she eats all of her evening meal, because she will be NPO after midnight.
   c. minimize the emotional impact of surgery by encouraging her to socialize with other patients.
   d. sit with her and provide an opportunity for her to talk about her concerns.

SHORT ANSWER

Read each statement carefully. Write your response in the space provided.

1. List four concepts that are key to understanding a steady state of dynamic balance: _____,
   _____, _____, and _____.

2. Define a *maladaptive* response to a stressor.
   _____

3. Explain why *hyperpnea*, after intense exercise, is considered an adaptive response to a physiologic stressor.
   _____

4. Give several examples of acute, *time-limited* stressors and chronic, *enduring* stressors.
   _____

5. Psychosocial stressors are classified as day-to-day occurrences (daily hassles), major events that affect large groups, and those infrequently occurring situations that directly affect a person. List two examples from your personal experiences that could be included under each classification.

   a. Day-to-day occurrences.
   _____
   _____

   b. Major events that affect large groups of people.
   _____
   _____

   c. Infrequently occurring major stressors.
   _____
   _____

6. Discuss the correlation between stress, illness, and critical life events.
   _____
   _____

7. Discuss how internal cognitive processes and external resources are used by an individual to manage stress.
   _____
   _____

8. Define stress according to Hans Selye's Theory of Adaptation (1976).
   _____
   _____

9. According to Hans Selye's Theory of Adaptation (1976), there are about 12 diseases of maladaptation.
   List six: _____, _____, _____, _____,
   _____, and _____.

10. List five bodily functions that are regulated by negative feedback mechanisms: _____,

_____, _____, _____, and _____.

11. List the five cardinal signs of inflammation: _____, _____,

_____, _____, and _____.

12. List four possible nursing diagnoses for individuals suffering from stress: _____,

_____, _____, and _____.

MATCHING

Match the primary category of stressors listed in column II with its associated stressors listed in column I.

Column I

1. _____ Anxieties
2. _____ Genetic disorders
3. _____ Hypoxia
4. _____ Infectious agents
5. _____ Life changes
6. _____ Nutritional imbalance
7. _____ Social relationships
8. _____ Trauma

Column II

a. Physiologic
b. Psychosocial

II. Critical Thinking Questions and Exercises

DISCUSSION AND ANALYSIS

Discuss the following topics with your classmates.

1. Discuss the concept of adaptation to a stressor at the cellular, tissue, and organ level.
2. Discuss the three levels of appraisal (primary, secondary, and reappraisal) that Lazarus (1991) suggests in his theory of cognitive appraisal.
3. Distinguish between physical, physiologic, and psychosocial stressors. Cite a personal example for each and explain how you were able to adapt or not adapt to the stressor.
4. Explain how a person with positive self-esteem, energy, and health (hardiness) typically responds to stressors in a positive way.
5. Discuss the cognitive process and emotional responses that you would experience in appraising a stressful event. Mention the steps involved in primary appraisal, secondary appraisal, and reappraisal.
6. Explain Hans Selye's Theory of Adaptation (1976), both the general and local adaptation syndromes.
7. Discuss several examples of adaptation to stressors, at the cellular level, by comparing hypertrophy to atrophy and hyperplasia to dysplasia and metaplasia.

CLINICAL SITUATIONS

Complete the flow chart. Fill in the physiologic reactions of the body that represent the sympathetic-adrenal-medullary response to stress. Provide the rationale for each reaction.

General Body Arousal	*Physiologic Reaction*	*Rationale*
↑ Norepinephrine and epinephrine	↑ _____	↑ _____
	↑ _____	↑ _____
	↑ _____	↑ _____
	↑ _____	↑ _____

↓

Effects on:

Skeletal muscles	_____	↑ _____
Pupils	_____	↑ _____
Ventilation	_____	_____

CASE STUDY: Hypertensive Heart Disease

Read the following case study. Fill in the blanks below.

The body is capable of integrated responses to stress mediated by the sympathetic nervous system and the hypothalamic-pituitary-adrenocortical axis (see Figure 6-2 in the text). Use the clinical diagnosis, hypertensive heart disease, as an example of the body's response to stress.

Renin secretion is compensatory to decreased renal blood flow. Renin indirectly leads to sodium and water retention by stimulating the release of aldosterone. This mechanism initially results in increased cardiac output. For each compensatory mechanism shown, list nursing implications (assessment, nursing diagnoses/collaborative problems, planning, implementation, and evaluation) and give a rationale for each.

Selected Compensatory Mechanisms	*Nursing Implications*	*Rationale*
a. Renal blood flow is decreased as a result of hypertensive heart disease.	Assessment _____ _____ _____	_____ _____ _____ _____
	Nursing Diagnoses _____ _____	_____ _____
	Collaborative Problems _____ _____	_____ _____
	Planning _____	_____
	Implementation _____	_____
	Evaluation _____	_____
b. Arteriole constriction occurs, resulting from renin secretion.		
c. Sodium and water retention occurs subsequent to aldosterone secretion.		
d. Increased cardiac output occurs as a result of increased extracellular fluid.		

IDENTIFYING PATTERNS

Complete the following flow chart.

The sympathetic-adrenal-medullary response and the hypothalamic-pituitary response to stressors are adaptive and protective mechanisms that maintain homeostasis in the body. Based on the information provided in the text, please complete the following flow chart. Fill in the rectangles, as appropriate, with the steps in the process. Fill in the triangles with the physiologic end responses. Use Figure 6-2 in the text as a guide.

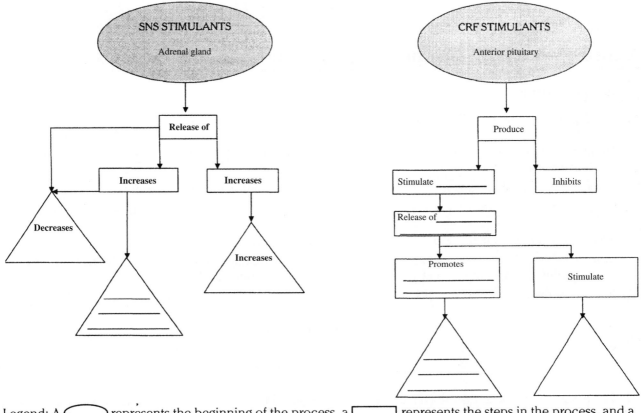

Legend: A ⬭ represents the beginning of the process, a ▭ represents the steps in the process, and a △ represents the physiologic end responses.

Individual and Family Considerations Related to Illness

I. Interpretation, Completion, and Comparison

MULTIPLE CHOICE

Read each question carefully. Circle your answer.

1. Compelling research has been established to show that the health of the immune system is correlated to the functioning of:
   a. the central nervous system.
   b. emotional moods and behavior.
   c. neuroendocrine responses.
   d. interconnections among all of the above.

2. To examine an individual's response to illness, a nurse should:
   a. analyze the way the patient thinks about stress, illness, and adaptive behavior.
   b. observe the patient's present behavior.
   c. obtain a description of the patient's previous coping mechanisms.
   d. do all of the above.

3. A person's perception of illness as a stressor is primarily influenced by:
   a. finances.
   b. intelligence.
   c. occupational status.
   d. previous coping experiences.

4. The basic initial system disturbance believed to be responsible for the symptoms of posttraumatic stress disorder (PTSD) is in the:
   a. cardiopulmonary system.
   b. neurologic system.
   c. renal system.
   d. respiratory system.

5. The incidence of PTSD in high-risk groups is approximately:
   a. 10% to 15%.
   b. 30%.
   c. 50%.
   d. 75% or greater.

6. In the United States, approximately what percentage of clinically depressed individuals are properly diagnosed?
   a. 5%
   b. 15%
   c. 30%
   d. 50%

7. Which of the following is *not* considered a risk for suicide?
   a. Altered body image.
   b. Family history of suicide.
   c. Female gender.
   d. Age 25 to 35 years.

8. It took Mr. A 3 months to admit that he was sick and in need of medical and nursing care and to accept his diagnosis of adenocarcinoma of the right kidney. An initial emotional response the nurse would expect to see associated with loss and grief is:

   a. shame.

   b. denial.

   c. guilt and shame.

   d. regression.

9. Nursing interventions to help a patient deal with denial include:

   a. allowing the patient to use denial when it serves an immediate purpose and is not harmful.

   b. challenging the patient's use of denial as a defense mechanism.

   c. encouraging the use of denial as a satisfactory method of dealing with illness.

   d. supporting the denial behavior, knowing that the patient needs this coping mechanism.

10. A communication breakdown will most probably occur if a nurse:

    a. anticipates barriers to communication and works out solutions in advance.

    b. clarifies facts about an illness with the patient during the patient's denial of that illness.

    c. plans a teaching session for a time when the patient is free from pain.

    d. presents a teaching program when the patient demonstrates a readiness to learn.

11. Mrs. Renton is hospitalized in the final states of metastatic carcinoma. She tells her physician that she will accept her prognosis if he can keep her alive until her grandchild is born in 3 months. Mrs. Renton is in that stage of dying identified by Kubler-Ross as:

    a. isolation.

    b. anger.

    c. bargaining.

    d. depression.

SHORT ANSWER

Read each statement carefully. Write your response in the space provided.

1. It is estimated that approximately _____% of consumers in the United States follow holistic health practices.

2. Write the most commonly accepted definition of a mental disorder.

   _____

3. Identify seven common emotional responses to posttraumatic stress disorder (PTSD).

   _____ _____

   _____ _____

   _____ _____

   _____

4. Three physiologic responses to PTSD are increased: _____, _____, and _____.

5. List four life events that are examples of occurrences that trigger symptoms of PTSD.

   _____ _____

   _____ _____

6. List two criteria that distinguish clinical depression from everyday sadness: _____ and

   _____.

7. Four of the seven leading somatic complaints of individuals struggling with depression are:

   _____, _____,

   _____, and _____.

8. Identify the five specific symptoms diagnostic of clinical depression: _____, _____,

   _____, _____, and _____.

9. List two common substance abuse problems: _____ and _____.

10. List the five major family functions described by Wright and Leahy (2005) that significantly influence an individual's response to illness.

    _____ _____

    _____ _____

    _____

11. List the four major tasks of the grieving process: _____, _____,

    _____, and _____.

II. Critical Thinking Questions and Exercises

DISCUSSION AND ANALYSIS

Discuss the following topics with your classmates.

1. Compare and contrast the characteristics associated with mental health to those characteristics associated with mental disorders.
2. Nurses need to be vigilant in assessing for signs of anxiety. List one indicator of anxiety for each

   classification: physiologic, emotional, relational, and spiritual: _____,

   _____, _____, _____, and

   _____.

3. Discuss at least five specific nursing interventions for helping patients manage anxiety:

   _____, _____, _____,

   _____, and _____.

4. Discuss several nursing approaches to assess a patient for possible substance

   abuse._____

   _____

5. Discuss two signs and symptoms of grieving that a nurse should assess for grieving for each of three indicators: physiologic, emotional, and behavioral.

_____ _____

_____ _____

_____ _____

RECOGNIZING CONTRADICTIONS

Rewrite each statement correctly. Underline the key concepts.

1. Since 1980, there has been a gradual decline in the number of individuals who seek holistic health care treatment.

2. The philosophical framework supporting holistic health care is emphasis on the spiritual domain of healing.

3. Clinical depression is a common response to health problems, especially for the young and the elderly.

4. A diagnosis of clinical depression requires repeated episodes of sadness over a 4-week period.

CLINICAL SITUATIONS

Read the following case studies. Circle the correct answer.

CASE STUDY: Hodgkin's Disease

Joan, a 29-year-old mother of two, works 20 hours a week as a secretary. She was diagnosed with Hodgkin's disease the week of her 29th birthday.

1. Joan's reaction to the diagnosis was to increase her working time to 40 hours per week and to increase her social activities. Joan's response is characteristic of the:
   a. first stage of illness.
   b. second stage of illness.
   c. third stage of illness.
   d. fourth stage of illness.

2. The most prominent emotion the nurse would expect Joan to experience at the time of her diagnosis is:
   a. acceptance.
   b. denial.
   c. depression.
   d. guilt.

3. Nursing intervention at the time of the diagnosis would *not* include:
   a. answering questions.
   b. listening to the patient ventilate.
   c. reinforcing reality.
   d. supporting denial.

CASE STUDY: Radical Mastectomy

Kathy, a 45-year-old, single executive with a major oil company, lives alone in a high-rise city apartment. She is recovering from a right radical mastectomy performed 3 days ago.

1. Kathy is firm about not bathing in the morning because her normal home routine involves a nightly relaxing tub bath. The nurse should:
   a. document in the plan of care that bathing is to take place near bedtime.
   b. explain the clinical routine to Kathy to help her understand the necessity for each patient to comply so that all patients will receive optimum care.
   c. gently remind Kathy that she is not in control in a hospital; the nurses decide when baths will be taken.
   d. give Kathy a choice of morning bath care or evening shower care, because staffing on the evening shift is not sufficient to meet her needs.

2. Kathy refuses to acknowledge that her breast was removed. She believes that her breast is intact under the dressings. The nurse should:
   a. call the physician to change the dressings so that Kathy can see the incision.
   b. recognize that Kathy is experiencing denial, a normal stage of the grieving process.
   c. reinforce Kathy's belief for several days, until her body can adjust to the stress of surgery.
   d. remind Kathy that she needs to accept her diagnosis so that she can begin rehabilitation exercises.

3. Kathy screams at her nurse because the nurse is 10 minutes late administering Kathy's pain medication. The nurse is aware that anger:
   a. is a maladaptive response to a stressful situation.
   b. is an anticipated reaction to a change in body appearance.
   c. should be reinforced to help reality orientation.
   d. should be repressed so that Kathy can gain control of her surroundings.

4. To help Kathy adjust to her altered body image, the nurse should:
   a. offer acceptance.
   b. reinforce Kathy's concept of self-worth.
   c. understand Kathy's emotional responses to her illness and her surgery.
   d. all of the above.

CHAPTER 8

Perspectives in Transcultural Nursing

I. Interpretation, Completion, and Comparison

MULTIPLE CHOICE

Read each question carefully. Circle your answer.

1. Choose the minority group in the United States that is not federally recognized as a minority.
   a. Asian/Pacific Islanders
   b. Hispanic Americans
   c. Native Americans
   d. Islamic

2. The most common non-English language spoken in the United States is:
   a. German.
   b. French.
   c. Italian.
   d. Spanish.

3. Madeline Leininger's theory of transcultural nursing supports providing care that:
   a. allows for restructuring.
   b. can be accommodated.
   c. is congruent.
   d. reflects all of the above characteristics.

4. Personal space is a culturally defined phenomenon. In comparing cultures, individuals who require the *most* personal space between themselves and others are from:
   a. Japan.
   b. Latin America.
   c. the Middle East.
   d. the United States.

5. Choose the culture that does *not* consider eye contact to be impolite when speaking with another:
   a. American.
   b. Arabian.
   c. Indo-Chinese.
   d. Native American.

6. The cultural group for which staring at the floor during conversation is considered behavior conveying respect is:
   a. Asian.
   b. Appalachian.
   c. Indo-Chinese.
   d. Native American.

7. The cultural group that maintains downcast eyes as a sign of appropriate deferential behavior toward others is:
   a. Asians.
   b. Hispanics.
   c. Indo-Chinese.
   d. Native Americans.

8. People from all of the following countries require the most personal space between themselves and others *except* for:
   a. Canada.
   b. Great Britain.
   c. Latin America.
   d. United States of America.

9. The cultural group that has a wide frame of reference for attitudes about time is:
   a. Hispanic.
   b. Arabian.
   c. Native American.
   d. Asian.

10. The nurse would expect that a woman from which of the following cultures would want only a female physician to examine her.
    a. Arabian
    b. Asian
    c. Japanese
    d. Latin American

11. For many in this cultural group, it is impolite to touch a person's head.
    a. Asian American
    b. Arabian
    c. Hispanic
    d. Japanese

12. Choose the religious group that shuns the use of caffeine-containing beverages.
    a. Hindu
    b. Jewish
    c. Mormon
    d. Seventh Day Adventist

13. Alcoholic beverages are shunned by all of the following religious groups *except*:
    a. Islam.
    b. Judaism.
    c. Mormonism.
    d. Seventh Day Adventism.

14. It is estimated that approximately . . . % of adults in the United States use alternative medicine?
    a. 15%
    b. 25%
    c. 35%
    d. 60%

15. The yin/yang theory of harmony and illness is rooted in which paradigm of health and illness?
    a. Biomedical
    b. Holistic
    c. Religious
    d. Scientific

SHORT ANSWER

Read each statement carefully. Write your response in the space provided.

1. The founder of transcultural nursing is: _____.

2. Name the four basic characteristics of all ethnic cultures:

   _____, _____,

   _____, and _____.

3. Three elements frequently used to identify diversity are: _____,

   _____, and _____.

4. Define the term *culturally competent nursing care*.

   _____

   _____

5. List four examples of American subcultures based on ethnicity: _____,

   _____, _____, and _____.

6. Give at least five examples of other groupings that can be used to identity subcultures.

   _____, _____, _____,

   _____, and _____.

7. The two underlying goals of transcultural nursing are to provide: _____ and

   _____ care.

8. Explain the concept of *culturally competent or congruent nursing care.*

   _____

   _____

9. List four strategies that individuals tend to use when communication has broken down.

   _____, _____,

   _____, and _____.

10. Name five religious groups that routinely incorporate fasting into their religious practices.

    _____, _____, _____,

    _____, and _____.

11. Explain the concept of yin/yang.

    _____

    _____

12. Three major paradigms are used to explain the causes of disease and illness. They are: _____,

    _____, and _____.

MATCHING

Match the classification of a complementary and alternative therapy listed in column II with a specific type of holistic care listed in column I. An answer can be used more than once.

Column I

1. _____ Hypnosis
2. _____ Reiki
3. _____ Acupuncture
4. _____ Chiropractic
5. _____ Dietary plans
6. _____ Ayurveda
7. _____ Therapeutic touch
8. _____ Homeopathic medicine
9. _____ Dance and music
10. _____ Qi gong

Column II

a. Alternative medical systems
b. Biologically based systems
c. Energy therapies
d. Manipulative methods
e. Mind–body interventions

II. Critical Thinking Questions and Exercises

DISCUSSION AND ANALYSIS

Discuss the following topics with your classmates.

1. Explain the goal of Madeleine Leininger's comprehensive research-based theory called "Culture Care Diversity and Universality."
2. Explain the concepts of culture care accommodation and culture care restructuring, according to Leininger's theory.
3. Distinguish between the terms *acculturation* and *cultural imposition*.
4. Discuss the meaning of the term *cultural blindness*.
5. Discuss several activities that a nurse could use to overcome language barriers when interacting with a patient from a different culture.
6. Explain the meaning of the term *general polymorphism*.
7. Distinguish between the five major categories of alternative medical interventions: alternative medical systems, mind–body interventions, biologically based therapies, manipulative and body-based methods, and energy therapies.

CHAPTER 9

Genetics and Genomics Perspectives in Nursing

I. Interpretation, Completion, and Comparison

MULTIPLE CHOICE

Read each question carefully. Circle your answer.

1. The study of all the genes in the human genome and their interactions is known as:
   a. genetics.
   b. genomics.
   c. meiosis.
   d. mitosis.

2. Chromosomes are located within the nucleus of a cell. The human body has _____ chromosomes.
   a. 23
   b. 46
   c. 69
   d. 92

3. Gene mutations have significant implications for health and illness. A mutation in protein structure that alters the configuration of hemoglobin is known as:
   a. fragile X syndrome.
   b. Huntington's disease.
   c. muscular dystrophy.
   d. sickle cell anemia.

4. *Trisomy* refers to a condition in which cellular division results in an extra chromosome. An example of trisomy is:
   a. Down syndrome.
   b. sickle cell anemia.
   c. Tay-Sachs disease.
   d. Turner's syndrome.

5. Stephanie has learned that her ovarian cancer syndrome is an autosomal dominant inherited condition. Stephanie knows that her daughter has . . . % of a chance of inheriting the gene mutation for this disease?
   a. 10% to 15%
   b. 25%
   c. 50%
   d. 60% to 80%

6. An example of an autosomal recessive inherited condition is:
   a. cystic fibrosis.
   b. hereditary breast cancer.
   c. Huntington's disease.
   d. familial hypercholesterolemia.

7. In autosomal recessive inheritance, each parent is a nonsymptomatic carrier and children have a 25% chance of inheriting the gene. All of the following are examples of autosomal recessive inheritance *except*:
   a. cystic fibrosis.
   b. Marfan's syndrome.
   c. phenylketonuria.
   d. sickle cell anemia.

8. An example of an X-linked, recessive inherited condition, in which a mother (carrier) has a 50% chance of passing the gene onto her son, is:

   a. cystic fibrosis.

   b. hemophilia.

   c. phenylketonuria.

   d. Tay-Sachs disease.

9. Katie has just been told that she has the *BRCA1* hereditary breast cancer gene mutation. At age 32, she knows that her risk of developing cancer by the age of 65 years is as high as:

   a. 25%.

   b. 50%.

   c. 80%.

   d. 100%.

10. Kurt and Kathy are carriers for thalassemia. They are thinking about starting a family. A nurse tells them that they have . . . % of a risk of having a child who will inherit the gene?

    a. 25%

    b. 50%

    c. 75%

    d. 100%

11. A multifactorial genetic condition that tends to cluster in families is:

    a. galactosemia.

    b. Duchenne muscular dystrophy.

    c. neurofibromatosis.

    d. neural tube defects.

12. When assessing patient information as part of genetic counseling, the nurse knows that Tay-Sachs disease is most common among:

    a. Ashkenazi Jews.

    b. Italian Americans.

    c. American Indians.

    d. African Americans.

SHORT ANSWER

Read each statement. Write your response in the space provided.

1. The term *genomic medicine* refers to:

   _____

   _____

2. The nurse uses a framework for integrating genetics into nursing practice when he or she:

   _____, _____, _____, and

   _____.

3. A person's individual genetic makeup (composed of 30,000 to 40,000 genes) is called a _____; the person's set of characteristics of physical appearance and other traits is called a _____.

4. Genes are working subunits of DNA. Genes are arranged in linear order within _____. Twenty-two pairs of chromosomes, also called _____, are the same in males and females. The 23rd pair, the _____, is composed of two _____ for the female and _____ for the male. At conception, the sex of a child is determined because each parent gives _____.

5. With autosomal dominant inheritance, a woman with the *BRCA1* hereditary breast cancer gene has a lifetime risk of _____% of acquiring breast cancer and a _____% chance of passing the gene to each child.

6. Cite five examples of multifactorial-inherited conditions: _____, _____, _____, _____, and _____.

7. Name the common chromosomal condition that occurs with greater frequency in pregnancies of women who are 35 years of age or older.

_____

8. The frequency of chromosomal abnormalities in newborns is _____; this accounts for a _____% of all spontaneous first-trimester pregnancy losses.

9. List three examples of adult-onset conditions that are believed to be the result of multifactorial genetic mutations. _____, _____, and _____.

10. The most common adult-onset condition in the Caucasian population that can be identified with parasymptomatic testing is:

_____.

11. Define the term *pharmacogenetics*.

_____

12. List five nursing activities in genetics-related nursing practice: _____, _____, _____, _____, and _____.

MATCHING

Match the genetic term listed in column II with its specific definition listed in column I.

Column I

1. _____ The number of chromosomes normally present in humans (N = 46)

2. _____ The presence of one extra chromosome (e.g., Down's syndrome)

3. _____ The genes and variations that a person inherits from his or her parents

4. _____ A single chromosome from any of the 22 pairs not involved in sex determination (XX or XY)

5. _____ A person's entire physiological and biological makeup as determined by genotype and environment

6. _____ Primary genetic material (DNA)

7. _____ A heterozygous person who carries two different alleles of a gene pair

8. _____ The microscopic cell nucleus that contains genetic information

Column II

a. Autosome
b. Carrier
c. Chromosome
d. Deoxyribonucleic acid
e. Diploid
f. Genotype
g. Phenotype
h. Trisomy

Match the age of adult onset in column II with the specific disorder listed in column I.

Column I

1. _____ Spinocerebellar ataxia, type 2

2. _____ Huntington's disease

3. _____ Early-onset familial Alzheimer's disease

4. _____ Hereditary hemochromatosis

5. _____ Spinocerebellar ataxia, type 3

6. _____ Polycystic kidney disease

7. _____ Familial hypercholesterolemia

8. _____ Amotrophic lateral sclerosis (ALS)

Column II

a. Mean age of 30 years

b. 30 to 40 years

c. 35 to 44 years

d. 40 to 60 years

e. 60 to 65 years

f. 50 to 70 years

II. Critical Thinking Questions and Exercises

DISCUSSION AND ANALYSIS

Discuss the following topics with your classmates.

1. Compare and contrast the characteristics of medical-era interventions to the genomic-era of personalized medicine.
2. Discuss the professional responsibilities and practices for nurses as recommended by the ANA (2006) in *"Essential Nursing Competencies and Curricula Guidelines for Genetics and Genomics."*
3. Developing self-awareness about attitudes, experiences, and assumptions regarding genetics can help the nurse apply a genetic framework to patient care. To understand your own attitudes, experiences, and assumptions, consider the following topics for discussion: (a) level of genetic knowledge; (b) past and current experiences with birth defects, chronic illnesses, and genetic conditions; (c) understanding of DNA; (d) beliefs about genetic testing; and (e) approach to those with disabilities.
4. Nursing assessment includes a family history to establish the presence of genetic conditions that are inherited (Mendelian conditions). Compare and contrast the types of Mendelian conditions: autosomal dominant, autosomal recessive, and X-linked.
5. Discuss the current availability of personalized genomic treatments.

CHAPTER 10

Chronic Illness and Disability

I. Interpretation, Completion, and Comparison

MULTIPLE CHOICE

Read each question carefully. Circle your answer.

1. In the United States (2006), chronic diseases account for what percentage of the leading causes of death?
   a. 20%
   b. 35%
   c. 50%
   d. 70%

2. The percentage of mortality in the United States (2002) directly attributed to chronic diseases was:
   a. 36%.
   b. 50%.
   c. 62%.
   d. 88%.

3. A medical condition, with associated symptoms or disabilities, is considered *chronic* when long-term management is required for a *minimum* of:
   a. 8 weeks.
   b. 3 months.
   c. 16 weeks.
   d. 6 months.

4. Currently the percentage of health care costs associated with chronic illness is approximately:
   a. 30%.
   b. 40%.
   c. 50%.
   d. 75%.

5. If preventable risk factors were eliminated, all of the following chronic illnesses would be eliminated *except*:
   a. 80% of heart disease.
   b. 40% of cancer.
   c. 80% of stroke incidences.
   d. 20% of diabetes.

6. Identify the chronic illness that is increasing rapidly and is directly related to an unhealthy lifestyle.
   a. Diabetes mellitus
   b. Breast cancer
   c. Emphysema
   d. Colorectal cancer

7. A major health-promoting behavior that can significantly improve the quality of life for those with a chronic condition is:
   a. diet.
   b. exercise.
   c. hydration.
   d. rest.

8. A person who is at risk for developing a chronic condition because of genetic factors is said to be in which phase of the Trajectory Model?
   a. Pretrajectory
   b. Trajectory
   c. Unstable
   d. Acute

9. Chronic illness can be monitored using the Trajectory Model. The phase in which a nursing diagnosis can help in care planning is known as:
   a. pretrajectory.
   b. trajectory.
   c. crisis.
   d. downward course.

10. Remission, after an exacerbation, represents the Trajectory Model phase known as:
    a. acute.
    b. crisis.
    c. comeback.
    d. downward course.

11. According to the most recent U.S. Census (2000), approximately what percentage of people has a disability and what percentage a severe disability?
    a. 10%; 5%
    b. 20%; 10%
    c. 30%; 15%
    d. 40%; 20%

12. An example of a developmental disability is:
    a. cerebral palsy.
    b. spinal cord injury.
    c. stroke.
    d. osteoarthritis.

13. Select the disability model that is most appropriate for nurses to use as a guide for planning care.
    a. Biopsychosocial Model
    b. Interface Model
    c. Medical and Rehabilitation Model
    d. Social Model

SHORT ANSWER

Read each statement carefully. Write your response in the space provided.

1. List the four preventable, by lifestyle changes, causes of major chronic illnesses: _____, _____, _____, and _____.

2. Three characteristics common to all forms of chronic illness are: _____, _____, and _____.

3. In 2000, approximately _____% of people in the United States had one or more chronic illnesses. In 2050, this percentage is expected to increase to _____%.

4. The three most frequently occurring chronic diseases that result from four preventable causes are: _____, _____, and _____.

5. Identify six of 11 challenges commonly associated with chronic conditions.

6. List six common medical and nursing management problems related to chronic conditions.

7. Define the concept of the Trajectory Model as it relates to chronic illness.

_____

_____

8. List three categories used to classify disabilities: _____, _____, and

_____.

II. Critical Thinking Questions and Exercises

DISCUSSION AND ANALYSIS

Discuss the following topics with your classmates.

1. Discuss the four major causes of the increased number of chronic conditions.
2. Select 5 of the 10 "Myths and Truths About Chronic Disease" (see Table 10-1 in the text) and discuss the role of nursing education in helping people understand the realities versus the perceptions of chronic disease.
3. Select 5 of the 11 "Characteristics of Chronic Conditions." Discuss the impact of these characteristics on chronic illness and the appropriate role for nursing in addressing these characteristics.
4. Discuss the difference between the terms _disability_ and _impairment_ according to the definitions approved by the World Health Organization's (1980) classification system.
5. Discuss the psychological and emotional reactions to chronic illness and those factors (e.g., lifestyle changes, financial resources) that affect adjustment.
6. Explain the differences between the Rehabilitation Act of 1973 and the Disabilities Act of 1990 and how they have helped protect disabled people from discrimination.
7. Discuss the importance of Senate bill (S. 1050), "Promoting Wellness for Individuals with Disabilities Act of 2007" proposed by Senator Harkin.

EXAMINING ASSOCIATIONS

Listed below are some characteristics of chronic illness. For each statement, write an explanation of how nursing care can improve the patient's and family's response to management and adaptation.

1. Managing chronic illness involves more than managing medical problems.

_____

_____

2. Chronic conditions are associated with different phases over a course of time.

_____

_____

3. Managing chronic conditions requires persistent adherence to a therapeutic regimen.

_____

_____

4. Chronic illness affects the whole family.

_____

_____

CLINICAL SITUATIONS

Read the case study below and follow the steps.

CASE STUDY: Applying the Nursing Process to the Trajectory Model of Chronic Illness

The focus of care for patients with chronic illness is determined by their phase of illness. Each of the nine phases can be correlated to a step in the nursing process. For each step below, discuss the role of nursing intervention. Use the example of a 32-year-old mother of one who works full-time as a teacher and has just been diagnosed with rheumatoid arthritis. She is in the Trajectory onset/stable phase of chronic illness.

Step 1: Using assessment, identify the specific problems and the Trajectory Phase.

_____

_____

Step 2: Establish and prioritize goals.

_____

_____

Step 3: Define a plan of action to achieve desired outcomes.

_____

_____

Step 4: Implement the plan and interventions.

_____

_____

Step 5: Follow-up and evaluate outcomes.

_____

_____

CHAPTER 11

Principles and Practices of Rehabilitation

I. Interpretation, Completion, and Comparison

MULTIPLE CHOICE

Read each question carefully. Circle your answer.

1. Rehabilitation, an integral part of nursing, should begin:
   a. after the patient feels comfortable in the clinical setting.
   b. after the physician has prescribed rehabilitative goals.
   c. when an exercise program has been initiated.
   d. with initial patient contact.

2. In the United States, approximately what percentage of Americans over age 5 have some form of disability and what percentage have a severe disability?
   a. 10%; 10%
   b. 20%; 10%
   c. 40%; 20%
   d. 60%; 30%

3. The most important member of the rehabilitation team is the:
   a. nurse.
   b. patient.
   c. physical therapist.
   d. physician.

4. The occurrence of spinal cord and traumatic brain injuries is directly associated with substance abuse, alcohol, and the use of illegal drugs. The percentage of patients who are under the influence of these at the time of injury is as high as:
   a. 50%.
   b. 75%.
   c. 80%.
   d. 95%.

5. The PULSES profile uses six components to evaluate self-care independence. The assessment of bladder control would be documented under:
   a. excretory function.
   b. lower system functions.
   c. physical condition.
   d. sensory functions.

6. The *least* common position used in positioning a patient in bed to prevent musculoskeletal complications is:
   a. prone.
   b. semi-Fowler's.
   c. side-lying.
   d. dorsal.

7. A nurse who wants to help a patient assume the side-lying position would:
   a. align the lower extremities in a neutral position.
   b. extend the legs with a firm support under the popliteal area.
   c. place the uppermost hip slightly forward in a position of slight abduction.
   d. position the trunk so that hip flexion is minimized.

8. A quick method used to measure for crutches is to use the patient's height and:
   a. add 6 in.
   b. add 12 in.
   c. subtract 8 in.
   d. subtract 16 in.

9. A pressure ulcer is associated with the presence of:
   a. dehydration and skin dryness.
   b. excessive skin moisture.
   c. inflammation and infection.
   d. small nutrient vessel compression.

10. Initial skin redness in a patient susceptible to pressure sores should be documented as tissue:
    a. anoxia.
    b. eschar.
    c. hyperemia.
    d. ischemia.

11. A patient at potential risk for a pressure ulcer is assessed by the nurse. A laboratory study the nurse should examine is:
    a. serum albumin.
    b. serum glucose.
    c. prothrombin time.
    d. sedimentation rate.

12. A diet recommended for hypoproteinemia that spares protein is one high in:
    a. carbohydrates.
    b. fats.
    c. minerals.
    d. vitamins.

13. Wound healing depends on collagen formation, which depends on vitamin:
    a. A.
    b. C.
    c. D.
    d. K.

14. To initiate a schedule of bladder training, the nurse should:
    a. encourage the patient to wait 30 minutes after drinking a measured amount of fluid before attempting to void.
    b. give up to 3,000 mL of fluid daily.
    c. teach bladder massage to increase intra-abdominal pressure.
    d. do all of the above.

15. Successful bowel training depends on:
    a. a daily defecation time that is within 15 minutes of the same time every day.
    b. an adequate intake of fiber-containing foods.
    c. fluid intake between 2 and 4 L/day.
    d. all of the above.

16. Sexual problems faced by the disabled include:
    a. impaired self-image.
    b. lack of opportunities to form friendships.
    c. limited access to information about sexuality.
    d. all of the above.

SHORT ANSWER

Read each statement carefully. Write your response in the space provided.

1. The three goals of rehabilitation are to: _____, _____, and _____.

2. List eight specialty rehabilitation programs accredited by the Commission for the Accreditation of Rehabilitation Facilities (CARF).

   _____   _____

   _____   _____

   _____   _____

   _____   _____

3. List five major goals for rehabilitation that are associated with the nursing diagnosis of self-care deficit in activities of daily living (ADL): bathing/hygiene, dressing/grooming, feeding, and toileting:

   _____, _____, _____, _____, and _____.

4. Five nursing diagnoses for patients with impaired physical mobility could be: _____, _____, _____, _____, and _____.

   Four major rehabilitative goals are: _____, _____, _____, and _____.

5. List four collaborative problems for a patient with impaired physical mobility:

   _____, _____, _____, and _____.

6. Three complications commonly associated with prolonged or impaired physical immobility are:

   _____, _____, and _____.

7. Two common musculoskeletal complications for patients who are in bed for prolonged periods are:

   _____ and _____.

8. Four factors that contribute to foot drop are: _____,

   _____, _____, and _____.

9. List five types of therapeutic exercises and describe the nursing activity required to support the exercise:

   Therapeutic Exercise Nursing Activity

   _____   _____

   _____   _____

   _____   _____

   _____   _____

   _____

10. To maintain use, a joint should be moved through its range of motion at least _____ times per day.

11. List 6 of 10 risk factors for pressure ulcer formation.

_____   _____

_____   _____

_____   _____

12. List 6 of a possible 12 areas susceptible to pressure ulcer formation.

_____   _____

_____   _____

_____   _____

13. A life-threatening complication of a stage IV pressure ulcer is: _____.

14. Eschar covering an ulcer should be removed surgically because: _____

15. Alkaline-producing beverages such as _____, _____, _____, _____, and _____ promote bacterial growth in the urine and should be avoided for patients who suffer from incontinence.

MATCHING

Match the explanations of range-of-motion techniques listed in column II with their associated terms in column I.

Column I

1. ____ Adduction
2. ____ Dorsiflexion
3. ____ Extension
4. ____ Inversion
5. ____ Pronation
6. ____ Abduction

Column II

a. Bending of the foot toward the leg
b. Increasing the angle of a joint
c. Movement away from the midline of the body
d. Movement that turns the sole of the foot inward
e. Movement toward the midline of the body
f. Rotating the forearm so that the palm is down

II. Critical Thinking Questions, Exercises, and Issues

DISCUSSION AND ANALYSIS

Discuss the following topics with your classmates.

1. Discuss the concerns of older adults facing disability; include personal, religious, and psychosocial concerns.
2. Compare and contrast activities of daily living (ADLs) and independent activities of daily living (IADLs) and discuss implications for nursing assessment for each.
3. Discuss several nursing interventions for patients who are experiencing one or more disability-triggered reactions or disability-associated coping strategies.
4. Compare and contrast four tools that are used to assess a patient's level of functional ability: the Functional Independence Measure (FIM), the PULSES profile, the Barthel Index, and the Patient Evaluation Conference System (PECS).
5. Discuss 14 indications of potential problems in function or movements that are needed to perform ADLs that a nurse should assess to determine a patient's level of self-care independence.
6. Discuss the nursing role for preparing patients to use crutches, a walker, and a cane. Review the directions needed for ambulation activities.

7. Explain the physiological basis for the development of a pressure ulcer.
8. Compare and contrast the physiological differences in pressure ulcers in stages I through IV.
9. Discuss three major nursing diagnoses and four major nursing goals for a patient with altered elimination patterns.

CLINICAL SITUATIONS

View Figures 11-5 and 11-6 and Charts 11-10 and 11-11 in the text, and answer the following clinically focused questions regarding impaired skin integrity.

1. Define the term *pressure ulcer.*

   _____

   _____

2. The initial sign of pressure is _____, which is caused by _____; unrelieved pressure results in _____ and _____.

3. Two areas that are the most susceptible to the effects of shear and therefore pressure ulcer formation are: the _____ and the _____.

4. Four microorganisms that contribute to infection in pressure ulcers are: _____, _____, _____, and _____.

5. Serum albumin levels less than _____ increase the risk of pressure ulcers. Therefore, a protein intake of _____ is recommended to promote ulcer healing.

6. Two assessment scales that nurses can use to quantify a patient's risk for pressure ulcer formation are the _____ and _____ scales.

7. Based on Pascal's law, explain why a gel-type flotation pad and an air-fluidized bed reduce pressure:

   _____

   _____

8. Explain why the shearing force is increased when the head of the bed is raised, even if only by a few centimeters.

   _____

   _____

Read the following case study. Circle the correct answers.

CASE STUDY: Assisted Ambulation: Crutches

Rita, a 17-year-old college student, is in a full leg cast because of a compound fracture of the left femur. Rita is to be discharged from the hospital in several days. She lives with her parents in a split-level house.

1. The exercises that the nurse would recommend to strengthen Rita's upper extremity muscles are:
   a. isometric exercises of the biceps.
   b. push-ups performed in a sitting position.
   c. gluteal setting.
   d. quadriceps setting.

2. Rita is 5 ft 5 in tall. Her crutches should measure:
   a. 45 in.
   b. 49 in.
   c. 54 in.
   d. 59 in.

3. Before teaching a crutch gait, the nurse directs Rita to assume the tripod position. In this basic crutch stance, the crutches are placed in front and to the side of Rita's toes, at an approximate distance of:
   a. 4 to 6 in.
   b. 6 to 8 in.
   c. 8 to 10 in.
   d. 10 to 12 in.

4. Because Rita is not allowed to bear weight on her casted leg, she should be taught the:
   a. two-point gait.
   b. three-point gait.
   c. four-point gait.
   d. swing-through gait.

CHAPTER 12

Health Care of the Older Adult

I. Interpretation, Completion, and Comparison

MULTIPLE CHOICE

Read each question carefully. Circle your answer.

1. The scientific study of the aging process is referred to as:
   a. ageism.
   b. geriatrics.
   c. gerontonics.
   d. gerontology.

2. The leading cause of morbidity and mortality in the aged is a disorder or dysfunction of which system?
   a. Cardiovascular
   b. Genitourinary
   c. Gastrointestinal
   d. Respiratory

3. Respiratory changes associated with aging include all of the following *except*:
   a. decreased residual volume.
   b. changes in the anteroposterior diameter of the chest.
   c. loss of elastic tissue surrounding the alveoli.
   d. reduced vital capacity.

4. All of the following statements concerning genitourinary system changes in the older adult are true *except*:
   a. the renal filtration rate decreases.
   b. the acid–base balance is restored more slowly.
   c. bladder capacity increases with advanced age.
   d. urinary frequency, urgency, and incontinence are common problems.

5. Dietary intake should emphasize fruits, vegetables, and fish. The daily intake of carbohydrates should be about:
   a. 20% to 25%.
   b. 40% to 45%.
   c. 55% to 60%.
   d. 70% to 75%.

6. Bone changes associated with aging frequently result from a loss of:
   a. calcium.
   b. magnesium.
   c. vitamin A.
   d. vitamin C.

7. Nervous system changes associated with aging include all of the following *except*:
   a. a decrease in brain weight subsequent to the destruction of brain cells.
   b. an increase in blood flow to the brain to compensate for the gradual loss of brain cells.
   c. atrophy of the convolutions of the brain surface.
   d. widening and deepening of the spaces between the convolutions of the brain.

8. Nursing measures to deal with sensory changes in the aged include:

   a. increasing room lighting without increasing glare.

   b. speaking louder than normal.

   c. suggesting appetite stimulants before meals.

   d. all of the above actions.

9. Drug dosages must be reduced in the elderly because:

   a. cardiac output is significantly reduced.

   b. the number of mucosal cells in the gastrointestinal tract is reduced.

   c. drug biotransformation takes longer in older persons.

   d. all of the above are true.

10. The medications that remain in the body longer in the elderly because of increased body fat are:

    a. anticoagulants.

    b. barbiturates.

    c. digitalis glycosides.

    d. diuretics.

11. The ninth leading cause of death in older persons is:

    a. accidents and injuries.

    b. drug toxicity.

    c. elder abuse.

    d. malnutrition.

12. The major source of federal funding that provides nursing home care for the poor elderly is:

    a. Medicaid.

    b. Medicare.

SHORT ANSWER

Read each statement carefully. Write your response in the space provided.

1. Define the term *geriatric syndromes*.

   _____

2. The four leading causes of death for people age 65 and older (2006) are: _____, _____, _____, and _____.

3. Age-related changes reduce the efficiency of the cardiovascular system. These changes include: _____, _____, and _____, which result in _____.

4. The primary cause of age-related vision loss in the elderly is: _____.

5. With aging, there is a gradual decline in _____ and _____; _____ skills tend to remain intact.

6. Two age-related alterations in metabolism are: _____ and _____.

7. The most common affective or mood disorder of old age is: _____.

8. List the five most common infections in the elderly: _____, _____, _____, _____, and _____.

9. The leading cause of injury in the elderly is: _____.

II. Critical Thinking Questions and Exercises

INTERPRETING DATA

Refer to Figure 12-1 in the text to answer the following questions.

1. In the decade between the years 2000 and 2010, the percentage of people older than 65 years of age was projected to increase by the following: _____%.
2. In the decade between 2010 and 2020, the projected increase in the number of people older than 65 years will be _____%, more than _____ that of the prior 10 years (2000–2010).
3. The percentage of people older than 65 years of age is projected to increase from 2020 to 2030 by _____%.
4. By the year 2020, it is projected that there will be approximately _____ million people over age 65. This number is projected to grow to _____ million by 2030, a _____% increase over 10 years.

RECOGNIZING CONTRADICTIONS

Rewrite each statement correctly. Underline the key concepts.

1. Osteoporosis, accelerated by the loss of estrogen, can be reversed with a high-calcium diet.

_____

2. If the symptoms of delirium go untreated, they will eventually decrease, and the person will regain his or her previous level of consciousness.

_____

3. Older persons should "take it easy" and avoid vigorous activity.

_____

4. Baseline body temperature is usually 1°F higher than normal in an older person because dehydration is common.

_____

DISCUSSION AND ANALYSIS

Discuss the following topics with your classmates.

1. Discuss age-related findings (subjective and objective) for the major body systems and nursing implications for health promotion strategies. Use Table 12-2 in the text as a guide.
2. Explain the concept of *continuing care retirement communities.*
3. Discuss several nursing interventions that can be used to help older adults with learning and memory.
4. Review a variety of nursing interventions that can be used to help patients manage their medications and improve compliance.
5. Compare and contrast the etiology, risk factors, symptoms, physical signs, and memory and personality changes for delirium and dementia.
6. Explain the statement, "Alzheimer's disease is a diagnosis of exclusion."
7. Discuss the purpose and services provided to the elderly as a result of the Older Americans Act.
8. Distinguish between the two major programs in the United States that finance health care: Medicare and Medicaid.
9. Explain the purpose and limitations of a living will and a durable power of attorney.
10. Explain the Patient Self-Determination Act (PSDA).

CLINICAL SITUATIONS

Read the following case studies. Circle the correct answer or fill in the blanks below.

CASE STUDY: Loneliness

Suzanne is an 80-year-old retired schoolteacher. She was recently widowed and lives alone. She is financially secure but socially isolated, because she has outlived most of her friends. Her children are self-sufficient and are very busy with their own lives.

1. Psychological threats that Suzanne may experience include:
   a. a deterioration of self-concept.
   b. a loss of self-esteem.
   c. extensive grief over frequently occurring losses.
   d. all of the above.

2. Suzanne is concerned about the dryness of her skin. Suggestions for skin care include:
   a. applying ointment to the skin several times a day.
   b. avoiding overexposure to the sun.
   c. patting the skin dry instead of rubbing it with a towel.
   d. all of the above measures.

3. Suzanne notices that food does not taste the same as before. She needs to be aware that this sensory change is most probably related to:
   a. a decrease in the number of taste buds.
   b. a loss of appetite associated with a decreased sense of smell.
   c. altered enzyme secretions.
   d. diminished gastric secretions.

4. An analysis of Suzanne's diet shows that it does not contain adequate protein. Her daily protein intake, for a body weight of 134 lb, should be about:
   a. 30 g.
   b. 40 g.
   c. 50 g.
   d. 60 g.

5. Most accidents among older people involve falls within the home. Preventive nursing measures include advising Suzanne to:
   a. avoid climbing and bending.
   b. keep personal items stored at a level between her hips and her eyes.
   c. make certain that all her shoes fit securely.
   d. do all of the above.

CASE STUDY: Alzheimer's Disease

Thomas, a 75-year-old retired bricklayer, lives at home with Anne, his 65-year-old wife, who is healthy and active. Lately Anne has noticed that Thomas is negative, hostile, and suspicious of her. He gets lost in his own home, and his conversations have been accompanied by forgetfulness. Recently, Thomas' physician has indicated a probable diagnosis of Alzheimer's disease.

1. Choose the statement that is *false* concerning Alzheimer's disease.
   a. It is found only in old persons.
   b. The disease process is irreversible.
   c. The probable cause is neuropathology and biochemical.
   d. The cells that are affected by the disease are the ones that use acetylcholine.

2. Physiologically, an enzyme that produces the neurotransmitter _____ is decreased and neural damage occurs primarily in the _____, causing decreased _____.

3. There is no cure and no way to delay the disease progression. However, there are five medications that treat the symptoms: _____, _____, _____, _____, and _____.

4. The nurse should suggest that Anne deal with Thomas' behavior by:
   a. reasoning with him.
   b. providing reality orientation.
   c. providing a calm and predictable environment.
   d. not structuring activities for him.

5. An important point to communicate to Anne is that:
   a. there are no realistic goals appropriate for Thomas.
   b. lists and written instructions will only tend to confuse Thomas.
   c. Thomas should be restrained when agitated.
   d. maintaining personal dignity and autonomy is still an important part of Thomas' life.

6. Caregivers of patients with Alzheimer's disease should be aware that:
   a. Alzheimer's support groups exist.
   b. Alzheimer's disease does not eliminate the need for intimacy.
   c. Socializing with old friends may be comforting.
   d. All of the above are appropriate.

7. The physician explains that there is no cure for the disease and no way to slow its progression, which intensifies symptoms. Eventually death occurs as a result of complications such as _____, _____, and _____.

CASE STUDY: Dehydration

Vera, an 89-year-old widow, was transferred from a nursing home to a hospital with a diagnosis of dehydration. Vera needs to be in bed because of her generalized weakness. She is occasionally confused and disoriented.

1. From knowledge of temperature regulation in the elderly, the nurse should:
   a. make sure that the environmental temperature is adequate.
   b. palpate Vera's skin periodically to assess for warmth.
   c. place extra blankets at Vera's bedside in case she becomes cold, especially in the evening.
   d. do all of the above.

2. The nurse initiates a 2-hour turning schedule for Vera, based on the knowledge that the underlying cause of all decubiti is:
   a. altered skin turgor.
   b. nutritional deficiency.
   c. pressure.
   d. vasoconstriction.

3. Vera has been incontinent of urine since admission. Nursing interventions include all of the following *except*:
   a. initiating a bladder-training program.
   b. offering fluids frequently to maintain a minimum daily intake of 2 to 3 L.
   c. providing means for limited daily exercises and ambulation.
   d. securing a physician's order for urethral catheterization.

4. The nurse suggests that Vera sit in a rocking chair for 20 minutes, four times a day. This suggestion is based on the knowledge that rocking:
   a. discourages hypostatic pulmonary congestion.
   b. increases pulmonary ventilation.
   c. improves venous return through contraction of the calf muscles.
   d. does all of the above.

CHAPTER 13

Pain Management

I. Interpretation, Completion, and Comparison

MULTIPLE CHOICE

Read each question carefully. Circle your answer.

1. Although the criterion is arbitrary, acute pain can be classified as chronic when it has persisted for:
   - a. 1 to 2 months.
   - b. 3 months.
   - c. 3 to 5 months.
   - d. longer than 6 months.

2. Acute pain may be described as having the following characteristic.
   - a. It does not usually respond well to treatment.
   - b. It is associated with a specific injury.
   - c. It serves no useful purpose.
   - d. It responds well to placebos.

3. A physiologic response not usually associated with acute pain is:
   - a. decreased cardiac output.
   - b. altered insulin response.
   - c. increased metabolic rate.
   - d. decreased production of cortisol.

4. Chronic pain may be described as:
   - a. attributable to a specific cause.
   - b. prolonged in duration.
   - c. rapidly occurring and subsiding with treatment.
   - d. separate from any central or peripheral pathology.

5. An example of chronic benign pain is:
   - a. a migraine headache.
   - b. an exacerbation of rheumatoid arthritis.
   - c. low back pain.
   - d. sickle cell crisis.

6. A chemical substance thought to inhibit the transmission of pain is:
   - a. acetylcholine.
   - b. bradykinin.
   - c. enkephalin.
   - d. histamine.

7. All of the following statements about endorphins are true *except*:
   - a. Their release inhibits the transmission of painful impulses.
   - b. They represent the same mechanism of pain relief as nonnarcotic analgesics.
   - c. They are endogenous neurotransmitters structurally similar to opioids.
   - d. They are found in heavy concentrations in the central nervous system.

8. The nurse assessing for pain should:
   a. believe a patient when he or she states that pain is present.
   b. doubt that pain exists when no physical origin can be identified.
   c. realize that patients frequently imagine and state that they have pain without actually feeling painful sensations.
   d. do all of the above.

9. When a nurse asks a patient to describe the quality of his or her pain, the nurse expects the patient to use a descriptive term such as:
   a. burning.
   b. chronic.
   c. intermittent.
   d. severe.

10. A physiologic indicator of acute pain is:
    a. diaphoresis.
    b. bradycardia.
    c. hypotension.
    d. lowered respiratory rate.

11. A nursing measure to manage anxiety during the anticipation of pain should include:
    a. focusing the patient's attention on another problem.
    b. teaching about the nature of the impending pain and associated relief measures.
    c. using an anxiety-reducing technique, such as desensitization.
    d. any or all of the above.

12. A nursing plan of care for pain management should include:
    a. altering factors that influence the pain sensation.
    b. determining responses to the patient's behavior toward pain.
    c. selecting goals for nursing intervention.
    d. all of the above.

13. Pain in the elderly requires careful assessment, because older people:
    a. are expected to experience chronic pain.
    b. have a decreased pain threshold.
    c. experience reduced sensory perception.
    d. have increased sensory perception.

14. Administration of analgesics to the elderly requires careful patient assessment, because older people:
    a. metabolize drugs more rapidly.
    b. have increased hepatic, renal, and gastrointestinal function.
    c. are more sensitive to drugs.
    d. have lower ratios of body fat and muscle mass.

15. The most serious side effect of opioid analgesic agents is:
    a. renal toxicity.
    b. respiratory depression.
    c. seizures.
    d. hypotension.

16. A preventive approach to pain relief with nonsteroidal anti-inflammatory drugs (NSAIDs) means that the medication is given:
    a. before the pain becomes severe.
    b. before the pain is experienced.
    c. when pain is at its peak.
    d. when the level of pain tolerance has been exceeded.

17. The nurse's major area of assessment for a patient receiving patient-controlled analgesia (PCA) is assessment of which system?
    a. Cardiovascular
    b. Integumentary
    c. Neurologic
    d. Respiratory

18. The advantage of using intraspinal infusion to deliver analgesics is:
    a. reduced side effects of systemic analgesia.
    b. reduced effects on pulse, respirations, and blood pressure.
    c. reduced need for frequent injections.
    d. all of the above.

19. This single-dose, extended-release drug is used for epidural administration for patients undergoing major surgical procedures:
    a. codeine.
    b. Demerol.
    c. Dilaudid.
    d. Depodur.

20. The most worrisome adverse effect of epidural opioids is:
    a. asystole.
    b. hypertension.
    c. bradypnea.
    d. tachycardia.

21. Cutaneous stimulation is helpful in reducing painful sensations, because it:
    a. provides distraction from the pain source and decreases awareness.
    b. releases endorphins.
    c. stimulates large-diameter nerve fibers and reduces the intensity of pain.
    d. accomplishes all of the above.

SHORT ANSWER

Read each statement carefully. Write your response in the space provided.

1. Pain can be defined according to its: _____, _____, and _____.

2. The three basic categories of pain are: _____, _____, and _____.

3. Pain can be categorized by its etiology. List four of eight pain syndromes: _____, _____, _____, and _____.

4. One pathophysiologic response to chronic pain is: _____.

5. List five algogenic substances that are released into the tissues and affect the sensitivity of nociceptors: _____, _____, _____, _____, and _____.

6. List seven factors that directly influence an individual's response to pain: _____, _____, _____, _____, _____, _____, and _____.

7. A person's reported intensity of pain is determined by an individual's _____ (the smallest stimulus where pain is felt) and _____ (the maximum amount of pain a person can tolerate).

8. Identify seven factors that a nurse needs to consider for complete pain assessment: _____, _____, _____, _____, _____, _____, and _____.

9. List eight common physiologic responses to pain: _____, _____, _____, _____, _____, _____, _____, and _____.

10. The only currently approved COX-2 inhibitor is: _____.

11. Define the term *balanced analgesia*.

_____.

12. After administration of an epidural opioid, the nurse needs to assess for _____, which may occur up to _____ hours but usually peaks between _____ hours.

13. Define the term *placebo effect*.

_____

14. List four of eight nonpharmacologic interventions for pain management: _____,

_____, _____, and _____.

MATCHING

Match the term listed in column II with its definition listed in column I.

Column I

1. _____ Pain receptors sensitive to noxious stimuli.

2. _____ Nonsteroidal agents that decrease inflammation.

3. _____ The only commercially available transdermal opioid medication.

4. _____ Significantly increases a person's response to pain.

5. _____ Chemicals known to inhibit the transmission or perception of pain.

6. _____ This substance, released in response to painful stimuli, causes vasodilation.

7. _____ An inactive substance given in place of pain medication.

8. _____ Medication administered directly into the subarachnoid space and cerebrospinal fluid.

9. _____ Transcutaneous stimulation of nonpain receptors in the same area of an injury.

10. _____ Term used to describe a pain's rhythm.

Column II

a. Fentanyl

b. Endorphins

c. Placebo

d. Waning

e. TENS

f. Nociceptors

g. Histamine

h. Anxiety

i. Epidural

j. NSAIDS

II. Critical Thinking Questions and Exercises

DISCUSSION AND ANALYSIS

Discuss the following topics with your classmates.

1. Explain the seven rights that patients have according to the Pain Care Bill of Rights, officially enacted by the state of California.
2. Distinguish among acute, chronic (persistent, nonmalignant), and cancer-related pain and cite an example of each.
3. Describe the transmission and awareness of pain (nociception system) by explaining the role of the central nervous system and the ascending and descending sensory pathways.
4. Describe the classic *Gate Control Theory* of pain as described by Melzack and Well in 1965.
5. Recognizing the value of your own culture, discuss feelings of pain with your classmates who might represent different cultures.
6. Using role-playing with a classmate, describe the sequence of nursing activities for assessing pain management for pharmacologic and nonpharmacologic interventions.

7. Discuss pain management strategies for those at the end of their life.
8. Compare and contrast the precautions and contraindications for the following opioids: morphine, codeine, Oxycodone, Demerol, Darvon, and Vicodin.
9. Describe nursing responsibilities for management of patient-controlled analgesia (PCA).
10. Explain how the technique of *distraction* works to relieve acute and chronic pain.

CLINICAL SITUATIONS

Read the following case study. Circle the correct answer.

CASE STUDY: Pain Experience

Courtney is a young, healthy adult who slipped off the stairs going down to the basement and struck her forehead on the cement flooring. Courtney did not lose consciousness but did sustain a mild concussion and a hematoma that was 5 cm in width and protruded outward about 6 cm. She experienced immediate acute pain at the site of injury plus a pounding headache.

1. An immediate assessment of the localized pain, based on the patient's description, is that it should be:
   a. brief in duration.
   b. mild in intensity.
   c. persistent after healing has occurred.
   d. recurrent for 3 to 4 months.

2. During the assessment process, the nurse attempts to determine Courtney's physiologic and behavioral responses to her pain experience. The nurse is aware that a patient can be in pain yet appear to be "pain free." A behavioral response indicative of acute pain is:
   a. an expressionless face.
   b. clear verbalization of details.
   c. muscle tension.
   d. physical inactivity.

3. The nurse uses distraction to help Courtney cope with her pain experience. A suggested activity is:
   a. promoting relaxation.
   b. playing music or using a videotape.
   c. using cutaneous stimulation.
   d. any or all of the above.

4. After treatment, Courtney is discharged to home while still in pain. The nurse should:
   a. clarify that Courtney knows what type of pain signals a problem.
   b. remind Courtney that acute pain may persist for several days.
   c. review methods of pain management.
   d. do all of the above.

CHAPTER 14

Fluids and Electrolytes: Balance and Disturbance

I. Interpretation, Completion, and Comparison

MULTIPLE CHOICE

Read each question carefully. Circle your answer.

1. The average daily urinary output in an adult is:
   a. 0.5 L.
   b. 1.0 L.
   c. 1.5 L.
   d. 2.5 L.

2. A febrile patient's fluid output is in excess of normal because of diaphoresis. The nurse should plan fluid replacement based on the knowledge that insensible losses in an *afebrile* person are normally not greater than:
   a. 300 mL/24 h.
   b. 600 mL/24 h.
   c. 900 mL/24 h.
   d. 1200 mL/24 h.

3. A patient's serum sodium concentration is within the normal range. The nurse estimates that the serum osmolality should be:
   a. less than 136 mOsm/kg.
   b. 275 to 300 mOsm/kg.
   c. greater than 408 mOsm/kg.
   d. 350 to 544 mOsm/kg.

4. The nurse expects that a decrease in serum osmolality would occur with:
   a. diabetes insipidus.
   b. hyperglycemia.
   c. renal failure.
   d. uremia.

5. A nurse can estimate that a patient has a serum osmolality of _____ if the patient's serum sodium is 140 mEq/L.
   a. 70 mOsm/kg
   b. 140 mOsm/kg
   c. 210 mOsm/kg
   d. 280 mOsm/kg

6. The nurse notes that a patient's urine osmolality is 980 mOsm/kg. The nurse knows to assess for the possible cause of:
   a. acidosis.
   b. fluid volume excess.
   c. diabetes insipidus.
   d. hyponatrenia.

7. One of the best indicators of renal function is:
   a. blood urea nitrogen.
   b. serum creatintine.
   c. specific gravity.
   d. urine osmolality.

8. A patient is hemorrhaging from multiple trauma sites. The nurse expects that compensatory mechanisms associated with hypovolemia would cause all of the following symptoms *except*:
   a. hypertension.
   b. oliguria.
   c. tachycardia.
   d. tachypnea.

9. A clinical manifestation *not* found in hypovolemia is:
   a. muscle weakness.
   b. oliguria.
   c. postural hypotension.
   d. bradycardia.

10. Laboratory findings consistent with hypovolemia in a female would include all of the following *except*:
    a. hematocrit level of >47%.
    b. BUN–serum creatinine ratio of >12:1.
    c. urine specific gravity of 1.027.
    d. urine osmolality of >450 mOsm/kg.

11. The nurse should expect that a patient with mild fluid volume excess would be prescribed a diuretic that blocks sodium reabsorption in the distal tubule, such as:
    a. Bumex.
    b. Demadex.
    c. HydroDIURIL.
    d. Lasix.

12. When assessing the weight of a patient who is on a sodium-restricted diet, the nurse knows that a weight gain of approximately 2 lb (2.2 lb = 1 kg) is equivalent to a gain of how much fluid?
    a. 0.5 L
    b. 1.0 L
    c. 1.5 L
    d. 2.0 L

13. Nursing intervention for a patient with a diagnosis of hyponatremia includes all of the following *except*:
    a. assessing for symptoms of nausea and malaise.
    b. encouraging the intake of low-sodium liquids, such as coffee or tea.
    c. monitoring neurologic status.
    d. restricting tap water intake.

14. A patient with abnormal sodium losses is receiving a house diet. To provide 1,600 mg of sodium daily, the nurse could supplement the patient's diet with:
    a. one beef cube and 8 oz of tomato juice.
    b. four beef cubes and 8 oz of tomato juice.
    c. one beef cube and 16 oz of tomato juice.
    d. one beef cube and 12 oz of tomato juice.

15. One of the dangers of treating hypernatremia is:
    a. red blood cell crenation.
    b. red blood cell hydrolysis.
    c. cerebral edema.
    d. renal shutdown.

16. A nurse is directed to administer a hypotonic intravenous solution. Looking at the following labeled solutions, she should choose:
    a. 0.45% sodium chloride.
    b. 0.90% sodium chloride.
    c. 5% dextrose in water.
    d. 5% dextrose in normal saline solution.

17. An isotonic solution that contains electrolytes similar to the concentration used in plasma is:
    a. 5% dextrose in water.
    b. lactated Ringer's solution.
    c. 3% NaCl solution.
    d. 5% NaCl solution.

18. A patient is admitted who has had severe vomiting for 24 hours. She states that she is exhausted and weak. The results of an admitting electrocardiogram (ECG) show flat T waves and ST-segment depression. Choose the most likely potassium (K^+) value for this patient.
    a. 4.0 mEq/L
    b. 8.0 mEq/L
    c. 2.0 mEq/L
    d. 2.6 mEq/L

19. The ECG change that is specific to hypokalemia is:
    a. a depressed ST segment.
    b. a flat T wave.
    c. an elevated U wave.
    d. an inverted T wave.

20. To supplement a diet with foods high in potassium, the nurse should recommend the addition of:
    a. fruits such as bananas and apricots.
    b. green leafy vegetables.
    c. milk and yogurt.
    d. nuts and legumes.

21. If a patient has severe hyperkalemia, it is possible to administer calcium gluconate intravenously to:
    a. immediately lower the potassium (K^+) level by active transport.
    b. antagonize the action of K^+ on the heart.
    c. prevent transient renal failure (TRF).
    d. accomplish all of the above.

22. Cardiac effects of hyperkalemia are usually present when the serum potassium level reaches:
    a. 5 mEq/L.
    b. 6 mEq/L.
    c. 7 mEq/L.
    d. 8 mEq/L.

23. The most characteristic manifestation of hypocalcemia and hypomagnesemia is:
    a. anorexia and nausea.
    b. constipation.
    c. lack of coordination.
    d. tetany.

24. A patient complains of tingling in his fingers. He has positive Trousseau's and Chvostek's signs. He says that he feels depressed. Choose the most likely serum calcium (Ca^{++}) value for this patient.
    a. 11 mg/dL
    b. 9 mg/dL
    c. 7 mg/dL
    d. 5 mg/dL

25. Management of hypocalcemia includes all of the following actions *except* administration of:
    a. fluid to dilute the calcium levels.
    b. the diuretic furosemide (Lasix), without saline, to increase calcium excretion through the kidneys.
    c. inorganic phosphate salts.
    d. intravenous phosphate therapy.

26. Cardiac arrest will probably occur with a serum calcium level of:
    a. 9 mg/dL.
    b. 12 mg/dL.
    c. 15 mg/dL.
    d. 18 mg/dL.

27. A patient is admitted with a diagnosis of renal failure. He also mentions that he has had stomach distress and has ingested numerous antacid tablets over the past 2 days. His blood pressure is 110/70 mm Hg, his face is flushed, and he is experiencing generalized weakness. Choose the most likely magnesium (Mg^{++}) value for this patient.
    a. 11 mEq/L
    b. 5 mEq/L
    c. 2 mEq/L
    d. 1 mEq/L

28. Management of the foregoing patient should include:
   a. a regular diet with extra fruits and green vegetables.
   b. potassium-sparing diuretics.
   c. discontinuance of any oral magnesium salts.
   d. all of the above measures.

29. A clinical indication of hypophosphatemia is:
   a. bone pain.
   b. paresthesia.
   c. seizures.
   d. tetany.

30. The most common buffer system in the body is the:
   a. plasma protein buffer system.
   b. hemoglobin buffer system.
   c. phosphate buffer system.
   d. bicarbonate–carbonic acid buffer system.

31. The kidneys regulate acid–base balance by all of the following mechanisms *except*:
   a. excreting hydrogen ions (H^+).
   b. reabsorbing or excreting HCO_3^- into the blood.
   c. reabsorbing carbon dioxide into the blood.
   d. retaining hydrogen ions (H^+).

32. The lungs regulate acid–base balance by all of the following mechanisms *except*:
   a. excreting HCO_3^- into the blood.
   b. slowing ventilation.
   c. controlling carbon dioxide levels.
   d. increasing ventilation.

33. Choose the condition that exhibits blood values with a low pH and a low plasma bicarbonate concentration.
   a. Respiratory acidosis
   b. Respiratory alkalosis
   c. Metabolic acidosis
   d. Metabolic alkalosis

34. The nursing assessment for a patient with metabolic alkalosis includes evaluation of laboratory data for all of the following *except*:
   a. hypocalcemia.
   b. hypoglycemia.
   c. hypokalemia.
   d. hypoxemia.

35. Choose the condition that exhibits blood values with a low pH and a high PCO_2.
   a. Respiratory acidosis
   b. Respiratory alkalosis
   c. Metabolic acidosis
   d. Metabolic alkalosis

36. A normal oxygen saturation value for arterial blood is:
   a. 65%.
   b. 75%.
   c. 85%.
   d. 95%.

SHORT ANSWER

Read each statement carefully. Write your response in the space provided.

1. About _____% of total body fluid is in the intracellular space; the major positively charged ion in intracellular fluid is _____. The extracellular space is divided into three compartments: _____, _____, and _____; the major positively charged ion in extracellular fluid is _____. About _____% of the _____ L of total blood volume is _____.

2. Define the term *osmotic pressure*.

   _____.

3. Distinguish between the terms urine specific gravity, BUN, and creatinine.

   _____.

4. Distinguish between the terms: baroreceptors and osmoreceptors.

   _____.

5. Calcium levels are primarily regulated by: _____.

6. The primary concentration of phosphorous (85%) is located in the _____, with about
   15% is located in _____.

7. The primary complication of hyperphosphatemia is: _____, which occurs
   when the calcium–magnesium product exceeds 70 mg/dL.

8. The normal blood pH is: _____.

9. The upper and lower blood pH levels that are incompatible with life are: _____ and

   _____.

10. Indicate which of the following factors contribute to *hyponatremia* by writing "Low" in the space
    provided, and indicate which contribute to *hypernatremia* by writing "High" in the space provided.
    a. _____ vomiting
    b. _____ diarrhea
    c. _____ watery diarrhea
    d. _____ inability to quench thirst
    e. _____ burns over a large surface area
    f. _____ diuretics
    g. _____ heat stroke
    h. _____ adrenal insufficiency
    i. _____ syndrome of inappropriate antidiuretic hormone
    j. _____ status post therapeutic abortion
    k. _____ diabetes insipidus with water restriction
    l. _____ excessive parenteral administration of dextrose and water solution

11. Indicate which of the following factors contribute to *hypokalemia* by writing "Low" in the space
    provided, and indicate which contribute to *hyperkalemia* by writing "High" in the space provided.
    a. _____ alkalosis
    b. _____ too tight a tourniquet when collecting a blood sample
    c. _____ vomiting
    d. _____ gastric suction
    e. _____ leukocytosis
    f. _____ anorexia nervosa
    g. _____ hyperaldosteronism
    h. _____ furosemide (Lasix) administration
    i. _____ steroid administration

    j. _____ renal failure

    k. _____ penicillin administration

    l. _____ adrenal steroid deficiency

12. Indicate which of the following factors contribute to *hypocalcemia* by writing "Low" in the space provided, and indicate which contribute to *hypercalcemia* by writing "High" in the space provided.

    a. _____ hyperparathyroidism

    b. _____ massive administration of citrated blood

    c. _____ malignant tumors

    d. _____ immobilization because of multiple fractures

    e. _____ pancreatitis

    f. _____ thiazide diuretics

    g. _____ renal failure

    h. _____ aminoglycoside administration

13. Indicate which of the following factors contribute to *hypomagnesemia* by writing "Low" in the space provided, and indicate which contribute to *hypermagnesemia* by writing "High" in the space provided.

    a. _____ alcohol abuse

    b. _____ renal failure

    c. _____ diarrhea

    d. _____ gentamicin administration

    e. _____ untreated ketoacidosis

14. Indicate which of the following factors contribute to *hypophosphatemia* by writing "Low" in the space provided, and indicate which contribute to *hyperphosphatemia* by writing "High" in the space provided.

    a. _____ hyperparathyroidism

    b. _____ renal failure

    c. _____ major thermal burns

    d. _____ alcohol withdrawal

    e. _____ neoplastic disease chemotherapy

15. For each of the following factors, indicate the probable cause by writing "M-ACID" for metabolic acidosis, "M-ALKA" for metabolic alkalosis, "R-ACID" for respiratory acidosis, or "R-ALKA" for respiratory alkalosis.

    a. _____ sedative overdose

    b. _____ lactic acidosis

    c. _____ ketoacidosis

    d. _____ severe pneumonia

    e. _____ hypoxemia

    f. _____ acute pulmonary edema

    g. _____ diarrhea

    h. _____ vomiting

    i. _____ hypokalemia

    j. _____ gram-negative bacterial infection

16. Write the mathematical formula that a nurse would use to approximate the value of serum osmolality.

17. Explain why the administration of a 3% to 5% sodium chloride solution requires intense monitoring.

_____

18. List four of six symptoms associated with air embolism, a complication of intravenous therapy:

_____, _____, _____, and _____.

II. Critical Thinking Questions and Exercises

DISCUSSION AND ANALYSIS

Discuss the following topics with your classmates.

1. Explain why decreased urine output, despite adequate fluid intake, is an early indicator of a third space fluid shift.
2. Explain the important role of two opposing forces, _hydrostatic pressure_ and _osmotic pressure_, in maintaining fluid movement through blood vessels.
3. Determine the normal daily urine output of an adult. Calculate the usual per hour output for adults with the following weights: 110 lb, 132 lb, and 176 lb.
4. Define the terms osmolality and osmolarity and explain how each is measured.
5. Distinguish between hypervolemia and hypovolemia (pathophysiology, clinical manifestations, assessment, diagnostic findings, medical, and nursing management).
6. Compare and contrast the clinical manifestations, assessment, diagnostic findings, medical and nursing management, and prevention and correction of hypokalemia and hyperkalemia.
7. Discuss why serum albumin levels and arterial pH must be considered when evaluating serum calcium levels.
8. Compare and contrast the clinical manifestations, assessment, diagnostic findings, medical and nursing management, and prevention and correction of hypochloremia and hyperchloremia.
9. Compare and contrast the clinical manifestations, assessment, diagnostic findings, medical and nursing management for acute and chronic metabolic acidosis and metabolic alkalosis.
10. Compare and contrast the clinical manifestations, assessment, diagnostic findings, medical and nursing management for acute and chronic respiratory acidosis and respiratory alkalosis.
11. Distinguish between the purposes of using isotonic, hypotonic, or hypertonic intravenous solutions.
12. Discuss the nursing care management for a patient receiving intravenous therapy.
13. Discuss the nurses' role in managing the common complications of intravenous therapy: infiltration, phlebitis, thrombophlebitis, hematoma, clotting, and obstruction.

APPLYING CONCEPTS

Examine Figure 14-1 in the text and answer the following questions.

1. Define the term _osmosis_, and explain how a fluid concentration gradient influences the movement between fluid compartments.

_____

_____

_____

2. Explain how the osmolality of a solution is determined.

_____

_____

_____

3. Explain the concept of tonicity and how it affects cell size.

_____.

_____.

_____.

4. Distinguish between osmotic pressure, oncotic pressure, and osmotic diuresis.

_____.

_____.

_____.

5. Clarify the differences between diffusion and filtration.

_____.

_____.

_____.

6. Give some examples of osmosis _____, diffusion _____,

and filtration _____.

EXAMINING ASSOCIATIONS

Examine each of the following relationship and answer each question.

1. Describe the interaction of sodium and potassium that is involved in the sodium–potassium pump.

_____.

_____.

_____.

2. Explain the interdependence of renin, angiotensin, and the aldosterone system on the fluid regulation cycle.

_____.

_____.

_____.

3. Correlate the associations between body fluid compartments. First, match the statement about body fluid listed in column III with its body fluid space listed in column II. Then match the fluid space in column II with an associated fact in column I. Write the associated Roman numeral and small letter in the space provided.

Body Fluid Compartments

Column I

1. _____ Third space fluid shift

2. _____ The smallest compartment of the extracellular fluid space

3. _____ Space where plasma is contained

4. _____ Comprises the intravascular, interstitial, and transcellular fluid

5. _____ Comprises about 60% of body fluid

6. _____ Comprises fluid surrounding cell

Column II

a. _____ Intracellular space

b. _____ Extracellular fluid compartment

c. _____ Intravascular space

d. _____ Transcellular space

e. _____ Interstitial space

f. _____ Intravascular fluid volume deficit

Column III

I. Comprises the cerebrospinal and pericardial fluids

II. Is equal to about 8 L in an adult

III. Signs include hypotension, edema, and tachycardia

IV. Found mostly in skeletal muscle mass

V. Comprises about one third of body fluid

VI. Comprises 50% of blood volume

EXTRACTING INFERENCES

Review Figure 14-4 in the text and answer the following questions.

1. Sodium, the most abundant electrolyte in extracellular fluid, is primarily responsible for maintaining fluid

   _____, which _____.

2. Sodium is regulated by _____, _____, and the

   _____ system.

3. Sodium establishes the electrochemical state necessary for _____ and the

   _____.

4. Signs of lethargy, increasing intracranial pressure, and seizures may occur when the serum sodium level reaches:

   a. 115 mEq/L.   c. 145 mEq/l.

   b. 130 mEq/L.   d. 160 mEq/L.

5. In a patient with excess fluid volume, hyponatremia is treated by restricting fluids to how many milliliters in 24 hours?

   a. 400   c. 800

   b. 600   d. 1,200

6. To return a patient with hyponatremia to normal sodium levels, it is safer to restrict fluid intake than to administer sodium:

a. in patients who are unconscious.

b. to prevent fluid overload.

c. to prevent dehydration.

d. in patients who show neurologic symptoms.

7. Hypernatremia is associated with a:

a. serum osmolality of 245 mOsm/kg.

b. serum sodium of 150 mEq/L.

c. urine specific gravity lower than 1.003.

d. combination of all of the above.

8. A semiconscious patient presents with restlessness and weakness. He has a dry, swollen tongue. His body temperature is 99.3°F, and his urine specific gravity is 1.020. Choose the most likely serum sodium (Na^+) value for this patient.

a. 110 mEq/L

b. 140 mEq/L

c. 155 mEq/L

d. 165 mEq/L

CLINICAL SITUATIONS

Read the following case studies. Circle the correct answer.

CASE STUDY: Extracellular Fluid Volume Deficit

Harriet, 30 years old, has been admitted to the burn treatment center with full-thickness burns over 30% of her upper body. Her diagnosis is consistent with extracellular fluid volume deficit (FVD).

1. The major indicator of extracellular FVD can be identified by assessing for:

a. a full and bounding pulse.

b. a drop in postural blood pressure.

c. an elevated temperature.

d. pitting edema of the lower extremities.

2. Manifestations of extracellular FVD include all of the following *except*:

a. collapsed neck veins.

b. decreased serum albumin.

c. elevated hematocrit.

d. weight loss.

3. A nursing plan of care for Harriet should include assessing blood pressure with the patient in the supine and upright positions. A diagnostic reading that should be recorded and reported is:

a. supine, 140/90; sitting, 120/80; standing, 110/70 mm Hg.

b. supine, 140/90; sitting, 130/90; standing, 130/90 mm Hg.

c. supine, 140/90; sitting, 140/85; standing, 135/85 mm Hg.

d. supine, 140/90; sitting, 140/90; standing, 130/90 mm Hg.

4. Nursing intervention for Harriet includes all of the following *except*:

a. monitoring urinary output to assess kidney perfusion.

b. placing the patient in the Trendelenburg position to maximize cerebral blood flow.

c. positioning the patient flat in bed with legs elevated to maintain adequate circulating volume.

d. teaching leg exercises to promote venous return and prevent postural hypotension when the patient stands.

CASE STUDY: Congestive Heart Failure

George, 88 years old, is suffering from congestive heart failure. He was admitted to the hospital with a diagnosis of extracellular fluid volume excess. He was frightened, slightly confused, and dyspneic on exertion.

1. During the assessment process, the nurse expects to identify all of the following *except*:
   a. a full pulse.
   b. decreased central venous pressure.
   c. edema.
   d. neck vein distention.

2. A manifestation of extracellular volume excess is:
   a. altered serum osmolality.
   b. hyponatremia.
   c. increased hematocrit when volume excess develops quickly.
   d. rapid weight gain.

3. A nursing plan of care for George should include:
   a. auscultating for abnormal breath sounds.
   b. inspecting for leg edema.
   c. weighing the patient daily.
   d. all of the above.

4. Nursing intervention for George should include all of the following *except*:
   a. administering diuretics, as prescribed, to help remove excess fluid.
   b. assisting the patient to a recumbent position to minimize his breathing effort.
   c. inspecting for sacral edema to note the degree of fluid retention.
   d. teaching dietary restriction of sodium to help decrease water retention.

CASE STUDY: Diabetes Mellitus

Isaac, 63 years old, was admitted to the hospital with a diagnosis of diabetes mellitus. On his admission, the nurse observed rapid respirations, confusion, and signs of dehydration.

1. Isaac's arterial blood gas values are pH, 7.27; HCO_3, 20 mEq/L; PaO_2, 33 mm Hg. These values are consistent with a diagnosis of compensated:
   a. metabolic acidosis.
   b. metabolic alkalosis.
   c. respiratory acidosis.
   d. respiratory alkalosis.

2. A manifestation *not* associated with altered acid–base balance is:
   a. bradycardia.
   b. hypertension.
   c. lethargy.
   d. hypokalemia.

3. In terms of cellular buffering response, the nurse should expect the major electrolyte disturbance to be:
   a. hyperkalemia.
   b. hypernatremia.
   c. hypocalcemia.
   d. hypokalemia.

4. The nurse should anticipate that the physician will attempt to reverse this acid–base imbalance by prescribing intravenous administration of:
   a. potassium chloride.
   b. potassium iodide.
   c. sodium bicarbonate.
   d. sodium chloride.

CASE STUDY: Intravenous Therapy

Jill, an 84-year-old woman, was admitted to the hospital for treatment for dehydration. The physician immediately ordered intravenous therapy, 1,000 mL of D5 W, q8 h.

1. The nurse knows that one of these four arm veins would be a recommended site: _____, _____, _____, and _____.

2. The nurse also knows that if a central vein is needed it would most likely include either the _____ or _____ vein.

3. Since the flow of the intravenous infusion is inversely proportional to the fluids viscosity, an infusion of blood would require _____ than that used for saline or water.

4. The formula to calculate flow rate at milliliter per hour (mL/h) is: _____.

5. A positive-pressure infusion pump maintains a steady infusion by overcoming vascular resistance caused by two things: the _____ and the _____.

6. Four systemic intravenous complications are: _____, _____, _____, and _____.

7. Five local complications of intravenous therapy are: _____, _____, _____, _____, and _____.

CHAPTER 15

Shock and Multiple Organ Dysfunction Syndrome

I. Interpretation, Completion, and Comparison

MULTIPLE CHOICE

Read each question carefully. Circle your answer.

1. Physiologic responses to all types of shock include all of the following *except*:
   a. activation of the inflammatory response.
   b. hypermetabolism.
   c. hypoperfusion of tissues.
   d. increased intravascular volume.

2. Calculate a patient's mean arterial pressure (MAP) when the blood pressure is 110/70 mm Hg.
   a. 65
   b. 73
   c. 83
   d. 91

3. Baroreceptors are a primary mechanism of blood pressure regulation which results from the initial stimulation of what type of receptors?
   a. Chemical
   b. Hormonal
   c. Neural
   d. Pressure

4. The stage of shock characterized by a normal blood pressure is the:
   a. initial stage.
   b. compensatory stage.
   c. progressive stage.
   d. irreversible stage.

5. The nurse knows to report an early indicator of compensatory shock that would be a pulse pressure of:
   a. 25 mm Hg.
   b. 40 mm Hg.
   c. 55 mm Hg.
   d. 70 mm Hg.

6. The nurse assesses a patient in compensatory shock whose lungs have decompensated. The nurse would *not* expect to find the following symptoms:
   a. a heart rate greater than 100 bpm.
   b. crackles.
   c. lethargy and mental confusion.
   d. respirations fewer than 15 breaths/min.

7. In progressive stage shock, clinical hypotension is present if the systematic blood pressure is:
   a. 85 mm Hg.
   b. 90 mm Hg.
   c. 95 mm Hg.
   d. 100 mm Hg.

8. Oliguria occurs in the progressive stage of shock because the kidneys decompensate. To verify this condition, the nurse should expect all of the following signs or symptoms *except*:

    a. acid–base imbalance.

    b. decreased capillary permeability and fluid and electrolyte shifts.

    c. increased blood urea nitrogen and serum creatinine.

    d. a mean arterial blood pressure greater than 70 mm Hg.

9. Hematologic system changes in progressive shock would be characterized by all of the following *except*:

    a. generalized hypoxemia.

    b. hypertension.

    c. metabolic acidosis.

    d. sluggish blood flow.

10. The hepatic effects of progressive shock would *not include*:

    a. lowered bilirubin levels.

    b. decreased lactic acid metabolism.

    c. impaired glycogenolysis.

    d. increased liver enzymes.

11. Depleted adenosine triphosphate (ATP) stores and multiple organ failure are characteristic of which stage of shock?

    a. Initial

    b. Compensatory

    c. Progressive

    d. Irreversible

12. Patients receiving fluid replacement should frequently be monitored for:

    a. adequate urinary output.

    b. changes in mental status.

    c. vital sign stability.

    d. all of the above.

13. Hypovolemic shock occurs when intravascular volume decreases by:

    a. 5% to 10%.

    b. 15% to 30%.

    c. 35% to 50%.

    d. more than 60%.

14. The most commonly used colloidal solution to treat hypovolemic shock is:

    a. blood products.

    b. 5% albumin.

    c. 6% dextran.

    d. 6% hetastarch.

15. Vasoactive agents are effective in treating shock if fluid administration fails because of their ability to:

    a. decrease blood pressure.

    b. decrease stroke volume.

    c. reverse the cause of dehydration.

    d. increase cardiac preload.

16. Coronary cardiogenic shock is seen primarily in patients with:

    a. cardiomyopathies.

    b. dysrhythmias.

    c. myocardial infarction.

    d. valvular damage.

17. In cardiogenic shock, decreased cardiac contractility leads to all of the following compensatory responses *except*:

    a. decreased stroke volume.

    b. decreased tissue perfusion.

    c. increased stroke volume.

    d. pulmonary congestion.

18. The primary goal in treating cardiogenic shock is to:
    a. improve the heart's pumping mechanism.
    b. limit further myocardial damage.
    c. preserve the healthy myocardium.
    d. treat the oxygenation needs of the heart muscle.

19. A common vasoactive agent used to improve cardiac contractility is:
    a. dopamine.
    b. epinephrine.
    c. nitroprusside.
    d. phenylephrine.

20. The drug of choice for cardiac pain relief is intravenous:
    a. codeine.
    b. Demerol.
    c. Dilaudid.
    d. morphine.

21. Sympathomimetic drugs increase cardiac output by all of the following measures *except*:
    a. decreasing preload and afterload.
    b. increasing myocardial contractility.
    c. increasing stroke volume.
    d. increasing cardiac output.

22. The nurse assesses for the negative effect of intravenous nitroglycerin (Tridil) for shock management, which is:
    a. reduced preload.
    b. reduced afterload.
    c. increased cardiac output.
    d. increased blood pressure.

23. The vasoactive effects of dopamine are diminished when high doses are given, because vasoconstriction increases cardiac workload. Doses are titrated for therapeutic range. A nontherapeutic drug dose for a 154-lb (70-kg) man would be:
    a. 210 mg/min.
    b. 350 mg/min.
    c. 490 mg/min.
    d. 630 mg/min.

24. Intra-aortic balloon counterpulsation (IABC) is a mechanical, assistive device used as a temporary means of improving the heart's pumping ability. IABC is primarily meant to:
    a. decrease cardiac work.
    b. decrease stroke volume.
    c. increase preload.
    d. maintain current coronary circulation.

25. The sequence of organ failure in multiple-organ dysfunction syndrome (MODS) usually begins in the:
    a. heart.
    b. kidneys.
    c. liver.
    d. lungs.

SHORT ANSWER

Read each statement. Write your response in the space provided.

1. The basic, underlying characteristic of shock is _____, which results in

   _____, _____, _____,

   _____, and _____.

2. Energy metabolism occurs in the cells, where _____ is primarily responsible for cellular

   energy in the form of _____.

3. To maintain an adequate blood pressure, three components of the circulatory system must respond

   effectively: the _____, _____, and _____.

4. The formula for calculating cardiac output is: cardiac output is the product of _____ times

   _____. Peripheral resistance is determined by the _____.

5. Define the term *mean arterial pressure (MAP).*

   _____

   _____

6. Baroreceptors are located in the _____ and _____,

   whereas chemoreceptors are located in the _____ and _____.

7. With the progression of shock, damage at the _____ and _____ level occurs when the blood
   pressure drops.

8. Two crystalloids commonly used for fluid replacement in hypovolemic shock are:

   _____ and _____.

9. Three medical management goals for cardiogenic shock are: _____, _____,

   and _____.

10. A new cardiac marker for ventricular dysfunction, _____, increases when the ventricle
    is overdistended. It is being used to assess the cardiovascular effects of shock.

11. Circulatory shock can be caused by: _____ and _____.

12. Neurogenic shock can be caused by: _____, _____,

    or _____.

MATCHING

Match the type of shock listed in column II with its associated cause listed in column I. An answer may be used more than once.

Column I

1. _____ Valvular damage
2. _____ Peritonitis
3. _____ Burns
4. _____ Bee sting allergy
5. _____ Immunosuppression
6. _____ Spinal cord injury
7. _____ Dysrhythmias
8. _____ Vomiting
9. _____ Pulmonary embolism
10. _____ Penicillin sensitivity

Column II

a. Hypovolemic, owing to an internal fluid shift
b. Hypovolemic, owing to an external fluid loss
c. Cardiogenic
d. Circulatory of a neurogenic nature
e. Circulatory of an anaphylactic nature
f. Circulatory of a septic nature
g. Noncoronary cardiogenic shock

II. Critical Thinking Questions and Exercises

DISCUSSION AND ANALYSIS

Discuss the following topics with your classmates.

1. Discuss the cellular changes that occur with shock, especially the movement of water and electrolytes through the membrane.
2. Compare and contrast the clinical findings in the three states of shock: compensatory, progressive, and irreversible.
3. Describe special assessments for recognizing shock in the elderly.
4. Distinguish between the advantages and disadvantages of administering crystalloid and/or colloid solutions as fluid replacement for shock.
5. Discuss nursing assessment activities to monitor possible complications of fluid administration.
6. Discuss the action and disadvantages of common vasoactive agents used to treat shock: sympathomimetics, vasodilators, and vasoconstrictors.
7. Discuss the risk factors and nursing management for anaphylactic shock.

IDENTIFYING PATTERNS

Chart the physiologic sequence of events.

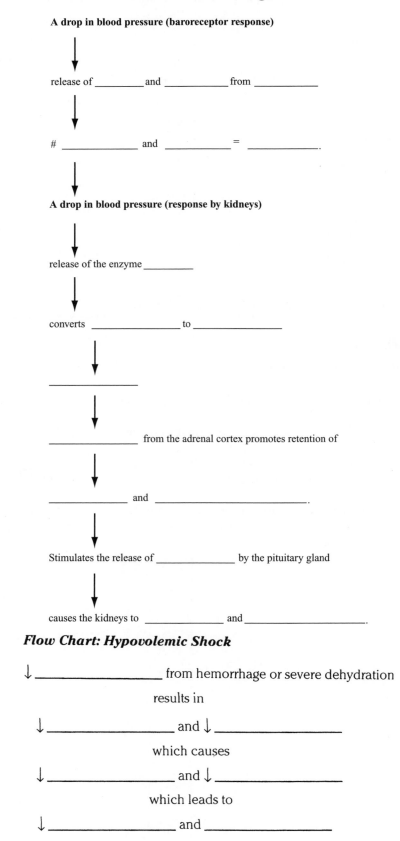

Flow Chart: Blood Pressure Regulation Shock

A drop in blood pressure (baroreceptor response)

release of _____ and _____ from _____

_____ and _____ = _____.

A drop in blood pressure (response by kidneys)

release of the enzyme _____

converts _____ to _____

_____

_____ from the adrenal cortex promotes retention of

_____ and _____.

Stimulates the release of _____ by the pituitary gland

causes the kidneys to _____ and _____.

Flow Chart: Hypovolemic Shock

↓ _____ from hemorrhage or severe dehydration

results in

↓ _____ and ↓ _____

which causes

↓ _____ and ↓ _____

which leads to

↓ _____ and _____

Study Guide for Brunner and Suddarth's Textbook of Medical-Surgical Nursing, 12th edition.

CLINICAL SITUATIONS

Read the following case studies. Fill in the blanks or circle the correct answer.

CASE STUDY: Hypovolemic Shock

Mr. Mazda is a 57-year-old, 154-lb (70-kg) patient who was received on the nursing unit from the recovery room after having a hemicolectomy for colon cancer. On initial assessment, Mr. Mazda was alert, yet anxious; his skin was cool, pale, and moist; and his abdominal dressings were saturated with bright red blood. Urinary output was 100 mL over 4 hours. The patient was receiving 1,000 mL of lactated Ringer's solution. Vital signs were blood pressure, 80/60 mm Hg; heart rate, 126 bpm; and respirations 40 breaths/min (baseline vital signs were 130/70, 84, and 22, respectively). The nurse assessed that the patient was experiencing hypovolemic shock.

1. The nurse understands that hypovolemic shock will occur with an intravascular volume reduction of 15% to 30%. Therefore, the nurse determines that Mr. Mazda, who weighs 70 kg, has probably lost:
   a. 150 to 250 mL of blood.
   b. 300 to 500 mL of blood.
   c. 500 to 600 mL of blood.
   d. 750 to 1500 mL of blood.

2. The nurse knows to monitor vital signs every 5 to 15 minutes and to be concerned about the patient's pulse pressure of _____.

3. The nurse knows that the progressive pattern of changes in vital signs is more important than the exact readings. A _____ in pulse rate, followed by a _____ in blood pressure, is indicative of shock.

4. The nurse understands that a systolic reading of 80 mm Hg is serious, because a systolic reading lower than _____ mm Hg in a normotensive person indicates well-advanced shock.

5. Urinary output will be measured hourly. An output less than _____ mL/h is indicative of decreased glomerular filtration.

6. Nursing interventions include notifying the physician, reinforcing the abdominal dressings, and treating the patient for shock by administering fluids ordered, such as: _____, _____, and _____.

CASE STUDY: Septic Shock

Mr. Dressler, a 43-year-old Caucasian, was admitted to the medical–surgical unit on the third postoperative day after a vertical bonded gastroplasty for morbid obesity. He had initially transferred to the intensive care unit from the recovery room. Mr. Dressler had a normal postoperative recovery period until his first afternoon on the unit. A registered nurse went into his room to assess 4:00 PM vital signs and noted that his temperature was 102°F, his HR was >90 bpm, his respirations were >20 breaths/min, and his systolic BP was <90 mm Hg. He was shaking with chills, his skin was warm and dry, yet his extremities were cool to the touch. The nurse, assessing that Mr. Dressler was probably experiencing septicemia, immediately notified the physician.

Answer the following questions based on your knowledge of septicemia and shock.

1. Septic shock has traditionally been caused by gram-negative organisms such as:

_____.

2. The nurse believes that Mr. Dressler may be experiencing a systemic inflammatory response syndrome (SIRS) that can be described as a:

   _____.

3. Mr. Dressler's condition may advance to severe sepsis which, in addition to the signs of sepsis, would

   include _____, _____, _____, _____, and

   _____.

4. The nurse knows that the mortality rate associated with septic shock is between _____% and _____%.

5. The nurse expects that the physician will request body fluid specimens for culture and sensitivity tests.

   The nurse prepares to collect specimens of: _____, _____, _____,

   and _____.

6. Aggressive fluid resuscitation is aimed to achieve a target CVP of _____ a MAP of

   _____, urine output of _____, and an $Sc\bar{v}O_2$ of _____.

7. The two most common and serious side effects of fluid replacement are: _____ and

   _____.

CHAPTER 16

Oncology: Nursing Management in Cancer Care

I. Interpretation, Completion, and Comparison

MULTIPLE CHOICE

Read each question carefully. Circle your answer.

1. As a cause of death in the United States, cancer ranks:
   a. first.
   (b.) second.
   c. third.
   d. fourth.

2. Cancer mortality in the United States is highest among:
   (a.) African Americans.
   b. American Indians.
   c. Caucasians.
   d. Hispanics.

3. The etiology of cancer can be associated with specific agents or factors such as:
   a. dietary and genetic factors.
   b. hormonal and chemical agents.
   c. viruses.
   (d.) all of the above.

4. David, age 67 years, is admitted for diagnostic studies to rule out cancer. He is white, has been employed as a landscaper for 40 years, and has a 36-year history of smoking one pack of cigarettes a day. David has three risk factors associated with the development of cancer. Choose the *least* significant risk factor among the following:
   a. age.
   b. sex.
   (c.) occupation.
   (d.) race.

5. Cancer cells can affect the immune system by:
   a. stimulating the release of T lymphocytes into the circulation.
   (b.) suppressing the patient's natural defenses.
   c. mobilizing macrophages.
   (d.) all of the above.

6. To reduce nitrate intake because of possible carcinogenic action, the nurse suggests that a patient decrease his or her intake of:
   a. eggs and milk.
   b. fish and poultry.
   (c.) ham and bacon.
   d. green, leafy vegetables.

7. An endoscopic procedure can be used to remove an entire piece of suspicious tissue growth. The diagnostic biopsy method used for this procedure is known as:
   (a.) excisional biopsy.
   b. incisional biopsy.
   c. needle biopsy.
   d. staging.

8. A patient is admitted for an excisional biopsy of a breast lesion. The nurse should do all of the following *except*:

   a. clarify information provided by the physician.

   b. provide aseptic care to the incision postoperatively.

   c. provide time for the patient to discuss her concerns.

   d. counsel the patient about the possibility of losing her breast.

9. A patient is scheduled for an outpatient procedure whereby liquid nitrogen is used to freeze a cervical cancer. The procedure is known as:

   a. chemosurgery.

   b. cryosurgery.

   c. laser surgery.

   d. radiofrequency ablation.

10. Surgery done to remove lesions that are likely to develop into cancer is known as:

    a. diagnostic.

    b. palliative.

    c. prophylactic.

    d. reconstructive.

11. An example of palliative surgery is a:

    a. colectomy.

    b. cordotomy. —*disables pain-conducting tracts in spinal cord to achieve loss of pain & temperature perception.*

    c. mastectomy.

    d. nephrectomy.

12. The *incorrect* rationale for the effectiveness of radiation therapy is its ability to:

    a. cause cell death.

    b. break the strands of the DNA helix.

    c. disrupt mitosis by slowing dividing cells.

    d. interrupt cellular growth when a nonsurgical approach is needed.

13. Radiation therapy for the treatment of cancer is administered over several weeks to:

    a. allow time for the patient to cope with the treatment.

    b. allow time for the repair of healthy tissue.

    c. decrease the incidence of leukopenia and thrombocytopenia.

    d. accomplish all of the above.

14. A patient with uterine cancer is being treated with internal radiation therapy. A primary nursing responsibility is to:

    a. explain to the patient that she will continue to emit radiation for approximately 1 week after the implant is removed.

    b. maintain as much distance as possible from the patient while in the room.

    c. alert family members that they should restrict their visiting to 5 minutes at any one time.

    d. wear a lead apron when providing direct patient care.

15. A major disadvantage of chemotherapy is that it:

    a. attacks cancer cells during their vulnerable phase.

    b. functions against disseminated disease.

    c. is systemic.

    d. targets normal body cells as well as cancer cells.

16. When a patient takes vincristine, a plant alkaloid, the nurse should assess for symptoms of toxicity affecting the:

    a. gastrointestinal system.

    b. nervous system.

    c. pulmonary system.

    d. urinary system.

17. Initial nursing action for extravasation of a chemotherapeutic agent includes all of the following *except*:
    a. applying warm compresses to the phlebitic area.
    b. immediately discontinuing the infusion.
    c. injecting an antidote, if required.
    d. placing ice over the site of infiltration.

18. Realizing that chemotherapy can result in renal damage, the nurse should:
    a. encourage fluid intake to dilute the urine.
    b. take measures to acidify the urine and thus prevent uric acid crystallization.
    c. withhold medication when the blood urea nitrogen level exceeds 20 mg/dL.
    d. limit fluids to 1,000 mL daily to prevent accumulation of the drugs' end products after cell lysis.

19. Allopurinol may be prescribed for a patient who is receiving chemotherapy to:
    a. stimulate the immune system against the tumor cells.
    b. treat drug-related anemia.
    c. prevent alopecia.
    d. lower serum and urine uric acid levels.

20. The use of hyperthermia as a treatment modality for cancer may cause:
    a. fatigue, nausea, and vomiting.
    b. hypotension, skin burn, and tissue damage.
    c. thrombophlebitis, diarrhea, and peripheral neuropathies.
    d. all of the above side effects.

21. Bacille Calmette-Guerin (BCG) is a nonspecific biologic response modifier that is a standard form of treatment for cancer of the:
    a. bladder.
    b. breast.
    c. lungs.
    d. skin.

22. The nurse should assess a cancer patient's nutritional status by:
    a. weighing the patient daily.
    b. monitoring daily calorie intake.
    c. observing for proper wound healing.
    d. doing all of the above.

23. The most frequently occurring gram-positive cause of infection in cancer patients is:
    a. *Candida albicans.*
    b. *Escherichia coli.*
    c. *Pseudomonas aeruginosa.*
    d. *Staphylococcus.*

24. The most common cause of bleeding in cancer patients is:
    a. anemia.
    b. coagulation disorders.
    c. hypoxemia.
    d. thrombocyotpenia.

SHORT ANSWER

Read each statement carefully. Write your response in the space provided.

1. List, in order of frequency, the three leading causes of cancer deaths in the United States: men (_lung_ , _prostate_ , and _colon_); women (_lung_ , _breast_ , and _colon_).

2. Define, in very simple language, the cause of cancer.
   abnormal cell-after transformed by DNA begins to proliferate abnormally.

3. The altered cell membranes of malignant cells contain tumor-specific antigens. List two examples:
   CEA and _PSA_ .

4. The two key ways by which cancer is spread are: the _lymph_ and the _blood_.

5. About _75_ % of all cancers are thought to be related to the environment.

6. The single most lethal chemical carcinogen that accounts for 30% of all cancer deaths is: _tobacco smoke_

7. Two examples of an inherited cancer susceptibility syndrome are: _breast & ovarian_ and _multiple endocrine neoplasia_

8. List four of seven cancers that are associated with an increased intake of alcohol: _mouth_, _larynx, pharynx, esophagus_, and _liver_, _colorectum, breast._

9. Three dietary substances (cruciferous vegetables) appear to reduce cancer risk: _cabbage_, _brocolli_, and _cauliflower_, whereas _fats_, _salt & smoked, meat_ _bacon_, and _red meats_ tend to increase the risk of cancer.

10. Identify five substances produced by the immune system in response to cancer cells: _B lymphocytes_, _lymphokines_, _macrophages_, _NK cells_, and _T lymphocytes_.

11. Toxicity occurs with radiation therapy. For each of the following, list three common side effects.

    1. Skin: _burns-erythema_, _alopecia_, and _desquamation_.

    2. Oral mucosal membrana: _stomatitis_, _xerostomia_, and _loss of taste_.

    3. Stomach or colon: _anorexia_, _nausea_, and _vomiting, diarrhea._

    4. Bone marrow-producing sites: _neutropenia_, _anemia_, and _thrombocytopenia._

12. List five of nine signs that indicate that an extravasation of an infusion of a cancer chemotherapeutic agent has occurred: _redness, pain, swelling_, _mottled appearance, phlebitis, loss of blood return,_ and _resistance to flow,_. _necrosis, damage to underlying tissues._

13. The two *most common* side effects of chemotherapy are: _nausea_ and _vomiting_.

14. Myelosuppression, caused by chemotherapeutic agents, results in _leukopenia, anemia, neutropenia, thrombocytopenia,_ and an increased risk of _infection_ and _bleeding_.

15. Three chemotherapeutic agents that are particularly toxic to the renal system are: _____, _____, and _____.

MATCHING

Match the term listed in column II with its associated definition listed in column I.

Column I

1. __A__ Growth of new capillaries from the host tissue
2. __B__ Innate process of programmed cell death
3. __F__ The use of thermal energy to destroy cancer cells
4. __e__ Point at which blood counts are their lowest
5. __d__ Target antibodies to destroy specific malignant cells
6. __g__ A substance that can cause tissue necrosis
7. __h__ A dry oral cavity caused by salivary gland dysfunction
8. __C__ Substances produced by the immune system cells to enhance the function of the immune system

Column II

a. Angiogenesis
b. Apoptosis
c. Cytokines
d. Monoclonal antibodies
e. Nadir
f. Radiofrequency ablation
g. Vesicant
h. Xerostomia

Match the type of neoplasm in column II with its associated description listed in column I.

Column I

1. __B__ Cells bear little resemblance to the normal cells of the tissue from which they arose
2. __A__ Rate of growth is usually slow
3. __A__ Tumor tissue is encapsulated – *enclosed*
4. __B__ Tumor spreads by way of blood and lymph channels to other areas of the body
5. __B__ Growth tends to recur when removed

Column II

a. Benign
b. Malignant

Match the drug category listed in column II with an associated antineoplastic agent listed in column I. For each drug, list a common side effect in column I. An answer may be used more than once. Refer to Table 16-6 in the text.

Column I

1. ____ Cisplatin _____
2. ____ 5-fluorouracil (5-FU) _____
3. ____ Estrogens _____
4. ____ Thiotepa _____
5. ____ Lomustine (CCNU) _____
6. ____ Doxorubicen _____
7. ____ Ifosfamide _____
8. ____ Methotrexate _____
9. ____ Vincristine (VCR) _____
10. ____ Iirinotecan _____
11. ____ Asparaginase _____

Column II

a. Alkylating agent
b. Nitrosourea
c. Antimetabolite
d. Antitumor antibiotic
e. Plant alkaloid/mitotic spindle
f. Hormonal agent
g. Miscellaneous agent
h. Topoisomerase 1 inhibitors

II. Critical Thinking Questions and Exercises

DISCUSSION AND ANALYSIS

Discuss the following topics with your classmates.

1. Distinguish between the terms *invasion* and *metastasis* as they relate to the spread of cancerous cells.
2. Distinguish between primary and secondary prevention of cancer, and provide an example of how nurses can participate in both types of prevention.
3. Compare and contrast 12 current diagnostic aids used today to detect cancer.
4. Explain the modes of action for the following two classifications of chemotherapeutic agents: cell cycle-specific and cell cycle-nonspecific.
5. Discuss the nursing role in responding to a hypersensitivity reaction to a chemotherapeutic agent.
6. Discuss the nurses' management of patients' pre- and post-bone marrow transplantation.
7. Describe the role of interferon in the treatment of cancer.
8. Describe the types and purposes of cancer vaccines.
9. Discuss the nurse's role in managing the side effects of chemotherapy.
10. Select at least three nursing diagnoses and collaborative problems for patients with cancer and discuss nursing interventions for treatment.
11. Describe the factors and underlying mechanisms that predispose a cancer patient to infection.

EXAMINING ASSOCIATIONS

Read each analogy. Write the best response in the space provided.

1. Primary cancer prevention : preventing or reducing the risk of cancer :: Secondary prevention : _____*screening*_____.

2. Staging of tumor cells : tumor size and existence of metastasis :: Grading : _*classification of tumor cells.*_

3. Excisional biopsy : malignant melanoma :: _____ biopsy : prostrate cancer.

4. An oophorectomy : prophylactic surgery :: abdominal shunt placement : _____ surgery.

5. Autologous bone marrow transplant : from the patient :: Syngeneic bone marrow transplant : _____.

6. Cytokines : interferons :: Lymphokines : _____.

7. Stomatitis : oral tissue inflammation :: Alopecia : _*hair loss*_.

8. Anorexia : loss of appetite :: Cachexia : _*weakness & wasting of body*_

9. Streptococcus : gram-positive :: _*e-coli*_ : gram-negative.

10. Avastin : metastatic colorectal cancer :: Mylotarg : _____.

CLINICAL SITUATIONS

Read the following case studies. Fill in the space or circle the correct answer.

CASE STUDY: Cancer of the Breast

Kim is a 45-year-old mother of four who, after a needle aspiration biopsy, is diagnosed as having a malignant breast tumor, stage III. She was scheduled for a modified radical mastectomy. On assessment, her breast tissue had a dimpling or "orange-peel" appearance. Nursing diagnoses included: (a) fear and ineffective coping related to the diagnosis and (b) disturbance in self-concept related to the nature of the surgery.

1. Realizing that Kim's mother died of breast cancer, the nurse correlates the cause of Kim's diagnosis to:
   a. environmental factors.
   b. genetics.
   c. dietary factors.
   d. chemical agents.

2. To assist Kim in adapting to the loss of her breast, the nurse should assess Kim's:
   a. attitude toward her body image.
   b. feelings of self-esteem.
   c. social and sexual values.
   d. attitudes and values regarding all of the above.

3. Kim's husband refuses to participate in any discussion about his wife's diagnosis. The nurse realizes that he is using the defense mechanism of:
   a. denial.
   b. depression.
   c. rationalization.
   d. repression. — *restraint, prevention, or inhibition of a feeling.*

4. Postoperatively, Kim experiences severe incisional pain. The nurse realizes that Kim's perception of pain is possibly influenced by:
   a. tissue manipulation during surgery.
   b. apprehension regarding the prognosis of her condition.
   c. anger stemming from her change in body image.
   d. all of the above.

5. Kim is scheduled to begin radiation therapy, followed by chemotherapy with 5-fluorouracil. Realizing the side effects of radiation therapy, the nurse should prepare Kim for all of the following *except*:
   a. her lungs may possibly produce more mucus.
   b. the skin at the treatment area may become red and inflamed.
   c. she may tire more easily and require additional rest periods.
   d. alopecia will occur as a result of the quickly growing hair follicles.

6. The nurse should teach Kim what she can do to protect her skin between radiation treatments. Measures include all of the following *except*:
   a. handle the area gently.
   b. avoid irritation with soap and water.
   c. use a heat lamp once a day directed to the radiation site to promote tissue repair.
   d. wear loose-fitting clothing.

7. After radiation therapy, Kim begins a regimen of chemotherapy with 5-fluorouracil. Three weeks after treatment begins, Kim develops a fever, sore throat, and cold symptoms. The nurse knows that Kim's symptoms could be due to all of the following *except*:
   a. hypercalcemia.
   b. bone marrow depression.
   c. altered nutrition.
   d. leukopenia.

8. Nursing assessment during Kim's chemotherapy includes observing for:
   a. evidence of stomatitis.
   b. renal and hepatic abnormalities.
   c. symptoms of infection owing to granulocytopenia.
   d. all of the above.

9. Kim is diagnosed as having thrombocytopenia. The nurse should assess for all of the following *except*:
   a. hematuria.
   b. fever.
   c. hematemesis.
   d. ecchymosis.

CASE STUDY: Cancer of the Lung

Mr. Donato is a 48-year-old accountant who has been a one-pack-a-day smoker for 23 years. He has had a persistent cough for 1 year that is hacking and nonproductive and has had repeated unresolved upper respiratory tract infections. He went to see his physician because he was fatigued, had been anorexic, and had lost 12 lb over the last 3 months. Diagnostic evaluation led to the diagnosis of a localized tumor with no evidence of metastatic spread. Mr. Donato is scheduled for a lobectomy in 3 days.

1. Because infection is the leading cause of mortality in the oncology population, the nurse preoperatively notes the significance of a(an):
   a. basophil count of 1.3%.
   b. eosinophil count of 4.5%.
   c. lymphocyte count of 23%.
   d. neutrophil count of 20%.

2. The nurse is concerned that the patient's nutritional status is compromised based on his recent weight loss. Impaired nutritional status contributes to: _disease progression_, _immune competence_ _increased infection_ _delayed tissue repair_; and _diminished functional ability_

3. List five factors that the nurse would assess to determine the patient's experience with pain, in order to develop a plan of care for pain management: _fear_, _apprehension_, _fatigue_, _anger_, and _social isolation_.

4. The nurse knows that a diagnosis of cancer is accompanied by grieving. Usually the first reaction in the grieving process is:
   a. bargaining.
   b. acceptance.
   c. denial.
   d. depression.

5. List four activities the nurse can do to support the patient and family during the grieving process: _answer ?s & concerns_, _identify resource & support persons_, _communicate & share concerns_, and _help frame ?s for physician._

6. The nurse knows that postoperative care needs to be directed toward the prevention of _infection_, the leading cause of death in cancer patients.

7. Two major gram-negative bacilli that cause infection in an immunosuppressed patient are: _p. aeruginosa_ and _e. coli_.

8. The nurse will also assess for the postoperative complication of septic shock, which is associated with all of the following *except*:
   a. dysrhythmias.
   b. hypertension.
   c. metabolic acidosis.
   d. oliguria.

CHAPTER 17

End-of-Life Care

I. Interpretation, Completion, and Comparison

MULTIPLE CHOICE

Read each question carefully. Circle your answer.

1. The major causes of death in this century are diseases of what type?
   a. Communicable
   b. Chronic degenerative
   c. Genetic
   d. Infectious

2. A common, initial patient response to the seriousness of a terminal illness is:
   a. acceptance.
   b. anger.
   c. denial.
   d. bargaining.

3. The first state in the United States that legalized assisted suicide in 1994 was:
   a. California.
   b. Colorado.
   c. Oregon.
   d. Vermont.

4. For a patient to use the Medicare Hospice Benefit, his or her life expectancy needs to be certified by a physician as approximately:
   a. 2 months.
   b. 4 months.
   c. 6 months.
   d. 8 to 10 months.

5. The median length of stay in a hospice program is:
   a. less than 1 month.
   b. 1 to 2 months.
   c. 4 months.
   d. 6 months or longer.

6. When a person authorizes another to make medical decisions on his or her behalf, the person has written:
   a. an advance directive.
   b. a living will.
   c. a standard addendum to a will.
   d. a proxy directive.

7. A dying patient wants to talk to the nurse about his fears. The patient states, "I know I'm dying, aren't I?" An appropriate nursing response would be:
   a. "This must be very difficult for you."
   b. "Tell me more about what's on your mind."
   c. "I'm so sorry. I know just how you feel."
   d. "You know you're dying?"

8. One of the most common and feared responses to terminal illness is:
   a. anorexia.
   b. cachexia.
   c. dyspnea.
   d. pain.

Study Guide for Brunner and Suddarth's Textbook of Medical-Surgical Nursing, 12th edition.

9. The anorexia–cachexia syndrome that is common toward the end-of-life is characterized by:

a. anemia.

b. alterations in carbohydrate metabolism.

c. endocrine dysfunction.

d. all of the above, plus altered fat and altered protein metabolism.

SHORT ANSWER

Read each statement carefully. Write your response in the space provided.

1. Dr. _____, who spearheaded a movement to increase an awareness of the dying process among health care practitioners, published a landmark book, _____ in 1969.

2. Distinguish between the terms *assisted suicide* and *physician-assisted suicide.*

3. Define the terms *palliative care* and *hospice care.* _____.

4. The first hospice program in the United States began in the state of _____ in the year _____.

5. The two most common primary hospice diagnoses for Medicare patients are: _____ and _____.

6. Two types of medications that are routinely used to treat the underlying obstructed pathology associated with dyspnea: _____ and _____.

7. List three medications that are commonly used to stimulate appetite in anorexic patients: _____, _____, and _____.

II. Critical Thinking Questions and Exercises

DISCUSSION AND ANALYSIS

Discuss the following topics with your classmates.

1. Discuss the clinical guidelines used to structure quality palliative and end-of-life programs identified by the National Consensus Project for Quality Palliative Care (NCP, 2004).
2. Discuss the major ethical question: "Because medical professionals can prolong life through a particular intervention, does it necessarily follow that they must do so?"
3. Explain how Dr. Keibler-Ross's work helped the medical and nursing community view the dying process in a more personalized way.
4. Explain the American Nurses Association's position on the role of nursing and assisted suicide.
5. Compare and contrast the different views about death for five religions: Hinduism, Judaism, Buddhism, Islam, and traditional Christianity.
6. Distinguish between the terms living will and durable power of attorney.
7. Explain the steps a nurse would follow, using the S-P-I-K-E-S strategy, to inform the patient and family that he or she was dying.
8. How a person and his or her family cope with the dying process is influenced by many cultural, psychological, and socioeconomic factors. Analyze the role of the nurse in assessing values, preferences, and practices for a patient influenced by the Western culture of autonomy over care decisions and for a patient influenced by an Eastern culture of interdependence with care decisions.

9. Consider a recent clinical experience involving a dying patient. Draft an outline of nursing interventions that were or could have been used to support the patient's ability to maintain "hope" within the context of realism for the patient.
10. Review the questions that a nurse would use to assess symptoms associated with a terminal illness.
11. Describe the nurse's role in managing dyspnea at the end-of-life.
12. Discuss the purpose and use of palliative sedation.
13. Describe the expected physiological changes that occur as death is approaching. Discuss one or more nursing interventions to help the patient and family cope with this process.
14. Review Dr. Kubler-Ross's five stages of dying and discuss nursing implications for each stage. Use some recent clinical examples if possible.

CHAPTER 18

Preoperative Concepts and Nursing Management

I. Interpretation, Comparison, and Completion

MULTIPLE CHOICE

Read each question carefully. Circle your answer.

1. An example of a surgical procedure classified as urgent is:
   a. an appendectomy.
   b. an exploratory laparotomy.
   c. a repair of multiple stab wounds.
   d. a face-lift.

2. A mammoplasty would be classified as surgery that is:
   a. urgent.
   b. optional.
   c. required.
   d. reconstructive.

3. An informed consent is required for:
   a. closed reduction of a fracture.
   b. insertion of an intravenous catheter.
   c. irrigation of the external ear canal.
   d. urethral catheterization.

4. Protein replacement for nutritional balance can be accomplished with a diet that:
   a. is high in carbohydrates.
   b. is high in protein.
   c. is low in fats.
   d. includes all of the above.

5. A significant mortality rate exists for those alcoholics who experience "delirium tremens" postoperatively. When caring for the alcoholic, the nurse should assess for symptoms of alcoholic withdrawal:
   a. within the first 12 hours.
   b. about 24 hours postoperatively.
   c. on the second or third day.
   d. 4 days after surgery.

6. It is recommended that those who smoke cigarettes should stop smoking how long before surgery?
   a. 2 months
   b. 3 months
   c. 2 weeks
   d. 3 weeks

7. Because liver disease is associated with a high surgical mortality rate, the nurse knows to alert the physician for:
   a. a blood ammonia concentration of 180 mg/dL.
   b. a lactate dehydrogenase concentration of 300 units.
   c. a serum albumin concentration of 5.0 g/dL.
   d. a serum globulin concentration of 2.8 g/dL.

8. Surgery would be contraindicated for a renal patient with:
   a. a blood urea nitrogen level of 42 mg/dL.
   b. a creatine kinase level of 120 U/L.
   c. a serum creatinine level of 0.9 mg/dL.
   d. a urine creatinine level of 1.2 mg/dL.

9. The chief life-threatening hazard for surgical patients with uncontrolled diabetes is:
   a. dehydration.
   b. hypertension.
   c. hypoglycemia.
   d. glucosuria.

10. The goal for the diabetic patient undergoing surgery is to maintain a blood glucose level of:
    a. 80 to 110 mg/dL.
    b. 150 to 240 mg/dL.
    c. 250 to 300 mg/dL.
    d. 300 to 350 mg/dL.

11. A nursing history of prior drug therapy is based on the particular concern that:
    a. phenothiazines may increase the hypotensive action of anesthetics.
    b. thiazide diuretics may cause excessive respiratory depression during anesthesia.
    c. tranquilizers may cause anxiety and even seizures if withdrawn suddenly.
    d. all of the above potential complications could occur.

12. The potential effects of medication therapy must be evaluated before surgery. A drug classification that may cause electrolyte imbalance is:
    a. corticosteroids.
    b. diuretics.
    c. phenothiazines.
    d. insulin.

13. Assessment of a gerontologic patient reveals bilateral dimmed vision. This information alerts the nurse to plan for:
    a. a safe environment.
    b. restrictions of the patient's unassisted mobility activities.
    c. probable cataract extractions.
    d. referral to an ophthalmologist.

14. Hazards of surgery for the geriatric patient are directly related to the:
    a. number of coexisting health problems.
    b. type of surgical procedure.
    c. severity of the surgery.
    d. all of the above.

15. Obesity is positively correlated with surgical complications of:
    a. the cardiovascular system.
    b. the gastrointestinal system.
    c. the pulmonary system.
    d. all of the systems listed.

16. The nursing goal of encouraging postoperative body movement is to:
    a. contribute to optimal respiratory function.
    b. improve circulation.
    c. prevent venous stasis.
    d. promote all of the above activities.

17. Food and water are usually withheld beginning at midnight of the surgical day. However, if necessary, water may be given up to:
    a. 8 hours before surgery.
    b. 6 hours before surgery.
    c. 4 hours before surgery.
    d. 2 hours before surgery.

18. The primary goal in withholding food before surgery is to prevent:
    a. aspiration.
    b. distention.
    c. infection.
    d. obstruction.

19. Expected patient outcomes for relief of anxiety related to a surgical procedure include all of the following *except*:
    a. understands the nature of the surgery and voluntarily signs an informed consent.
    b. verbalizes an understanding of the preanesthetic medication.
    c. requests a visit with a member of the clergy.
    d. questions the anesthesiologist about anesthesia-related concerns.

20. Choose a statement that indicates that a patient is knowledgeable about his or her impending surgery. The patient:
    a. participates willingly in the preoperative preparation.
    b. discusses stress factors that are making him or her depressed.
    c. expresses concern about postoperative pain.
    d. verbalizes his or her fears to family.

21. Hidden fears may be indicated when a patient:
    a. avoids communication.
    b. repeatedly asks questions that have previously been answered.
    c. talks incessantly.
    d. does all of the above.

22. Choose the appropriate response to the statement, "I'm so nervous about my surgery."
    a. "Relax. Your recovery period will be shorter if you're less nervous."
    b. "Stop worrying. It only makes you more nervous."
    c. "You needn't worry. Your doctor has done this surgery many times before."
    d. "You seem nervous about your surgery."

23. The purpose of preoperative skin preparation is to:
    a. reduce the number of microorganisms.
    b. remove all resident bacteria.
    c. render the skin sterile.
    d. accomplish all of the above.

24. The *least* desirable method of hair removal is use of:
    a. electric clippers.
    b. a depilatory cream in nonsensitive patients.
    c. a razor with an extruded blade.
    d. scissors for long hair (more than 3 mm).

25. Purposes of preanesthetic medication include all of the following *except*:
    a. facilitation of anesthesia induction.
    b. lowering of the dose of the anesthetic agent used.
    c. potentiation of the effects of anesthesia.
    d. reduction of preoperative pain.

SHORT ANSWER

Read each statement carefully. Write your response in the space provided.

1. The preoperative phase begins _____ and ends when the patient _____.

2. The intraoperative phase begins when the patient _____ and ends when _____.

3. The hazards of surgery for the elderly are directly proportional to _____ and _____.

4. The leading causes of postoperative morbidity and mortality in older adults are _____ and _____ complications.

5. Informed consent for a surgical procedure is necessary when a procedure meets the following four conditions: _____, _____, _____, and _____.

6. Diabetics undergoing surgery are at risk for four complications: _____, _____, _____, and _____.

7. Aspirin is withheld _____ days prior to surgery, if possible, because it acts by _____.

8. List three significant nutritional concerns for the elderly surgical patient: _____, _____, and _____.

9. Name three primary goals necessary to promote postoperative mobility: _____, _____, and _____.

MATCHING

Match the nutrient in column II with its associated rationale for use in column I.

Column I

1. _____ Essential for normal blood clotting
2. _____ Allows collagen deposition to occur
3. _____ Necessary for DNA synthesis
4. _____ Increases inflammatory response in wounds
5. _____ Vital for capillary formation

Column II

a. Protein
b. Vitamin C
c. Vitamin A
d. Vitamin K
e. Zinc

II. Critical Thinking Questions and Exercises

DISCUSSION AND ANALYSIS

Discuss the following topics with your classmates.

1. Discuss several examples of nursing activities in the perioperative phases of care.
2. Discuss the criteria for valid informed consent.
3. Discuss nursing interventions for at least 10 risk factors for surgical complications.
4. Discuss at least 8 of 13 patient safety goals as identified by the "2009 National Patient Safety Goals" and "The Joint Commission (2008)."

EXAMINING ASSOCIATIONS

Medication Administration

For each drug classification, list the potential effects of interaction with anesthetics.

1. Anticoagulants _____
2. Antiseizure agents _____

3. Corticosteroids _____

4. Diuretics _____

5. Insulin _____

6. Phenothiazines _____

7. Tranquilizers _____

8. Monoamine oxidase inhibitors (MAO) _____

Preoperative Nursing

For each essential preoperative nursing activity, write an appropriate nursing goal. An example is provided.

1. (Example) Restriction of nutrition and fluids <u>Prevent aspiration</u>

2. Intestinal preparation _____

3. Preoperative skin preparation (cleansing) _____

4. Urinary catheterization _____

5. Administration of preoperative medications _____

6. Transportation of patient to presurgical suite _____

CLINICAL APPLICATIONS

Please refer to Chart 18-5 in the text. List five preoperative teaching points the nurse would cover to instruct a patient (1) how to splint the chest while coughing correctly and (2) how to perform leg exercises to prevent postoperative complication.

Splinting when coughing

1. _____

2. _____

3. _____

4. _____

5. _____

Leg exercises

1. _____

2. _____

3. _____

4. _____

5. _____

CHAPTER 19

Intraoperative Nursing Management

I. Interpretation, Completion, and Comparison

MULTIPLE CHOICE

Read each question carefully. Circle your answer.

1. The circulating nurse's responsibilities, in contrast to the scrub nurse's responsibilities, include:
   a. assisting the surgeon.
   b. coordinating the surgical team.
   c. setting up the sterile tables.
   d. all of the above functions.

2. Preoperatively, an anesthesiologist is responsible for:
   a. assessing pulmonary status.
   b. inquiring about preexisting pulmonary infections.
   c. knowing the patient's history of smoking.
   d. all of the above.

3. There are four stages to general anesthesia. An unconscious patient with normal pulse and respirations is considered to be in the stage known as:
   a. beginning anesthesia.
   b. excitement.
   c. surgical anesthesia.
   d. medullary depression.

4. A nurse knows that perioperative risks increase with age because:
   a. ciliary action decreases, reducing the cough reflex.
   b. fatty tissue increases, prolonging the effects of anesthesia.
   c. liver size decreases, reducing the metabolism of anesthetics.
   d. all of the above biologic changes exist.

5. Currently, the *most commonly* used volatile liquid anesthetic agent is:
   a. ethrane.
   b. florane.
   c. nitrous oxide.
   d. ultrane.

6. The nurse should know that, postoperatively, a general anesthetic is primarily eliminated by:
   a. the kidneys.
   b. the lungs.
   c. the skin.
   d. all of these routes.

7. An example of a stable and safe nondepolarizing muscle relaxant is:
   a. anectine (succinylcholine chloride).
   b. norcuron (vercuronium bromide).
   c. pavulon (pancuronium bromide).
   d. syncurine (decamethonium).

8. An intravenous anesthetic that has a powerful respiratory depressant effect sufficient to cause apnea and cardiovascular depression is:
   a. amidate.
   b. ketalar.
   c. pentothal.
   d. versed.

9. Postoperative nursing assessment for a patient who has received a depolarizing neuromuscular blocking agent includes careful monitoring of the:
   a. cardiovascular system.
   b. endocrine system.
   c. gastrointestinal system.
   d. genitourinary system.

10. A factor involved in postspinal anesthesia headaches is the:
    a. degree of patient hydration.
    b. leakage of spinal fluid from the subarachnoid space.
    c. size of the spinal needle used.
    d. combination of the above mechanisms.

11. Epinephrine is often used in combination with a local infiltration anesthetic, because it:
    a. causes vasoconstriction.
    b. prevents rapid absorption of the anesthetic drug.
    c. prolongs the local action of the anesthetic agent.
    d. does all of the above.

12. A local infiltration anesthetic can last for up to:
    a. 1 hour.
    b. 3 hours.
    c. 5 hours.
    d. 7 hours.

13. Recent research has indicated that inadvertent hypothermia in gerontologic patients can be effectively and inexpensively prevented by:
    a. placing the patient on a hyperthermia blanket.
    b. maintaining environmental temperature at 37°C.
    c. covering the top of the patient's head with an ordinary plastic shower cap during anesthesia.
    d. frequent massage of the extremities with warmed skin lotion.

14. The nurse caring for a patient who is at risk for malignant hyperthermia subsequent to general anesthesia would assess for the *most common* early sign of:
    a. hypertension.
    b. muscle rigidity ("tetany-like" movements).
    c. oliguria.
    d. tachycardia.

15. If an operating room nurse is to assist a patient to the Trendelenburg position, he or she would place him:
    a. flat on his back with his arms next to his sides.
    b. on his back with his head lowered so that the plane of his body meets the horizontal on an angle.
    c. on his back with his legs and thighs flexed at right angles.
    d. on his side with his uppermost leg adducted and flexed at the knee.

SHORT ANSWER

Read each statement carefully. Write your response in the space provided.

1. Describe *malignant hyperthermia.* _____

2. Explain why anesthesia dosage is reduced with age. _____.

3. List four primary responsibilities of a Registered Nurse First Assistant (RNFA):

   _____, _____, _____,

   and _____.

4. Five health hazards associated with the surgical environment are: _____, _____, _____, _____, and _____.

5. The type of anesthesia most likely to be used for a patient undergoing a colonoscopy is _____, and the most frequently used agents are _____ and _____.

6. The anesthetic most commonly used for general anesthesia by intravenous injection is _____, which can cause _____ as a serious, toxic side effect.

7. Spinal anesthesia is a conduction nerve block that occurs when a local anesthetic is injected into _____.

8. The conduction block anesthesia commonly used in labor is the _____.

9. What nursing assessment indicates that a patient has recovered from the effects of spinal anesthesia? _____

10. List five potential intraoperative complications: _____, _____, _____, _____, and _____.

11. With malignant hypothermia, the core body temperature can increase 1° to 2° every 5 minutes, reaching or exceeding a body temperature of _____ degrees in a short amount of time.

MATCHING

Match the inhalation anesthetic agent list in column II with its associated nursing implication found in column I.

Column I
1. _____ Monitor for chest pain and stroke
2. _____ Monitor blood pressure frequently
3. _____ Observe for respiratory depression
4. _____ Monitor respirations closely
5. _____ Monitor for malignant hypothermia

Column II
a. Ethrane
b. Fluothane
c. Forane
d. Nitrous oxide
e. Suprane

Match the commonly used intravenous medication in column II with its associated common usage in column I.

Column I
1. _____ Sedation with regional anesthesia
2. _____ Hypnotic and anxiolytic; adjunct to induction
3. _____ Epidural infusion for postoperative analgesia
4. _____ Maintenance of relaxation
5. _____ Skeletal muscle relaxation for orthopedic surgery

Column II
a. Fentanyl
b. Midazolam
c. Pancuronium
d. Propofol
e. Succinylcholine

II. Critical Thinking Questions and Exercises

DISCUSSION AND ANALYSIS

Discuss the following topics with your classmates.

1. Distinguish between the purposes for three types of anesthesia: epidural, general, and local.
2. Discuss at least 10 potential adverse effects of surgery and anesthesia and their associated causes.
3. Explain why the elderly are at a higher risk of complications from anesthesia because of biologic changes that occur in later life.
4. Discuss, in detail, the role and responsibilities of the circulating nurse.
5. Briefly describe the basic guidelines for maintaining surgical asepsis.
6. Discuss the risks to be avoided when lasers are used in the surgical environment.
7. Explain what is meant by "anesthesia awareness."
8. Identify and discuss several nursing diagnoses for a patient during surgery.

RECOGNIZING CONTRADICTIONS

Rewrite each statement correctly. Underline the key concepts.

1. Older patients need more anesthetic agent to produce anesthesia, because they eliminate anesthetic agents more quickly.

_____

2. A scrub nurse controls the operating room environment, coordinates the activities of other personnel, and monitors the patient.

_____

3. If there is any doubt about the sterility of an area, it is considered sterile.

_____

4. A draped table is considered sterile from the top to the edge of the drapes.

_____

5. Only the circulating nurse can extend an arm over the sterile area to deliver sterile supplies.

_____

CLINICAL SITUATIONS

Read the following case studies. Circle the correct answer.

CASE STUDY: General Anesthesia

Anne, age 34, is in excellent health and is scheduled for open reduction of a fractured femur. The general anesthetic drugs to be used include enflurane and nitrous oxide.

1. The nurse knows that the advantages of enflurane (Ethrane) include all of the following *except:*
   a. fast recovery.
   b. low incidence of respiratory depression.
   c. potent analgesia.
   d. rapid induction.

2. The major disadvantage of nitrous oxide is its ability to cause:
   a. hypertension.
   b. hypoxia.
   c. liver damage.
   d. nausea and vomiting.

3. The major postoperative nursing assessment after administration of Ethrane is observation for:
   a. anuria.
   b. laryngospasm.
   c. respiratory depression.
   d. tachycardia.

CASE STUDY: Intravenous Anesthesia

Brian is scheduled to have a wisdom tooth extracted. The anesthetic agent of choice is thiopental sodium (Pentothal).

1. The nurse anticipates that the route of administration will be:
   a. by inhalation.
   b. by mask.
   c. intramuscular.
   d. intravenous.

2. The nurse is aware that after anesthetic administration, Brian will be unconscious in:
   a. 30 seconds.
   b. 60 seconds.
   c. 2 minutes.
   d. 3 minutes.

3. The chief danger with thiopental sodium is its:
   a. beta-adrenergic blocking action.
   b. depressant action on the respiratory system.
   c. nephrotoxicity.
   d. rapid onset and prolonged duration.

CHAPTER **20**

Postoperative Nursing Management

I. Interpretation, Completion, and Comparison

MULTIPLE CHOICE

Read each question carefully. Circle your answer.

1. The primary nursing goal in the immediate postoperative period is maintenance of pulmonary function and prevention of:
   a. laryngospasm.
   b. hyperventilation.
   c. hypoxemia and hypercapnia.
   d. pulmonary edema and embolism.

2. Unless contraindicated, any unconscious patient should be positioned:
   a. flat on his or her back, without elevation of the head, to facilitate frequent turning and minimize pulmonary complications.
   b. in semi-Fowler's position, to promote respiratory function and reduce the incidence of orthostatic hypotension when the patient can eventually stand.
   c. in Fowler's position, which most closely simulates a sitting position, thus facilitating respiratory as well as gastrointestinal functioning.
   d. on his or her side with a pillow at the patient's back and his or her chin extended, to minimize the dangers of aspiration.

3. A major postoperative nursing responsibility is assessing for cardiovascular function by monitoring:
   a. arterial blood gases.
   b. central venous pressure.
   c. vital signs.
   d. all of the above.

4. In the immediate postoperative period, a nurse should immediately report:
   a. a systolic blood pressure lower than 90 mm Hg.
   b. a temperature reading between 97°F and 98°F.
   c. respirations between 20 and 25 breaths/min.
   d. all of the above assessments.

5. Patients remain in the recovery room or postanesthesia care unit (PACU) until they are fully recovered from anesthesia. This is evidenced by:
   a. a patient airway.
   b. a reasonable degree of consciousness.
   c. a stable blood pressure.
   d. indication that all of the above have occurred.

6. When a PACU room scoring guide is used, a patient can be transferred out of the recovery room with a minimum score of:
   a. 5.
   b. 6.
   c. 7.
   d. 8.

114

7. With the PACU room scoring guide, a nurse would give a patient an admission cardiovascular score of 2 if the patient's blood pressure is what percentage of his or her preanesthetic level?
   a. 20%
   b. 30% to 40%
   c. 40% to 50%
   d. Greater than 50%

8. When vomiting occurs postoperatively, the most important nursing intervention is to:
   a. measure the amount of vomitus to estimate fluid loss, in order to accurately monitor fluid balance.
   b. offer tepid water and juices to replace lost fluids and electrolytes.
   c. support the wound area so that unnecessary strain will not disrupt the integrity of the incision.
   d. turn the patient's head completely to one side to prevent aspiration of vomitus into the lungs.

9. Postoperatively, the nurse monitors urinary function. An abnormal outcome that should be reported to the physician is a 2-hour output that is:
   a. less than 30 mL.
   b. between 75 and 100 mL.
   c. between 100 and 200 mL.
   d. greater than 200 mL.

10. Most surgical patients are encouraged to be out of bed:
    a. within 6 to 8 hours after surgery.
    b. between 10 and 12 hours after surgery.
    c. as soon as it is indicated.
    d. on the second postoperative day.

11. One of the most common postoperative respiratory complications in elderly patients is:
    a. pleurisy.
    b. pneumonia.
    c. hypoxemia.
    d. pulmonary edema.

12. A nurse documents the presence of granulation tissue in a healing wound. She describes the tissue as:
    a. necrotic and hard.
    b. pale yet able to blanch with digital pressure.
    c. pink to red and soft, noting that it bleeds easily.
    d. white with long, thin areas of scar tissue.

13. A physician's admitting note lists a wound as healing by second intention. The nurse expects to see:
    a. a deep, open wound that was previously sutured.
    b. a sutured incision with a little tissue reaction.
    c. a wound with a deep, wide scar that was previously resutured.
    d. a wound in which the edges were not approximated.

14. A wound that has hemorrhaged carries an increased risk of infection, because:
    a. reduced amounts of oxygen and nutrients are available.
    b. the tissue becomes less resilient.
    c. retrograde bacterial contamination may occur.
    d. dead space and dead cells provide a culture medium.

15. Postoperative abdominal distention seems to be directly related to:
    a. a temporary loss of peristalsis and gas accumulation in the intestines.
    b. beginning food intake in the immediate postoperative period.
    c. improper body positioning during the recovery period.
    d. the type of anesthetic administered.

16. The characteristic sign of a paralytic ileus is:
    a. abdominal tightness.
    b. abdominal distention.
    c. absence of peristalsis.
    d. increased abdominal girth.

17. Nursing measures to prevent thrombophlebitis include:
    a. assisting the patient with leg exercises.
    b. encouraging early ambulation.
    c. avoiding placement of pillows or blanket rolls under the patient's knees.
    d. all of the above.

18. One of the major dangers associated with deep venous thrombosis is:
    a. pulmonary embolism.
    b. immobility because of calf pain.
    c. marked tenderness over the anteromedial surface of the thigh.
    d. swelling of the entire leg owing to edema.

19. One of the most effective nursing procedures for reducing nosocomial infections is:
    a. administration of prophylactic antibiotics.
    b. aseptic wound care.
    c. control of upper respiratory tract infections.
    d. proper hand-washing techniques.

20. It is estimated that health-care associated infections occur in the surgical site in what percentage of surgical patients?
    a. 5% to 10% of surgical patients.
    b. 14% to 16% of surgical patients.
    c. 20% to 30% of surgical patients.
    d. Approximately 57% of surgical patients.

21. The nurse recognizes that a clean-contaminated wound has a relative probability of infection of:
    a. 1% to 3%.
    b. 7% to 16%.
    c. 3% to 7%.
    d. more than 16%.

22. A nursing measure for evisceration is to:
    a. apply an abdominal binder snugly so that the intestines can be slowly pushed back into the abdominal cavity.
    b. approximate the wound edges with adhesive tape so that the intestines can be gently pushed back into the abdomen.
    c. carefully push the exposed intestines back into the abdominal cavity.
    d. cover the protruding coils of intestines with sterile dressings moistened with sterile saline solution.

SHORT ANSWER

Read each statement carefully. Write your response in the space provided.

1. List five areas of concern for a recovery room PACU nurse who has just received a patient from the operating room: _____, _____, _____, _____, and _____.

2. The primary nursing objective during the immediate postoperative assessment is to maintain _____ and prevent _____.

3. Five types of shock are: _____, _____, _____, _____, and _____.

4. Distinguish among the three classifications of hemorrhage (primary, intermediary, and secondary) and include the defining characteristics of each.

   Primary: _____

   Intermediary: _____

   Secondary: _____

5. The *most serious* and *most frequent* postoperative complications involve the _____ system.

6. Explain patient-controlled analgesia (PCA). _____.

7. Explain why the postoperative complications of atelectasis and hypostatic pneumonia are reduced as a result of early ambulation.

   _____

8. Two potential postoperative complications following abdominal surgery are: _____ and

   _____.

9. The return of peristalsis in the postoperative period can be determined by the presence of _____ and _____, both of which are assessed by the nurse.

10. Distinguish between wound *dehiscence* and *evisceration*.

    _____

    _____

II. Critical Thinking Questions and Exercises

DISCUSSION AND ANALYSIS

Discuss the following topics with your classmates.

1. Explain the type of information that a nurse should receive when a patient is transferred to the PACU from the operating room.
2. Demonstrate the steps a nurse would take to prevent hypopharyngeal obstruction, postanesthesia.
3. Describe the nursing assessment to detect any of the eight classic signs of hypovolemic shock.
4. Discuss the system assessment that a nurse would need to perform in determining a patient's readiness for discharge from the PACU.
5. Review common nursing diagnoses and collaborative problems for the postoperative patient.
6. Describe three postoperative conditions that put a patient at risk for common respiratory complications.
7. Explain how various factors (age, edema, nutritional deficits, oxygen deficit, medications, and systemic disorders) affect the progress of wound healing.
8. Describe nursing assessment activities and interventions to detect postoperative deep vein thrombosis and pulmonary embolism.

IDENTIFYING PATTERNS

Read the case study. Fill in the spaces provided.

CASE STUDY: Postoperative Pain

Mr. Flynn's pain medication was frequently delayed because his staff nurses were busy with other patients. As a nursing supervisor, you emphasized the necessity of preventing or managing postoperative pain, knowing that there is a positive correlation between pain experience and the frequency of complications. Support your argument by filling in these blank spaces.

1. Pain stimulates _____, which increases _____ and

   _____.

2. Noxious impulses stimulate _____, which increases _____ and

   _____.

3. Hypothalamic stress responses increase _____ and _____,

   which can lead to _____ and _____.

CLINICAL SITUATIONS

Read the following case studies. Circle the correct answer.

CASE STUDY: Hypovolemic Shock

Mario is admitted to the emergency department with a diagnosis of hypovolemic shock secondary to a 30% blood volume loss resulting from a motorcycle accident.

1. A primary nursing objective is to:
   a. administer vasopressors.
   b. ensure a patent airway.
   c. minimize energy expenditure.
   d. provide external warmth.

2. With a diagnosis of hypovolemic shock, the nurse expects to assess all of the following *except*:
   a. a decreased and concentrated urinary output.
   b. an elevated central venous pressure reading.
   c. hypotension with a small pulse pressure.
   d. tachycardia and a thready pulse.

3. The nurse takes blood pressure readings every 5 minutes. She knows that shock is well advanced when the systolic pressure drops to less than:
   a. 90 mm Hg.
   b. 100 mm Hg.
   c. 110 mm Hg.
   d. 120 mm Hg.

4. A urinary catheter is inserted to measure hourly output. The nurse knows that inadequate volume replacement is reflected by an output of less than:
   a. 30 mL/h.
   b. 50 mL/h.
   c. 80 mL/h.
   d. 100 mL/h.

5. The physician prescribes crystalloid solution to be administered to restore blood volume. The nurse knows that a crystalloid solution is:
   a. a blood transfusion.
   b. lactated Ringer's solution.
   c. plasma or a plasma substitute.
   d. serum albumin.

CASE STUDY: Hypopharyngeal Obstruction

Deana is unconscious when she is transferred to the recovery room. She has experienced prolonged anesthesia, and all her muscles are relaxed.

1. During the initial assessment, the nurse diagnosed hypopharyngeal obstruction. This difficulty is signaled by:
   a. choking.
   b. cyanosis.
   c. irregular respirations.
   d. all of the above.

2. To treat hypopharyngeal obstruction, the nurse would:
   a. flex the neck and pull the lower jaw down toward the chest.
   b. hyperextend the neck and push forward on the angle of the lower jaw.
   c. raise the head and open the mouth as far as possible.
   d. rotate the head to either side and unclench the teeth.

3. The nurse knows that the most accurate way to determine whether Deana is breathing is to:
   a. auscultate for breath sounds.
   b. inspect for diaphragmatic movement.
   c. palpate for thoracic changes.
   d. place his or her palm over Deana's nose and mouth.

4. The anesthesiologist chose to leave a plastic airway in Deana's mouth. The nurse knows that an airway should not be removed:
   a. without a physician's order.
   b. until the patient's secretions have been aspirated.
   c. until signs indicate that reflexes are returning.
   d. until arterial blood gas measurements indicate adequate PO_2 levels.

CASE STUDY: Wound Healing

Elizabeth is returned from the recovery room to a patient care area after a routine cholecystectomy.

1. The nurse expects that the inflammatory phase of wound healing should last for about:
   a. 1 day.
   b. 3 days.
   c. 5 days.
   d. 4 days.

2. When both sides of the wound approximate within 24 to 48 hours, the healing is said to be by:
   a. first intention.
   b. second intention.
   c. third intention.
   d. spontaneous intention.

3. Those clinical manifestations associated with the inflammatory phase of wound healing that the nurse would expect to see postoperatively are:
   a. pain.
   b. redness.
   c. warmth.
   d. all of the above.

4. Nursing measures to promote adequate tissue oxygenation during the inflammatory phase of wound healing include:
   a. applying warm compresses to the incision every 4 hours for 2 to 3 days to stimulate vasodilation.
   b. encouraging coughing and deep breathing to enhance pulmonary and cardiovascular functions.
   c. helping Elizabeth stay in bed for 4 to 6 days to prevent unnecessary strain on the suture line.
   d. leaving soiled dressings in place to prevent airborne microorganisms from entering the wound and setting up a localized infection.

CHAPTER 21

Assessment of Respiratory Function

I. Interpretation, Completion, and Comparison

MULTIPLE CHOICE

Read each question carefully. Circle your answer.

1. The purpose of the cilia is to:
   a. produce mucus.
   b. phagocytize bacteria.
   c. contract smooth muscle.
   d. move the mucus back to the larynx.

2. A patient with sinus congestion points to the area on the inside of the eye as a point of pain. The nurse knows that the patient is referring to which sinus?
   a. Frontal
   b. Ethmoidal
   c. Maxillary
   d. Sphenoidal

3. The lungs are enclosed in a serous membrane called the:
   a. diaphragm.
   b. mediastinum.
   c. pleura.
   d. xiphoid process.

4. The left lung, in contrast to the right lung, has:
   a. one less lobe.
   b. one more lobe.
   c. the same number of lobes.
   d. two more lobes.

5. The divisions of the lung lobe proceed in the following order, beginning at the mainstem bronchi:
   a. lobar bronchi, bronchioles, segmented bronchi, subsequent bronchi.
   b. segmented bronchi, subsegmented bronchi, lobar bronchi, bronchioles.
   c. lobar bronchi, segmented bronchi, subsegmented bronchi, bronchioles.
   d. subsegmented bronchi, lobar bronchi, bronchioles, segmented bronchi.

6. Choose the initial part of the respiratory tract that is *not considered* part of the gas-exchange airways.
   a. Bronchioles
   b. Respiratory bronchioles
   c. Alveolar duct
   d. Alveolar sacs

7. Choose the alveolar cells that secrete surfactant.
   a. Type I cells
   b. Type II cells
   c. Type III cells
   d. Types I and II cells

8. Gas exchange between the lungs and blood and between the blood and tissues is called:
   a. active transport.
   b. respiration.
   c. ventilation.
   d. cellular respiration.

9. The maximum volume of air that can be inhaled after a normal inhalation is known as:
   a. inspiratory reserve volume.
   b. expiratory reserve volume.
   c. tidal volume.
   d. residual volume.

10. Tidal volume, which may not significantly change with disease, has a normal value of approximately:
    a. 300 mL.
    b. 500 mL.
    c. 800 mL.
    d. 1,000 mL.

11. The exchange of oxygen and carbon dioxide from the alveoli into the blood occurs by:
    a. active transport.
    b. diffusion.
    c. osmosis.
    d. pinocytosis.

12. Airflow into the lungs during inspiration depends on all of the following *except*:
    a. contraction of the muscles of respiration.
    b. enlargement of the thoracic cavity.
    c. lowered intrathoracic pressure.
    d. relaxation of the diaphragm.

13. The pulmonary circulation is considered a:
    a. high-pressure, high-resistance system.
    b. low-pressure, low-resistance system.
    c. high-pressure, low-resistance system.
    d. low-pressure, high-resistance system.

14. Gerontologic changes in the respiratory system include all of the following *except*:
    a. decreased alveolar duct diameter.
    b. decreased gag reflex.
    c. increased presence of collagen in alveolar walls.
    d. decreased presence of mucus.

15. The symbol used to identify the partial pressure of oxygen is:
    a. PO_2.
    b. PAO_2.
    c. PaO_2.
    d. $PV\text{-}O_2$.

16. Uneven perfusion of the lung is primarily due to:
    a. pulmonary artery pressure.
    b. gravity.
    c. alveolar pressure.
    d. all of the above.

17. A nurse caring for a patient with a pulmonary embolism understands that a high ventilation–perfusion ratio may exist. This means that:
    a. perfusion exceeds ventilation.
    b. there is an absence of perfusion and ventilation.
    c. ventilation exceeds perfusion.
    d. ventilation matches perfusion.

18. A nurse understands that a safe but low level of oxygen saturation provides for adequate tissue saturation but allows no reserve for situations that threaten ventilation. A safe but low oxygen saturation level is:
    a. 40 mm Hg.
    b. 75 mm Hg.
    c. 80 mm Hg.
    d. 95 mm Hg.

19. When taking a respiratory history, the nurse should assess:
    a. the previous history of lung disease in the patient or family.
    b. occupational and environmental influences.
    c. smoking and exposure to allergies.
    d. all of the above.

20. Bacterial pneumonia can be indicated by the presence of all of the following *except*:
    a. green, purulent sputum.
    b. thick, yellow sputum.
    c. thin, mucoid sputum.
    d. rusty sputum.

21. Nursing assessment for a patient with chest pain includes:
    a. determining whether there is a relationship between the pain and the patient's posture.
    b. evaluating the effect of the phases of respiration on the pain.
    c. looking for factors that precipitate the pain.
    d. all of the above.

22. Chest pain described as knifelike on inspiration would most likely be diagnostic of:
    a. bacterial pneumonia.
    b. bronchogenic carcinoma.
    c. lung infarction.
    d. pleurisy.

23. Hemoptysis, a symptom of cardiopulmonary disorders, is characterized by all of the following *except*:
    a. a coffee ground appearance.
    b. an alkaline pH.
    c. a sudden onset.
    d. bright red bleeding mixed with sputum.

24. A patient exhibits cyanosis when how much hemoglobin is unoxygenated?
    a. 0.77 g/dL
    b. 2.3 g/dL
    c. 15.0 g/dL
    d. 5.0 g/dL

25. The nurse inspects the thorax of a patient with advanced emphysema. The nurse expects chest configuration change consistent with a deformity known as:
    a. barrel chest.
    b. funnel chest.
    c. kyphoscoliosis.
    d. pigeon chest.

26. Breath sounds that originate in the smaller bronchi and bronchioles and are high-pitched, sibilant, and musical are called:
    a. wheezes.
    b. rhonchi.
    c. rales.
    d. crackles.

27. Crackles, noncontiguous breath sounds, would be assessed for a patient with:
    a. asthma.
    b. bronchospasm.
    c. collapsed aleveoli.
    d. pulmonary fibrosis.

28. During a preadmission assessment, the nurse would expect to find decreased tactile fremitus and hyper-resonant percussion sounds with a diagnosis of:
    a. bronchitis.
    b. emphysema.
    c. atelectasis.
    d. pulmonary edema.

29. The arterial blood gas measurement that best reflects the adequacy of alveolar ventilation is the:
    a. PaO_2.
    b. $PaCO_2$.
    c. pH.
    d. SaO_2.

30. Nursing directions to a patient from whom a sputum specimen is to be obtained should include all of the following *except* directing the patient to:
    a. initially clear his or her nose and throat.
    b. spit surface mucus and saliva into a sterile specimen container.
    c. take a few deep breaths before coughing.
    d. use diaphragmatic contractions to aid in the expulsion of sputum.

31. A physician wants a study of diaphragmatic motion because of suspected pathology. The physician would most likely order a:
    a. barium swallow.
    b. bronchogram.
    c. fluoroscopy.
    d. tomogram.

32. Nursing instructions for a patient who is scheduled for a perfusion lung scan should include informing the patient that:
    a. a mask will be placed over his or her nose and mouth during the test.
    b. he or she will be expected to lie under the camera.
    c. the imaging time will amount to 20 to 40 minutes.
    d. all of the above will occur.

33. The nurse should advise the patient who is scheduled for bronchoscopy that he or she will:
    a. have his or her nose sprayed with a topical anesthetic.
    b. be required to fast before the procedure.
    c. receive preoperative medication.
    d. experience all of the above.

SHORT ANSWER

Read each statement carefully. Write your response in the space provided.

1. Distinguish between the terms *ventilation* and *respiration*.

   _____

2. Describe the function of the epiglottis.

   _____

3. List four conditions that cause low compliance or distensibility of the lungs: _____,
   _____, _____, and _____.

4. Define the term *partial pressure*.

   _____.

5. Name two centers in the brain that are responsible for the neurologic control of ventilation:
   _____ and _____.

6. The alveoli begin to lose elasticity at about age _____ years, resulting in decreased gas diffusion.

7. List six major signs and symptoms of respiratory disease.

   _____   _____

   _____   _____

   _____   _____

8. List four conditions that are influenced by genetic factors that affect respiratory function:
   _____, _____, _____, and _____.

9. Explain the breathing pattern characterized as Cheyne–Stokes respirations.

   _____

II. Critical Thinking Questions and Exercises

DISCUSSION AND ANALYSIS

Discuss the following topics with your classmates.

1. Explain the process of gas exchange known as respiration.
2. Describe four common phenomena that can alter bronchial diameter.
3. Discuss the description and significance of the various lung volumes and capacities.
4. Explain the difference between the terms *diffusion* and *pulmonary perfusion*.
5. Describe the age-related structural and functional changes in the respiratory system.
6. Explain how oxygen is carried in the blood.
7. Explain the pathophysiological changes that occur with dyspnea.
8. Compare and contrast the description of three types of adventitious breath sounds: crackles, wheezes, and friction rubs.
9. Distinguish between three voice sounds: bronchophony, egophony, and whispered pectoriloquey.

CLINICAL SITUATIONS

Read the following case studies. Circle the correct answer.

CASE STUDY: Bronchoscopy

Mr. Kecklin is scheduled for a bronchoscopy for the diagnostic purpose of locating a pathologic process.

1. Because a bronchoscopy was ordered, the nurse knows that the suspected lesion *was not* in the:
   a. bronchus.
   b. larynx.
   c. pharynx.
   d. trachea.

2. Nursing measures before the bronchoscopy include:
   a. obtaining an informed consent.
   b. supplying information about the procedure.
   c. withholding food and fluids for 6 hours before the test.
   d. all of the above.

3. The nurse is aware that possible complications of bronchoscopy include all of the following *except*:
   a. aspiration.
   b. gastric perforation.
   c. infection.
   d. pneumothorax.

4. After the bronchoscopy, Mr. Kecklin must be observed for:
   a. dyspnea.
   b. hemoptysis.
   c. tachycardia.
   d. all of the above.

5. After the bronchoscopy, Mr. Kecklin:
   a. can be given ice chips and fluids after he demonstrates that he can perform the gag reflex.
   b. should immediately be given a house diet to alleviate the hunger resulting from the required fast.
   c. should initially be given iced ginger ale to prevent vomiting and possible aspiration of stomach contents.
   d. will need to remain NPO for 6 hours to prevent pharyngeal irritation.

CASE STUDY: Thoracentesis

Mrs. Lomar is admitted to the clinical area for a thoracentesis. The physician wants to remove excess air from the pleural cavity.

1. Nursing responsibilities before the thoracentesis should include:
   a. informing Mrs. Lomar about pressure sensations that will be experienced during the procedure.
   b. making sure that chest roentgenograms ordered in advance have been completed.
   c. seeing that the consent form has been explained and signed.
   d. all of the above.

2. For the thoracentesis, the patient is assisted to any of the following positions *except*:
   a. lying on the unaffected side with the bed elevated 30 to 40 degrees.
   b. lying prone with the head of the bed lowered 15 to 30 degrees.
   c. sitting on the edge of the bed with her feet supported and her arms and head on a padded overbed table.
   d. straddling a chair with her arms and head resting on the back of the chair.

3. Nursing intervention includes exposing the entire chest even though the thoracentesis site is normally in the midclavicular line between the:
   a. first and second intercostal spaces.
   b. second and third intercostal spaces.
   c. third and fourth intercostal spaces.
   d. fourth and fifth intercostal spaces.

4. Nursing observations after the thoracentesis include assessment for:
   a. blood-tinged mucus.
   b. signs of hypoxemia.
   c. tachycardia.
   d. all of the above.

5. A chest x-ray film is usually ordered after the thoracentesis to rule out:
   a. pleurisy.
   b. pneumonia.
   c. pneumothorax.
   d. pulmonary edema.

INTERPRETING DATA

Review the figure below and explain in your own words what the oxyhemoglobin dissociation curve depicts. Also explain expected changes with clinical conditions.

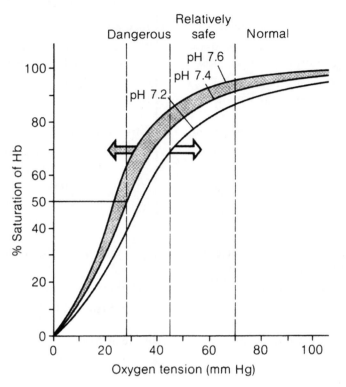

The oxyhemoglobin dissociation curve is marked to show three oxygen levels: (1) normal levels (PaO$_2$ above 70 mm Hg), (2) relatively safe levels (PaO$_2$ 45 to 70 mm Hg), and (3) dangerous levels (PaO$_2$ below 40 mm Hg). The normal (middle) curve shows that 75% saturation occurs at a PaO$_2$ of 40 mm Hg. If the curve shifts to the right, the same saturation (75%) occurs at the higher PaO$_2$ of 57 mm Hg. If the curve shifts to the left, 75% saturation occurs at a PaO$_2$ of 25 mm Hg.

Explain the concepts supporting the basis for the oxyhemoglobin dissociation curve in your own words. Interpret the relevance of the data depicted in the oxyhemoglobin dissociation curve above.

_____

_____

_____

_____

_____

CHAPTER 22

Management of Patients With Upper Respiratory Tract Disorders

I. Interpretation, Completion, and Comparison

MULTIPLE CHOICE

Read each question carefully. Circle your answer.

1. Nursing measures associated with the uncomplicated common cold include all of the following *except*:
   a. administering prescribed antibiotics to decrease the severity of the viral infection.
   b. informing the patient about the symptoms of secondary infection, the major complication of a cold.
   c. suggesting adequate fluid intake and rest.
   d. teaching people that the virus is contagious for 2 days before symptoms appear and during the first part of the symptomatic phase.

2. Health teaching for viral rhinitis (common cold) includes advising the patient to:
   a. blow his or her nose gently to prevent spread of the infection.
   b. blow through both nostrils to equalize the pressure.
   c. rest, to promote overall comfort.
   d. do all of the above.

3. Acyclovir, an antiviral agent, is recommended for:
   a. herpes simplex infection.
   b. rhinitis.
   c. sinusitis.
   d. bronchitis.

4. About 60% of cases of acute rhinosinusitis are caused by bacterial organisms. The antibiotic of choice is:
   a. Augmentin.
   b. Amoxil.
   c. erythromycin.
   d. septra.

5. Nursing suggestions for a patient with acute or chronic rhinosinusitis include:
   a. adequate fluid intake.
   b. increased humidity.
   c. local heat applications to promote drainage.
   d. all of the above.

6. Acute pharyngitis of a bacterial nature is *most commonly* caused by:
   a. group A, beta-hemolytic streptococci.
   b. gram-negative *Klebsiella*.
   c. *Pseudomonas*.
   d. *Staphylococcus aureus*.

7. A complication of acute pharyngitis can be:
   a. mastoiditis.
   b. otitis media.
   c. peritonsillar abscess.
   d. all of the above.

8. Nursing management for a patient with acute pharyngitis includes:

   a. applying an ice collar for symptomatic relief of a severe sore throat.

   b. encouraging bed rest during the febrile stage of the illness.

   c. suggesting a liquid or soft diet during the acute stage of the disease.

   d. all of the above measures.

9. The most common bacterial pathogen associated with tonsillitis and adenoiditis is:

   a. group A, beta-hemolytic streptococcus.

   b. gram-negative *Klebsiella*.

   c. *Pseudomonas*.

   d. *Staphylococcus aureus*.

10. Potential complications of enlarged adenoids include all of the following *except*:

    a. bronchitis.

    b. nasal obstruction.

    c. allergies.

    d. acute otitis media.

11. To assess for an upper respiratory tract infection, the nurse should palpate:

    a. the frontal and maxillary sinuses.

    b. the trachea.

    c. the neck lymph nodes.

    d. all of the above areas.

12. To assess for an upper respiratory tract infection, the nurse should inspect:

    a. the nasal mucosa.

    b. the frontal sinuses.

    c. the tracheal mucosa.

    d. all of the above.

13. Airway clearance in a patient with an upper airway infection is facilitated by all of the following *except*:

    a. decreasing systemic hydration.

    b. humidifying inspired room air.

    c. positional drainage of the affected area.

    d. administering prescribed vasoconstrictive medications.

14. Nursing intervention for a patient with a fractured nose includes all of the following *except*:

    a. applying cold compresses to decrease swelling and control bleeding.

    b. assessing respirations to detect any interference with breathing.

    c. observing for any clear fluid drainage from either nostril.

    d. packing each nostril with a cotton pledget to minimize bleeding and help maintain the shape of the nose during fracture setting.

15. Surgical reduction of nasal fractures is usually performed how long after the fracture?

    a. Within 24 hours

    b. 3 to 7 days

    c. 2 to 3 weeks

    d. 2 months

16. Angioedema as a risk factor that leads to laryngeal obstruction is usually caused by:

    a. heavy alcohol use.

    b. a history of airway problems.

    c. the presence of foreign body.

    d. the use of ACE inhibitors.

17. To correctly perform the Heimlich maneuver, a person should forcefully apply pressure against the victim's:

    a. abdomen.

    b. diaphragm.

    c. lungs.

    d. trachea.

18. An early sign of cancer of the larynx in the glottic area (66% of cases) is:

    a. affected voice sounds.

    b. burning of the throat when hot liquids are ingested.

    c. enlarged cervical nodes.

    d. dysphagia.

19. A patient with a total laryngectomy would no longer have:
    a. natural vocalization.
    b. protection of the lower airway from foreign particles.
    c. a normal effective cough.
    d. all of the above mechanisms.

20. Patient education for a laryngectomy includes:
    a. advising that large amounts of mucus can be coughed up through the stoma.
    b. cautioning about preventing water from entering the stoma.
    c. telling the patient to expect a diminished sense of taste and smell.
    d. doing all of the above.

SHORT ANSWER

Read each statement carefully. Write your response in the space provided.

1. Explain how rhinitis can lead to rhinosinusitis.

   _____

2. Name four bacterial organisms that account for more than 60% of all cases of acute rhinosinusitis:
   _____, _____, _____, and _____.

3. If untreated, chronic rhinosinusitis can lead to severe complications. List four: _____,
   _____, _____, and _____.

4. The most serious complication of a tonsillectomy is: _____.

5. The most common cause of laryngitis is _____, with symptoms including _____,
   _____, and _____.

6. List four possible nursing diagnoses for a patient with an upper airway infection: _____,
   _____, _____, and _____.

7. List five potential complications of an upper airway infection: _____, _____,
   _____, _____, and _____.

8. List the clinical manifestations that are used to diagnose obstructive sleep apnea.

   _____

9. List three types of alaryngeal communication: _____, _____, and
   _____.

II. Critical Thinking Questions and Exercises

DISCUSSION AND ANALYSIS

Discuss the following topics with your classmates.

1. Discuss nursing considerations for upper respiratory tract disorders in the elderly.
2. Compare and contrast the pathophysiology, clinical manifestations, medical interventions, and nursing management for acute and chronic pharyngitis.
3. Discuss the latest medical treatment for epistaxis.

CLINICAL SITUATIONS

Read the following case studies. Fill in the blanks or circle the correct answer.

CASE STUDY: Tonsillectomy and Adenoidectomy

Isabel, a 14-year-old girl, has just undergone a tonsillectomy and adenoidectomy. The staff nurse assists her with transport from the recovery area to her room.

1. On the basis of knowledge about tonsillar disease, the nurse knows that Isabel must have experienced symptoms that required surgical intervention. Clinical manifestations may have included:
   a. hypertrophy of the tonsils.
   b. repeated attacks of otitis media.
   c. suspected hearing loss secondary to otitis media.
   d. all of the above.

2. The nurse assesses Isabel's postoperative vital signs and checks for the most significant postoperative complication of:
   a. epiglottis.
   b. eustachian tube perforation.
   c. hemorrhage.
   d. oropharyngeal edema.

3. The nurse maintains Isabel in the recommended postoperative position of:
   a. prone with her head on a pillow and turned to the side.
   b. reverse Trendelenburg with the neck extended.
   c. semi-Fowler's position with the neck flexed.
   d. supine with her neck hyperextended and supported with a pillow.

4. Isabel is to be discharged the same day of her tonsillectomy. The nurse makes sure that her family knows to:
   a. encourage her to eat a house diet to build up her resistance to infection.
   b. offer her only clear liquids for 3 days, to prevent pharyngeal irritation.
   c. offer her soft foods for several days to minimize local discomfort and supply her with necessary nutrients.
   d. supplement her diet with orange and lemon juices because of the need for vitamin C to heal tissues.

CASE STUDY: Epistaxis

Gilberta, a 14-year-old high school student, is sent with her mother to the emergency department of a local hospital for uncontrolled epistaxis.

1. Describe what the school nurse should tell Gilberta to manage the bleeding site while being transported to the hospital.

2. Initial nursing measures in the emergency department that can be used to stop the nasal bleeding include:

    a. compressing the soft outer portion of the nose against the midline septum continuously for 5 to 10 minutes.

    b. keeping Gilberta in the upright position with her head tilted forward to prevent swallowing and aspiration of blood.

    c. telling Gilberta to breathe through her mouth and to refrain from talking.

    d. all of the above.

3. The nurse expects that emergency medical treatment may include insertion of a cotton pledget moistened with:

    a. an adrenergic blocking agent.

    b. a topical anesthetic.

    c. protamine sulfate.

    d. vitamin K.

4. The nurse can advise the mother that nasal packing used to control bleeding can be left in place:

    a. no longer than 2 hours.

    b. an average of 12 hours.

    c. an average of 24 hours.

    d. anywhere from 2 to 6 days.

CASE STUDY: Cancer of the Larynx

Brenda, a 64-year-old with a long-term history of smoking, recently retired from the chemical laboratory department of a large company. After months of complaining of a persistent cough, sore throat, pain, and burning in the throat, Brenda was admitted to the hospital with a diagnosis of cancer of the larynx.

1. During her assessment, the nurse knows that a number of risk factors are associated with laryngeal cancer. List 10 of 20 possible factors.

    1. _____
    2. _____
    3. _____
    4. _____
    5. _____
    6. _____
    7. _____
    8. _____
    9. _____
    10. _____

2. The most common form of cancer of the larynx is: _____.

3. Assessment of a patient admitted for laryngeal carcinoma includes:

    a. palpation of the frontal and maxillary sinuses to detect infection or inflammation.

    b. palpation of the neck for swelling.

    c. inspection of the nasal mucosa for polyps.

    d. all of the above techniques.

4. The nurse advises Brenda that the likelihood of lymph node involvement is less than _____%.

    Without lymph node metastasis, recovery is expected in _____% of patients.

5. The nurse knows that Brenda's stage I cancer will most likely be treated by

_____.

6. The nurse advises Brenda to be vigilant about her follow-up care because the highest risk for laryngeal

cancer is in the first _____ to _____ years.

CASE STUDY: Laryngectomy

Jerome, a 52-year-old widower, is admitted for a laryngectomy owing to a malignant tumor.

1. Before developing a care plan, the nurse needs to know whether Jerome's voice will be preserved. The surgical procedure that *would not damage* the voice box is a:
   a. partial laryngectomy.
   b. supraglottic laryngectomy.
   c. thyrotomy.
   d. total laryngectomy.

2. Jerome is scheduled for a total laryngectomy. Preoperative education includes:
   a. informing him that there are ways he will be able to carry on a conversation without his voice.
   b. making sure that he knows he will require a permanent tracheal stoma.
   c. reminding him that he will not be able to sing, whistle, or laugh.
   d. all of the above.

3. Postoperative nutrition is usually maintained by way of a nasogastric catheter. The nurse needs to tell Jerome that oral feedings usually begin after:
   a. 24 hours.
   b. 2 to 3 days.
   c. 5 to 6 days.
   d. 1 week.

4. The nurse knows to assess for the most common postoperative complications of: _____,

_____, _____, _____, _____, and

_____.

5. Postoperative nursing measures to promote respiratory effectiveness include:
   a. assisting with turning and early ambulation.
   b. positioning Jerome in semi- to high-Fowler's position.
   c. reminding Jerome to cough and take frequent deep breaths.
   d. all of the above.

6. List at least four signs of postoperative infection that the nurse should monitor: _____,

_____, _____, and _____.

7. Jerome needs to know that the laryngectomy tube will be removed when:
   a. esophageal speech has been perfected.
   b. he requests that it be removed.
   c. oral feedings are initiated.
   d. the stoma is well healed.

8. A lethal complication of wound breakdown is: _____.

APPLYING CONCEPTS

Examine Chart 22-6 in the text and answer the following questions.

A woman is signaling that she is chocking. The nurse is performing an abdominal thrust maneuver (the Heimlich Maneuver). List the eight steps suggested by the AHA to dislodge the foreign object.
Steps to dislodge object

1. _____
2. _____
3. _____
4. _____
5. _____
6. _____
7. _____
8. _____

CHAPTER 23

Management of Patients With Chest and Lower Respiratory Tract Disorders

I. Interpretation, Comprehension, and Comparison

MULTIPLE CHOICE

Read each question carefully. Circle your answer.

1. Nursing management for a person diagnosed as having acute tracheobronchitis includes:
   a. increasing fluid intake to remove secretions.
   b. encouraging the patient to remain in bed.
   c. using cool-vapor therapy to relieve laryngeal and tracheal irritation.
   d. all of the above.

2. The nurse knows that a sputum culture is necessary to identify the causative organism for acute tracheobronchitis. If the culture identifies a fungal agent, the nurse knows it would most likely be:
   a. *Aspergillus.*
   b. *Haemophilus.*
   c. *Mycoplasma pneumoniae.*
   d. *Streptococcus pneumoniae.*

3. In the United States, the most common causes of death from infectious diseases are influenza and:
   a. atelectasis.
   b. pulmonary embolus.
   c. pneumonia.
   d. tracheobronchitis.

4. *Streptococcus pneumoniae* is the most common organism responsible for which of the following types of pneumonia?
   a. Hospital-acquired
   b. Immunocompromised
   c. Aspiration-specific
   d. Community-acquired

5. Characteristics of the *Mycobacterium tuberculosis* include all of the following *except*:
   a. it can be transmitted only by droplet nuclei.
   b. it is acid-fast.
   c. it is able to lie dormant within the body for years.
   d. it survives in anaerobic conditions.

6. It is estimated that *Mycobacterium tuberculosis* infects about what percentage of the world's population?
   a. 10%
   b. 25%
   c. 35%
   d. 50%

7. For the tubercle bacillus to multiply and initiate a tissue reaction in the lungs, it must be deposited in:
   a. the alveoli.
   b. the bronchi.
   c. the trachea.
   d. all of the above.

8. A Mantoux skin test is considered *not significant* if the size of the induration is:
   a. 0 to 4 mm.
   b. 5 to 6 mm.
   c. 7 to 8 mm.
   d. 9 mm.

9. Prophylactic isoniazid (INH) drug treatment is necessary for about how many months?
   a. 3 months
   b. 3 to 5 months
   c. 6 to 12 months
   d. 13 to 18 months

10. Diagnostic confirmation of a lung abscess is made by:
    a. chest x-ray.
    b. bronchoscopy.
    c. sputum culture.
    d. evaluating all of the above studies.

11. The most diagnostic clinical symptom of pleurisy is:
    a. dullness or flatness on percussion over areas of collected fluid.
    b. dyspnea and coughing.
    c. fever and chills.
    d. stabbing pain during respiratory movement.

12. A pleural effusion results when fluid accumulation in the pleural space is greater than:
    a. 5 mL.
    b. 10 mL.
    c. 15 mL.
    d. 20 mL.

13. Auscultation can be used to diagnose the presence of pulmonary edema when the following adventitious breath sounds are present:
    a. crackles in the lung bases.
    b. low-pitched rhonchi during expiration.
    c. pleural friction rub.
    d. sibilant wheezes.

14. Acute respiratory failure (ARF) occurs when oxygen tension (PaO_2) falls to less than _____ mm Hg (hypoxemia) and carbon dioxide tension ($PaCO_2$) rises to greater than _____ mm Hg (hypercapnia).
    a. 50 and 50
    b. 60 and 60
    c. 75 and 75
    d. 80 and 80

15. The pathophysiology of ARF is directly related to:
    a. decreased respiratory drive.
    b. chest wall abnormalities.
    c. dysfunction of lung parenchyma.
    d. all of the above mechanisms.

16. Neuromuscular blockers are given to patients who are on ventilators in ARF to accomplish all of the following *except*:
    a. maintain positive end-expiratory pressure (PEEP).
    b. maintain better ventilation.
    c. increase the respiratory rate.
    d. keep the patient from fighting the ventilator.

17. A key characteristic feature of adult respiratory distress syndrome (ARDS) is:
    a. unresponsive arterial hypoxemia.
    b. diminished alveolar dilation.
    c. tachypnea.
    d. increased PaO_2.

18. A 154-lb, 60-year-old woman is being treated for ARDS. The nurse knows that the minimum daily caloric requirement to meet normal requirements is:
    a. 1,200 to 1,800 calories.
    b. 1,800 to 2,200 calories.
    c. 2,000 to 2,400 calories.
    d. 2,500 to 3,000 calories.

19. A nurse knows to assess a patient with pulmonary arterial hypertension for the primary symptom of:
    a. ascites.
    b. dyspnea.
    c. hypertension.
    d. syncope.

20. Clinical manifestations directly related to cor pulmonale include all of the following *except*:
    a. dyspnea and cough.
    b. diminished peripheral pulses.
    c. distended neck veins.
    d. edema of the feet and legs.

21. The nurse assesses a patient for a possible pulmonary embolism. The nurse looks for the most frequent sign of:
    a. cough.
    b. hemoptysis.
    c. syncope.
    d. tachypnea.

22. Anticoagulant therapy with heparin is administered in an attempt to maintain the International Normalized Ratio (INR) in a therapeutic range of:
    a. 0.5 to 1.0.
    b. 1.5 to 2.5.
    c. 2.0 to 2.5.
    d. 3.0 to 3.5.

23. Nursing measures to assist in the prevention of pulmonary embolism in a hospitalized patient include all of the following *except*:
    a. a liberal fluid intake.
    b. assisting the patient to do leg elevations above the level of the heart.
    c. encouraging the patient to dangle his or her legs over the side of the bed for 30 minutes, four times a day.
    d. the use of elastic stockings, especially when decreased mobility would promote venous stasis.

24. To assess for a positive Homans' sign, the nurse should:
    a. dorsiflex the foot while the leg is elevated to check for calf pain.
    b. elevate the patient's legs for 20 minutes and then lower them slowly while checking for areas of inadequate blood return.
    c. extend the leg, plantar flex the foot, and check for the patency of the dorsalis pedis pulse.
    d. lower the patient's legs and massage the calf muscles to note any areas of tenderness.

25. As a cause of death among men and women in the United States, lung cancer ranks:
    a. first.
    b. second.
    c. third.
    d. fourth.

26. More than 80% of all lung cancers are primarily caused by:
    a. cigarette smoking.
    b. fibrosis.
    c. inhalation of environmental carcinogens.
    d. tuberculosis.

27. The most prevalent lung carcinoma that is peripherally located and frequently metastasizes is:
    a. adenocarcinoma.
    b. bronchioalveolar.
    c. large cell.
    d. squamous cell.

28. The most frequent symptom of lung cancer is:
    a. copious sputum production.
    b. coughing.
    c. dyspnea.
    d. severe pain.

29. The nurse is aware that the most common surgical procedure for a small, apparently curable tumor of the lung is a:
    a. lobectomy.
    b. pneumonectomy.
    c. segmentectomy.
    d. wedge resection.

30. Paradoxical chest movement is associated with which chest disorder?
    a. Pneumothorax
    b. Flail chest
    c. ARDS
    d. Tension pneumothorax

31. An initial characteristic symptom of a simple pneumothorax is:
    a. ARDS.
    b. severe respiratory distress.
    c. sudden onset of chest pain.
    d. tachypnea and hypoxemia.

SHORT ANSWER

Read each statement carefully. Write your response in the space provided.

1. Atelectasis, which refers to closure or collapse of alveoli, may be chronic or acute in nature. List 10 possible causes of atelectasis in the postoperative patient.

2. Name seven possible clinical manifestations of atelectasis.

3. Identify eight nursing measures that can be used to prevent atelectasis.

4. The diagnosis of hospital-acquired pneumonia is usually associated with the presence of one of three conditions: _____, _____, and _____.

5. Name three common pathogens that cause aspiration pneumonia: _____, _____, and _____.

6. Pneumonia tends to occur in patients with one or more of these five underlying disorders:

   _____, _____, _____,

   _____, and _____.

7. Three severe complications of pneumonia are: _____, _____,

   and _____.

8. Explain the meaning of the term *superinfection*.

   _____

9. List four respiratory system mechanisms that can lead to acute respiratory failure (ARF):

   _____, _____, _____, and

   _____.

10. The mortality rate with ARDS is as high as _____%. The major cause of death is usually

    _____.

11. A characteristic and diagnostic feature of ARDS is: _____.

12. Define the etiology of cor pulmonale. _____.

13. The 5-year survival rate for lung cancer is: _____%.

II. Critical Thinking Questions and Exercises

DISCUSSION AND ANALYSIS

Discuss the following topics with your classmates.

1. Explain the pathophysiology of atelectasis.
2. Discuss a variety of risk factors and associated preventive measures for pneumonia, e.g., immunosuppression, age, smoking, sedation.
3. Describe the clinical picture of a patient who has developed an aspiration pneumonia.
4. Describe the etiology and clinical characteristics of severe acute respiratory syndrome (SARS).
5. Explain the medical and nursing management for a patient with an empyema.
6. In simple terms, explain the pathophysiology of pulmonary edema.
7. Discuss at least six etiologic factors and nursing assessments for patients with ARDS.
8. Discuss the risk factors and nursing assessments for patients with a pulmonary embolism.
9. Distinguish between the pathophysiology and clinical manifestations of sarcoidosis and pneumoconiosis.
10. Compare and contrast the etiology, clinical manifestations, and medical and nursing management for three types of pneumothorax: simple, traumatic, and tension.

INTERPRETING PATTERNS

Fill out the following flow charts according to the directions.

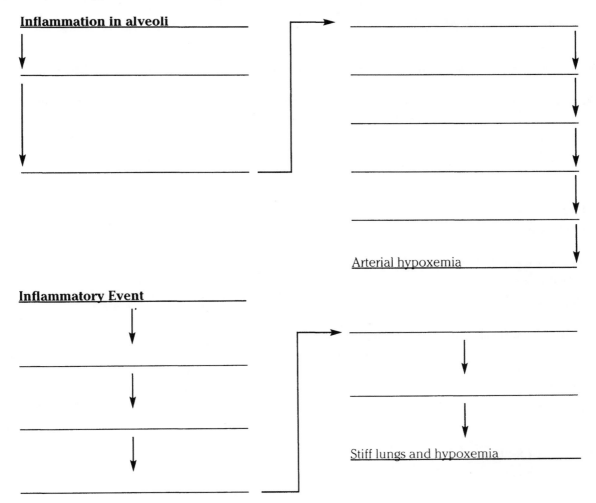

APPLYING CONCEPTS

Examine Figure 23-2 in the text and answer the following two questions.

1. Look at the right lobes of the lung and explain how the figure illustrates lobar pneumonia.

2. Look at the left lobes and explain how the figure illustrates bronchopneumonia.

CLINICAL SITUATIONS

Read the following case studies. Circle the correct answer.

CASE STUDY: Community-Acquired Pneumonia

Theresa, a 20-year-old college student, lives in a small dormitory with 30 other students. Four weeks into the spring semester, she was diagnosed as having bacterial pneumonia and was admitted to the hospital.

1. The nurse is informed that Theresa has the strain of bacteria most frequently found in community-acquired pneumonia. The nurse suspects that the infecting agent is:
   a. *Haemophilus influenza.*
   b. *Klebsiella.*
   c. *Pseudomonas aeruginosa.*
   d. *Streptococcus pneumoniae.*

2. All of the following are manifestations of bacterial pneumonia *except*:
   a. fever.
   b. bradycardia.
   c. stabbing or pleuritic chest pain.
   d. tachypnea.

3. The nurse expects that Theresa will be medicated with the usual antibiotic of choice, which is:
   a. cephalosporin.
   b. clindamycin.
   c. erythromycin.
   d. penicillin G.

4. The nurse is aware that Theresa may develop arterial hypoxemia, because:
   a. bronchospasm causes alveolar collapse, which decreases the surface area necessary for perfusion.
   b. mucosal edema occludes the alveoli, thereby producing a drop in alveolar oxygen.
   c. venous blood is shunted from the right to the left side of the heart.
   d. all of the above are true.

5. Theresa is expected to respond to antibiotic therapy:
   a. within 6 hours.
   b. between 1 and 2 days.
   c. by the fourth day.
   d. after 7 days.

6. Nursing management includes assessment for complications such as:
   a. atelectasis.
   b. hypotension and shock.
   c. pleural effusion.
   d. all of the above.

CASE STUDY: Tuberculosis

Mr. Carrera, a 67-year-old retired baker and pastry chef, is admitted to the clinical area for confirmation of suspected tuberculosis. He is anorexic and fatigued and suffers from "indigestion." His temperature is slightly elevated every afternoon.

1. Mr. Carrera's Mantoux tuberculin test yields an induration area of 6 to 10 mm. This result is interpreted as indicating that:
   a. active disease is present.
   b. he has been exposed to *M. tuberculosis* or has been vaccinated with BCG.
   c. preventive treatment should be initiated.
   d. the reaction is doubtful and should be repeated.

2. After Mr. Carrera has undergone a series of additional tests, the diagnosis is confirmed by:

a. a chest radiograph.

b. the ELISA test.

c. a positive multiple-puncture skin test.

d. repeated Mantoux tests that yield indurations of 10 mm or greater.

3. Mr. Carrera is started on a multiple-drug regimen. Nursing management includes observing for hepatotoxicity when which drug is used?

a. Ethambutol

b. Isoniazid

c. Rifampin

d. Pyrazinamide

4. Mr. Carrera needs to know that the initial intensive treatment is usually given daily for:

a. 2 weeks.

b. 2 to 4 weeks.

c. 2 months.

d. 4 to 6 months.

5. Mr. Carrera is informed that he will no longer be considered infectious after:

a. repeat Mantoux test results are negative.

b. serial chest radiographs show improvement.

c. two consecutive sputum specimens are negative.

d. all of the above parameters are met.

CASE STUDY: Acute Respiratory Distress Syndrome

Anne, 71 years of age and single, is admitted to the unit with a diagnosis of ARDS. She was receiving treatment at home for viral pneumonia and had appeared to be improving until yesterday.

1. During assessment, the nurse notes symptoms positively correlated with ARDS, including:

a. dysrhythmias and hypotension.

b. contraction of the accessory muscles of respiration.

c. tachypnea and tachycardia.

d. all of the above.

2. The nurse also observes symptoms of cerebral hypoxia, including:

a. drowsiness.

b. confusion.

c. irritability.

d. all of the above.

3. The nurse observes that Anne is receiving oxygen by way of a nasal cannula at 6 L/min. The nurse knows that Anne's FiO_2 is:

a. 24%.

b. 34%.

c. 44%.

d. 54%.

4. Indications for ventilator support for ARDS include all of the following *except*:

a. O_2 saturation greater than 90%.

b. PaO_2 greater than 60%.

c. respiratory rate greater than 35 breaths/min.

d. vital capacity equal to 60 mL/kg of body weight.

5. It is decided that Anne needs a ventilator to help her breathe. Her physician prescribes PEEP. When PEEP is used, all of the following occur *except*:

a. improved arterial oxygenation.

b. improved ventilation–perfusion.

c. increased alveolar dilation.

d. increased functional residual capacity.

CASE STUDY: Pulmonary Embolism

Sandy, a 37-year-old woman recovering from multiple fractures sustained in a car accident, was admitted to the intensive care unit for treatment of a pulmonary embolism. Before admission, she was short of breath after walking up a flight of stairs.

1. On the basis of Sandy's medical history, the nurse suspects that a predisposing condition may have been:
   a. hypercoagulability.
   b. postoperative immobility.
   c. venous stasis.
   d. all of the above factors.

2. As part of her assessment information, the nurse knows that the majority of pulmonary emboli originate in the:
   a. deep leg veins.
   b. lung tissue.
   c. pelvic area.
   d. right atrium of the heart.

3. The most common symptom of pulmonary embolism is:
   a. chest pain.
   b. dyspnea.
   c. fever.
   d. hemoptysis.

4. The nurse knows that treatment must be immediate since death from a pulmonary embolism can occur:
   a. within 1 hour.
   b. within 24 hours.
   c. in the first 48 hours.
   d. in 3 to 5 days.

5. On the basis of Sandy's diagnosis, the nurse knows to look for a decrease in:
   a. alveolar dead space.
   b. cardiac output.
   c. pulmonary arterial pressure.
   d. right ventricular work load of the heart.

6. A primary nursing problem for Sandy would be:
   a. atelectasis.
   b. bradycardia.
   c. dyspnea.
   d. hypertension.

7. The nurse knows that Sandy's diagnosis was probably confirmed by:
   a. a bronchogram.
   b. a chest roentgenogram.
   c. an electrocardiogram.
   d. a lung scan.

CHAPTER 24

Management of Patients With Chronic Pulmonary Disease

I. Interpretation, Completion, and Comparison

MULTIPLE CHOICE

Read each question carefully. Circle your answer.

1. As a cause of death in the United States, chronic obstructive pulmonary disease (COPD) ranks:
   - a. second.
   - b. third.
   - c. fourth.
   - d. fifth.

2. The new definition of COPD leaves only one disorder under its classification. That is:
   - a. asthma.
   - b. bronchiectasis.
   - c. cystic fibrosis.
   - d. emphysema.

3. The underlying pathophysiology of COPD is:
   - a. inflamed airways that obstruct airflow.
   - b. mucus secretions that block airways.
   - c. overinflated alveoli that impair gas exchange.
   - d. characterized by variations of all of the above.

4. The abnormal inflammatory response in the lungs occurs primarily in the:
   - a. airways.
   - b. parenchyma.
   - c. pulmonary vasculature.
   - d. areas identified in all of the above.

5. Two diseases common to the etiology of COPD are:
   - a. asthma and atelectasis.
   - b. chronic bronchitis and emphysema.
   - c. pneumonia and pleurisy.
   - d. tuberculosis and pleural effusions.

6. For a patient with chronic bronchitis, the nurse expects to see the major clinical symptoms of:
   - a. chest pain during respiration.
   - b. sputum and a productive cough.
   - c. fever, chills, and diaphoresis.
   - d. tachypnea and tachycardia.

7. The most important environmental risk factor for emphysema is:
   - a. air pollution.
   - b. allergens.
   - c. infectious agents.
   - d. cigarette smoking.

8. The pathophysiology of emphysema is directly related to airway obstruction. The end result of deterioration is:
   - a. diminished alveolar surface area.
   - b. hypercapnia resulting from decreased carbon dioxide elimination.
   - c. hypoxemia secondary to impaired oxygen diffusion.
   - d. respiratory acidosis due to airway obstruction.

9. The primary presenting symptom of emphysema is:

   a. chronic cough.

   b. dyspnea.

   c. tachypnea.

   d. wheezing.

10. A nurse notes that the FEV_1/FVC ratio is less than 70% for a patient with COPD. The nurse documents that the patient is in stage:

   a. 0.

   b. I.

   c. II.

   d. III.

11. Nursing assessment of a patient with bronchospasm associated with COPD would include assessment for:

   a. compromised gas exchange.

   b. decreased airflow.

   c. wheezes.

   d. all of the above.

12. A commonly prescribed methylxanthine used as a bronchodilator is:

   a. albuteral.

   b. levalbuteral.

   c. theophylline.

   d. terbutaline.

13. The physician orders a beta-2 adrenergic agonist agent (bronchodilator) that is short-acting and administered only by inhaler. The nurse knows this would probably be:

   a. Alupent.

   b. Brethine.

   c. Foradil.

   d. Isuprel.

14. The nurse should be alert for a complication of bronchiectasis that results from a combination of retained secretions and obstruction that leads to the collapse of alveoli. This complication is known as:

   a. atelectasis.

   b. emphysema.

   c. pleurisy.

   d. pneumonia.

15. Histamine, a mediator that supports the inflammatory process in asthma, is secreted by:

   a. eosinophils.

   b. lymphocytes.

   c. mast cells.

   d. neutrophils.

16. Obstruction of the airway in the patient with asthma is caused by all of the following *except*:

   a. thick mucus.

   b. swelling of bronchial membranes.

   c. destruction of the alveolar wall.

   d. contraction of muscles surrounding the bronchi.

17. A commonly prescribed mast cell stabilizer used for asthma is:

   a. albuterol.

   b. budesonide.

   c. cromolyn sodium.

   d. theophylline.

18. The nurse understands that a patient with status asthmaticus will likely initially evidence symptoms of:

   a. metabolic acidosis.

   b. metabolic alkalosis.

   c. respiratory acidosis.

   d. respiratory alkalosis.

SHORT ANSWER

Read each statement carefully. Write your response in the space provided.

1. Chronic airway inflammation in COPD results in: _____.

2. Define the term *emphysema.* _____.

3. A genetic risk factor for COPD is: _____.

4. The three *primary symptoms* associated with the progressive disease of COPD are:
   _____, _____, and _____.

5. List at least five of the nine major factors that determine the clinical course and survival of patients with
   COPD. _____, _____, _____, _____, and _____.

6. The *single most cost-effective* intervention to reduce the risk of developing COPD or slow its progression
   is: _____.

7. List the three ways that bronchodilators relieve bronchospasm: _____, _____,
   and _____.

8. Primary causes for an acute exacerbation of COPD are: _____ and
   _____.

9. To help prevent infections in patients with COPD, the nurse should recommend vaccination against two
   bacterial organisms: _____ and _____.

10. The strongest predisposing factor for asthma is: _____; the three most
    common symptoms are: _____, _____, and
    _____.

11. Complications of asthma may include: _____, _____,
    _____, and _____.

12. The median survival age for individuals diagnosed with cystic fibrosis is now _____ years.

II. Critical Thinking Questions and Exercises

DISCUSSION AND ANALYSIS

Discuss the following topics with your classmates.

1. Outline a health education teaching plan for a program at your local YMCA to present and explain the
   risk factors associated with COPD.
2. Compare and contrast the therapeutic issues and nursing teaching concerns for five aerosol delivery
   devices: metered-dose inhalers, breath-activated MDIs, dry powder inhalers, spacer or valved holding
   chambers, and nebulizers.
3. Explain how too much oxygen for COPD patients who have chronic hypercapnia can result in the
   retention of carbon dioxide.

4. Explain the pathophysiology of asthma.
5. Discuss the nursing considerations and teaching opportunities for asthma patients receiving beta-2 adrenergic agonists, anticholinergics, and corticosteroids.
6. Describe the clinical picture of a person during a status asthmaticus episode.

IDENTIFYING PATTERNS

Fill out the following flow charts according to the directions.

1. Chart the sequence of events that illustrate the pathophysiology of chronic bronchitis.

Smoke and environmental pollutants irritate the airways

_____

_____

Constant irritation

_____

_____

Bronchial wall thickening

_____

_____

Adjacent alveoli may become damaged and fibrosed

_____

_____

Respiratory infections (viral, bacterial, and mycoplasmal)

2. Chart the sequence of events that illustrate the pathophysiology of emphysema.

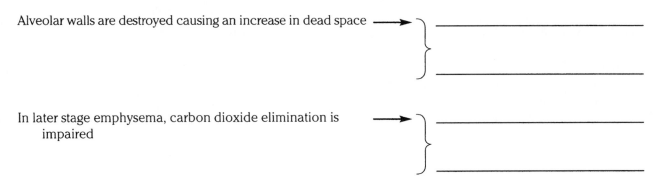

Alveolar walls are destroyed causing an increase in dead space ⟶

In later stage emphysema, carbon dioxide elimination is impaired ⟶

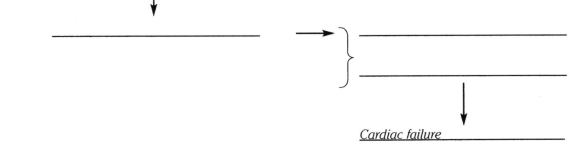

As the alveolar walls break down, the pulmonary capillary bed is reduced, causing increased pulmonary blood flow

Cardiac failure

CLINICAL SITUATIONS

Read the following case study. Circle the correct answers.

CASE STUDY: Emphysema

Lois, who has had emphysema for 25 years, is admitted to the hospital with a diagnosis of bronchitis.

1. During assessment, the nurse notes the presence of a "barrel chest," which the nurse knows is caused by:
   a. a compensatory expansion of the bronchial airway.
   b. a decrease in intrapleural pressure.
   c. "air trapping" in the lungs.
   d. a progressive increase in vital capacity.

2. The nurse recognizes the need to be alert for the major presenting symptom of emphysema, which is:
   a. bradypnea.
   b. dyspnea.
   c. expiratory wheezing.
   d. fatigue.

3. Arterial blood gas measurements that are consistent with a diagnosis of emphysema are:
   a. pH, 7.32; PaO_2, 70 mm Hg; $PaCO_2$, 50 mm Hg.
   b. pH, 7.37; PaO_2, 90 mm Hg; $PaCO_2$, 42 mm Hg.
   c. pH, 7.39; PaO_2, 80 mm Hg; $PaCO_2$, 35 mm Hg.
   d. pH, 7.40; PaO_2, 85 mm Hg; $PaCO_2$, 42 mm Hg.

4. Lois is being medicated with a bronchodilator to reduce airway obstruction. Nursing actions include observing for the side effect of:
   a. dysrhythmias.
   b. central nervous system excitement.
   c. tachycardia.
   d. all of the above.

5. Diaphragmatic breathing is recommended for Lois because it does all of the following *except*:
   a. decrease respiratory rate.
   b. decrease tidal volume.
   c. increase alveolar ventilation.
   d. reduce functional residual capacity.

6. Oxygen is prescribed for Lois. The nurse knows that the most effective delivery system is:
   a. a rebreathing bag that delivers oxygen at a concentration greater than 60%.
   b. an oxygen mask set a 8 L/min.
   c. a nasal cannula set at 6 L/min.
   d. a Venturi mask that delivers a predictable oxygen flow at about 24%.

CHAPTER 25

Respiratory Care Modalities

I. Interpretation, Completion, and Comparison

MULTIPLE CHOICE

Read each question carefully. Circle your answer.

1. The nurse knows that hypoxemia can be detected by noting a decrease in:
   a. PaO_2.
   b. P_AO_2.
   c. pH.
   d. PCO_2.

2. A patient with bradycardia and hypotension would most likely exhibit:
   a. anemic hypoxia.
   b. circulatory hypoxia.
   c. histotoxic hypoxia.
   d. hypoxic hypoxia.

3. Carbon monoxide poisoning results in:
   a. anemic hypoxia.
   b. histotoxic hypoxia.
   c. hypoxic hypoxia.
   d. stagnant hypoxia.

4. Decreased gas exchange at the cellular level resulting from a toxic substance is classified as:
   a. circulatory.
   b. histotoxic.
   c. hypoxemic.
   d. hypoxic.

5. Oxygen therapy administered to a pulmonary patient who retains carbon dioxide:
   a. can cause a dangerous rise in $PaCO_2$ levels.
   b. can suppress ventilation.
   c. should bring the patient's PO_2 level to 60 to 70 mm Hg.
   d. is able to accomplish all of the above mechanisms.

6. When oxygen therapy is being used, "No Smoking" signs are posted, because oxygen:
   a. is combustible.
   b. is explosive.
   c. prevents the dispersion of smoke particles.
   d. supports combustion.

7. A patient has been receiving 100% oxygen therapy by way of a nonrebreather mask for several days. He complains of tingling in his fingers and shortness of breath. He is extremely restless and states that he has pain beneath his breastbone. The nurse should suspect:
   a. oxygen-induced hypoventilation.
   b. oxygen toxicity.
   c. oxygen-induced atelectasis.
   d. all of the above.

8. Oxygen concentrations of 70% can usually be delivered with the use of:
   a. a nasal cannula.
   b. an oropharyngeal catheter.
   c. a partial rebreathing mask.
   d. a Venturi mask.

9. The method of oxygen administration primarily used for patients with chronic obstructive pulmonary disease (COPD) is:
   a. a nasal cannula.
   b. an oropharyngeal catheter.
   c. a nonrebreathing mask.
   d. a Venturi mask.

10. Intermittent positive-pressure breathing differs from incentive spirometry in all the following ways *except*:
   a. it is a mechanical aid to lung expansion.
   b. it is used to encourage hyperinflation.
   c. it produces a forced flow of air into the lungs during inhalation.
   d. it provides for the breathing of air or oxygen.

11. To help a patient use a mini-nebulizer, the nurse should encourage the patient to do all of the following *except*:
   a. hold his or her breath at the end of inspiration for a few seconds.
   b. cough frequently.
   c. take rapid, deep breaths.
   d. frequently evaluate his or her progress.

12. To assist a patient with the use of an incentive spirometer, the nurse should:
   a. make sure the patient is in a flat, supine position.
   b. tell the patient to try not to cough during and after each session, because doing so will cause pain.
   c. set an unrealistic goal so that the patient will try to maximize effort.
   d. encourage the patient to take approximately 10 breaths per hour, while awake.

13. Nursing actions associated with postural drainage include:
   a. encouraging the patient to cough after the procedure.
   b. auscultating the lungs before and after the procedure.
   c. encouraging the patient to exhale through pursed lips.
   d. all of the above.

14. When using percussion to aid in secretion removal, the nurse should avoid:
   a. the sternum and spine.
   b. the liver and kidneys.
   c. the spleen and female breast area.
   d. all of the above areas.

15. Percussion is accomplished by continuing the process for:
   a. 3 to 5 minutes while the patient uses diaphragmatic breathing.
   b. 10 to 15 minutes while the patient uses diaphragmatic breathing.
   c. 3 to 5 minutes while the patient breathes normally.
   d. 10 to 15 minutes while the patient breathes normally.

16. When vibrating the patient's chest, the nurse applies vibration:
   a. while the patient is inhaling.
   b. during both inhalation and exhalation.
   c. while the patient is exhaling.
   d. while the patient is holding his or her breath.

17. The purpose of pursed lips during exhalation is to:
   a. prolong exhalation.
   b. slow down the respiratory rate to allow for maximum lung expansion during inspiration.
   c. widen the airways.
   d. do all of the above.

18. Signs of an upper airway obstruction include:
    a. drawing in of the upper chest, sternum, and intercostal spaces.
    b. prolonged contraction of the abdominal muscles.
    c. tracheal tug.
    d. all of the above.

19. The suggested sequence of nursing actions for management of an upper airway obstruction is:
    a. clear airway, hyperextend head, lift jaw, use cross-finger technique, and perform a Heimlich maneuver.
    b. hyperextend neck, lift jaw, clear airway using cross-finger technique, and perform a Heimlich maneuver.
    c. hyperextend head, clear airway, lift jaw, and insert airway.
    d. lift jaw, clear airway, and perform a Heimlich maneuver.

20. Nursing management of a patient with an endotracheal tube includes:
    a. ensuring oxygen administration with high humidity.
    b. repositioning the patient every 2 hours.
    c. suctioning the oropharynx as needed.
    d. all of the above.

21. When suctioning secretions from a tracheostomy tube, it is helpful to first instill:
    a. less than 1 mL of sterile normal saline solution.
    b. 1 to 2 mL of sterile normal saline solution.
    c. 3 to 5 mL of sterile normal saline solution.
    d. 6 to 8 mL of sterile normal saline solution.

22. When suctioning a tracheostomy tube, the nurse needs to remember that each aspiration should not exceed:
    a. 15 seconds.
    b. 30 seconds.
    c. 45 seconds.
    d. 60 seconds.

23. Choose the blood gas sequence that indicates a need for mechanical ventilation.
    a. Decreasing PO_2, decreasing PCO_2, normal pH.
    b. Increasing PO_2, decreasing PCO_2, increasing pH.
    c. Decreasing PO_2, increasing PCO_2, decreasing pH.
    d. Increasing PO_2, decreasing PCO_2, decreasing pH.

24. The most commonly used positive-pressure ventilator currently is the:
    a. chest cuirass.
    b. time-cycled ventilator.
    c. pressure-cycled ventilator.
    d. volume-cycled ventilator.

25. With positive-pressure ventilation, positive intrathoracic pressure:
    a. increases venous return and decreases cardiac output.
    b. decreases venous return and increases cardiac output.
    c. decreases venous return and decreases cardiac output.
    d. increases venous return and increases cardiac output.

26. The sigh mechanism on an assist-control ventilator needs to be adjusted to provide _____ sigh(s) per hour at a rate that is _____ times the tidal volume.
    a. 1 and 1
    b. 1 to 2 and 2
    c. 1 to 3 and 1.5
    d. 3 to 6 and 3.5

27. The term used to describe thoracic surgery in which an entire lung is removed is:
    a. lobectomy.
    c. segmentectomy.
    b. pneumonectomy.
    d. wedge resection.

28. Preoperatively, the patient who is scheduled for thoracic surgery needs to know that postoperatively:
    a. chest tubes and drainage bottles may be necessary.
    c. oxygen will be administered to facilitate breathing if the need arises.
    b. he or she will be turned frequently and will be asked to cough and breathe deeply.
    d. all of the above treatments will be incorporated into a plan of care.

29. The water seal used in a disposable chest drainage system is effective if the water seal chamber is filled to the level of:
    a. 0.5 cm H_2O.
    c. 1.5 cm H_2O.
    b. 1.0 cm H_2O.
    d. 2.0 cm H_2O.

SHORT ANSWER

Read each statement carefully. Write your response in the space provided.

1. Oxygen transport to the tissues is dependent on four factors: _____, _____, _____, and _____.

2. Oxygen toxicity may occur when oxygen concentration at greater than _____% is administered for _____ (length of time).

3. List five signs and symptoms of oxygen toxicity: _____, _____, _____, _____, and _____.

4. For a patient with COPD, the stimulus for respiration is: _____.

5. Five examples of low-flow oxygen delivery systems are: _____, _____, _____, _____, and _____.

6. The oxygen flow rate for a nasal cannula should not exceed ____L/min.

7. List three goals of chest physiotherapy (CPT): _____, _____, and _____.

8. Cuff pressure for an endotracheal tube should be maintained at _____ mm Hg and be checked every _____ hours.

9. List three types of negative-pressure ventilators: _____, _____, and _____.

10. Explain how positive-pressure ventilators work.

_____

11. Explain what is meant when the patient is said to be "bucking the ventilator."

_____

12. List four nursing diagnoses for a patient receiving mechanical ventilation: _____,

_____, _____, and _____.

13. For a patient to be safely weaned from a ventilator, the vital capacity should be _____mL/kg; the minute ventilation should be _____L/m; and the tidal volume should be _____mL/kg.

14. List seven postoperative risk factors for atelectasis and pneumonia.

_____   _____

_____   _____

_____   _____

_____

COMPLETE THE CHART

Look at the following figure of a disposable chest drainage system, and label the figure using the terms provided.

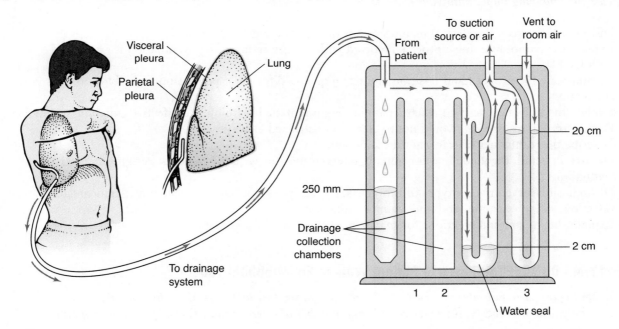

Suction control
Water seal
Vent
Drainage collection chambers
Suction source
Ventilation source

II. Critical Thinking Questions and Exercises

EXAMINING ASSOCIATIONS

Read each analogy. Write the best response in the space provided.

1. Hypoxia: decreased oxygen supply to the tissues :: Hypoxemia : _____.

2. Arterial oxygen pressure (PaO_2) : 60 to 95 mm Hg :: Oxygen saturation : _____%.

3. Partial rebreather mask : a flow rate of 8 to 11 L/min and 50% to 75% oxygen concentration :: Nonrebreather mask : a flow rate of _____ and a _____% oxygen concentration.

4. Anemic hypoxia : decreased effective hemoglobin concentration :: Circulatory hypoxia:

   _____.

5. Ventilator tidal volume : 6 to 12 mL/kg (IBW) :: Ventilator rate : _____.

DISCUSSION AND ANALYSIS

Discuss the following topics with your classmates.

1. Distinguish between the clinical manifestations of *hypoxia* and *hypoxemia*.
2. Explain the pathophysiologic process involved with oxygen-induced hypoventilation for a patient with COPD.
3. Demonstrate the proper hand position and technique used for chest percussion and vibration on a classmate.
4. Explain the steps necessary to teach a patient diaphragmatic breathing and effective coughing techniques.
5. Demonstrate the steps you would use to clear an obstructed airway.
6. Describe the techniques of tracheal tube suctioning.
7. Discuss, in detail, the guidelines for nursing interventions for weaning patients from mechanical ventilation.
8. Distinguish between the six types of thoracic surgeries: pneumonectomy, lobectomy, segmentectomy, wedge resection, sleeve resection, and lung volume reduction.
9. Explain the nursing interventions for managing a chest drainage system.

APPLYING CONCEPTS: Care of a Patient With an Endotracheal Tube

Examine Figure 25-6 and refer to Charts 25-7 and 25-8 in the text to answer the following questions. Immediately after intubation, the nurse completes a number of interventions. Consider each activity and explain the nursing role.

1. Check symmetry of chest expansion. To do this, the nurse would do four things: _____,

   _____, _____, and _____ to verify tube placement every 8 hours.

2. To ensure high humidity, the nurse would:

   _____.

3. Describe how the tube would be secured to prevent displacement.

   _____.

4. To prevent the patient from biting the tube, the nurse would:

   _____.

5. The patient would be repositioned every 2 hours for the purpose of:

   _____.

6. Describe the suctioning technique.

   _____.

7. List at least 5 of 10 interventions that a nurse would do to prevent complications:

   _____, _____, _____,

   _____, and _____.

CLINICAL SITUATIONS

Read the following case studies. Circle the correct answer.

CASE STUDY: Pneumonectomy: Preoperative Concerns

Mrs. Miley, a 66-year-old widow, is admitted to the clinical area as a preoperative patient scheduled for a pneumonectomy for lung cancer.

1. Nursing assessment during the admission history and physical examination includes obtaining data about the patient's:
   a. breathing patterns during exertion.
   b. cardiac status during exercise.
   c. smoking history.
   d. history relevant to all of the above.

2. The nurse knows that medical clearance for surgery is based primarily on evaluation of the:
   a. cardiopulmonary system.
   b. endocrine system.
   c. neurologic system.
   d. renal—urinary system.

3. A battery of preoperative tests are ordered. The nurse evaluates the serum creatinine level because it reflects:
   a. cardiac status.
   b. endocrine status.
   c. pulmonary function.
   d. renal function.

4. The nurse knows that Mrs. Miley's functional lung capacity can be assessed by evaluating:
   a. arterial blood gases.
   b. blood urea nitrogen levels.
   c. chest x-rays.
   d. serum protein levels.

CASE STUDY: Pneumonectomy: Postoperative Concerns

Mrs. Miley is returned to the clinical area after being in the intensive care unit. She is recovering from a right pneumonectomy.

1. The major postoperative nursing objective is to:
   a. maintain a patent airway.
   b. provide for maximum remaining lung expansion.
   c. provide rehabilitative measures.
   d. recognize early indicators of complications.

2. Mrs. Miley had a central venous pressure line in place. Readings are to be taken to detect:
   a. hypothermia.
   b. hypovolemia.
   c. hypoxemia.
   d. hypoxia.

3. Pulmonary edema is a potential danger owing to the possible rapid infusion of intravenous fluids and a reduced vascular bed. Early symptoms of pulmonary edema include:
   a. dyspnea.
   b. frothy sputum.
   c. crackles (rales).
   d. all of the above.

4. The nurse should always be alert for signs of impending respiratory insufficiency, which would include all of the following *except*:
   a. bradycardia.
   b. dyspnea.
   c. hypertension.
   d. tachypnea.

CASE STUDY: Ventilator Patient

Mr. Brown, a 25-year-old man with a drug overdose, has been maintained on a volume-cycled ventilator for 3 weeks.

1. A major nursing assessment for Mr. Brown would be:
   a. breath sounds.
   b. nutritional needs.
   c. psychological status.
   d. spontaneous ventilatory efforts.

2. Positive-pressure ventilation can alter cardiac function. The nurse assesses for indicators of hypoxia and hypoxemia, which would include all of the following *except*:
   a. bradycardia and bradypnea.
   b. diaphoresis and oliguria.
   c. restlessness and confusion.
   d. transient hypertension.

3. A primary nursing intervention for Mr. Brown is maintaining optimal gas exchange. This can be accomplished by:
   a. conservative use of analgesics so that pain is relieved, yet the respiratory drive is not decreased.
   b. daily monitoring of fluid balance to prevent fluid overload.
   c. frequent repositioning to diminish the pulmonary effects of immobility.
   d. all of the above measures.

4. The nurse wants to determine early whether Mr. Brown is "bucking" his ventilator (breathing out during the ventilator's mechanical inspiratory phase) so that he can initiate preventive measures if necessary. The nurse should assess for signs and symptoms related to:
   a. hypercarbia.
   b. hypoxia.
   c. inadequate minute volume.
   d. all of the above.

CASE STUDY: Weaning from Ventilator

Mr. O'Day, a 71-year-old trauma victim, is to be weaned from his ventilator.

1. Before weaning, Mr. O'Day's ventilatory capacity should be such that he:
   a. can maintain an inspiratory force of at least 20 cm H_2O pressure.
   b. has a PaO_2 greater than 60% and an FiO_2 lower than 40%.
   c. is able to generate a minimum vital capacity of 10 to 15 mL/kg of body weight.
   d. is capable of all of the above.

2. Criteria to determine whether Mr. O'Day's endotracheal tube can be removed include:
   a. active pharyngeal and laryngeal gag reflexes.
   b. adequate spontaneous ventilation.
   c. voluntary cough mechanisms.
   d. all of the above.

3. Mr. O'Day will be weaned from oxygen when he can breathe room air and maintain a PaO_2 in the range of:
   a. 40 to 50 mm Hg.
   b. 50 to 60 mm Hg.
   c. 60 to 70 mm Hg.
   d. 70 to 100 mm Hg.

CHAPTER 26

Assessment of Cardiovascular Function

I. Interpretation, Completion, and Comparison

MULTIPLE CHOICE

Read each question carefully. Circle your answer.

1. The nurse who is caring for a patient with pericarditis understands that there is inflammation involving the:
   - a. thin fibrous sac encasing the heart.
   - b. inner lining of the heart and valves.
   - c. heart's muscle fibers.
   - d. exterior layer of the heart.

2. The coronary arteries arise from the:
   - a. aorta near the origin of the left ventricle.
   - b. pulmonary artery at the apex of the right ventricle.
   - c. pulmonary vein near the left atrium.
   - d. superior vena cava at the origin of the right atrium.

3. The pacemaker for the entire myocardium is the:
   - a. atrioventricular junction.
   - b. bundle of His.
   - c. Purkinje fibers.
   - d. sinoatrial node.

4. The intrinsic pacemaker rate of ventricular myocardial cells is:
   - a. more than 80 bpm.
   - b. 60 to 80 bpm.
   - c. 40 to 60 bpm.
   - d. fewer than 40 bpm.

5. An example of a beta-blocker that is administered to decrease automaticity is:
   - a. Cardizem.
   - b. Cordarone.
   - c. Lopressor.
   - d. Rythmol.

6. So that blood may flow from the right ventricle to the pulmonary artery, which of the following conditions is *not required*?
   - a. The atrioventricular valves must be closed.
   - b. The pulmonic valve must be open.
   - c. Right ventricular pressure must be less than pulmonary arterial pressure.
   - d. Right ventricular pressure must rise with systole.

7. Heart rate is stimulated by all of the following *except*:
   - a. excess thyroid hormone.
   - b. increased levels of circulating catecholamines.
   - c. the sympathetic nervous system.
   - d. the vagus nerve.

8. Stroke volume of the heart is determined by:

   a. the degree of cardiac muscle strength (precontraction).

   b. the intrinsic contractility of the cardiac muscle.

   c. the pressure gradient against which the muscle ejects blood during contraction.

   d. all of the above factors.

9. Changes in cardiac structure associated with aging would include all of the following *except*:

   a. elongation of the aorta.

   b. endocardial fibrosis.

   c. increased sensitivity to baroreceptors.

   d. the increased size of the left atrium.

10. A nonmodifiable risk factor for atherosclerosis is:

    a. stress.

    b. obesity.

    c. positive family history.

    d. hyperlipidemia.

11. The difference between the systolic and the diastolic pressure is called the:

    a. pulse pressure.

    b. auscultatory gap.

    c. pulse deficit.

    d. Korotkoff sound.

12. The nurse assessing a patient for postural hypotension recognizes that the following is a positive sign:

    a. a heart rate of 5 to 20 bpm above the resting rate.

    b. an unchanged systolic pressure.

    c. an increase of 10 mm Hg reading.

    d. an increase of 5 mm Hg in diastolic pressure.

13. If the sphygmomanometer cuff is too small for the patient, the blood pressure reading will probably be:

    a. falsely elevated.

    b. falsely decreased.

    c. an accurate reading.

    d. significantly different with each reading.

14. The first heart sound is generated by:

    a. closure of the aortic valve.

    b. closure of the atrioventricular valves.

    c. opening of the atrioventricular valves.

    d. opening of the pulmonic valve.

15. Exercise stress testing is a noninvasive procedure that can be used to assess certain aspects of cardiac function. After the test, the patient is instructed to:

    a. rest for a time.

    b. avoid stimulants.

    c. avoid extreme temperature changes.

    d. do all of the above.

16. Postcatheterization nursing measures for a patient who has had a cardiac catheterization include:

    a. assessing the peripheral pulses in the affected extremity.

    b. checking the insertion site for hematoma formation.

    c. evaluating temperature and color in the affected extremity.

    d. all of the above.

SHORT ANSWER

Read each statement carefully. Write your response in the space provided.

1. List the five categories of cardiovascular disease (CVD): _____HTN_____,

   _____CAD_____, _____HF_____,

   _____Stroke_____, and _____congenital cardio vascular defects_____

2. Distinguish between the functions of the atrioventricular and the semilunar valves.

   _____

3. Briefly explain depolarization as it relates to cardiac physiology.

   _____

4. List the three factors that determine stroke volume: _preload_ , _afterload_ and _contractility_

5. Estimate the cardiac output, per beat, for an adult heart rate of 76 bpm with an average stroke volume of 70 mL per beat.

   _76 X 70 = 5320mL_ _5.32L_

6. Describe Starling's law of the heart.

   _____

7. List four physiologic effects on the cardiovascular system that are associated with the aging process: _↓ size Ht vent._ , _↓ elasticity & widening_, _thick cardiac valves_ , and _↑CT in SA & AV nodes & bundle branches of aorta_

8. List three major cardiovascular risk factors: _hyperlipidemia_ , _HTN_ , and _diabetes mellitus_ .

9. If coronary artery disease (CAD) is present, the American Heart Association (AHA) recommends the following laboratory measurements: low-density lipoprotein (LDL), _____; blood pressure (BP), _____; serum glucose concentration, _____; and a body mass index (BMI) of _____.

10. To assess the apical pulse, the nurse would find the following location:

    _____.

11. The two most specific enzymes traditionally used to analyze an acute myocardial infarction (MI) are _CK_ and _CK-MB_ ; two new biomarkers, _T + T_ and _myoglobin_ , are early indicators of a myocardial infarction (MI).

12. List several purposes of cardiac catheterization.
    √ pressures in chambers; check O₂ in blood & assess patency of pts coronary arteries & determine readiness for bypass surgery

13. Describe selective angiography. _contrast to outline ♡ & vessels._

    _____

14. Discuss the implications of a low central venous pressure reading.

    indicates pt. has hypovolemia

15. Identify four of seven possible complications of pulmonary artery monitoring: _____,

_____, _____, and _____.

MATCHING

Match the anatomic term in column II with its associated function in column I.

Column I

1. __C__ Separates the right and left atria

2. __e__ Is located at the juncture of the superior vena cava and the right atrium

3. __A__ Supports the heart in the mediastinum

4. __D__ Sits between the right ventricle and the pulmonary artery

5. __B__ Distributes venous blood to the lungs

6. __f__ Is embedded in the right atrial wall near the tricuspid valve

Column II

a. Parietal pericardium

b. Pulmonary artery

c. Bicuspid valve

d. Pulmonic valve

e. Sinatrial node

f. Atrioventricular node

Match the terminology associated with coronary atherosclerosis in column II with its function/characteristic listed in column I.

Column I

1. __D__ A principal blood lipid

2. __G__ A risk factor that causes pulmonary damage

3. __A__ The functional lesion of atherosclerosis

4. __F__ Biochemical substances, soluble in fat, that accumulate within a blood vessel

5. __I__ A risk factor that is endocrine in origin

6. __K__ A risk factor associated with a type A personality

7. __B__ A risk factor related to weight gain

8. __J__ A recommended dietary restriction that is a risk factor for heart disease

9. __C__ A symptom of myocardial ischemia

10. __H__ Myocardial manifestation of coronary artery disease

11. __e__ A lifestyle habit that is considered a modifiable risk factor for heart disease

Column II

a. Atheroma

b. Obesity

c. Chest pain

d. Cholesterol

e. Inactivity

f. Lipids

g. Smoking

h. Dysrhythmias

i. Diabetes

j. Fat

k. Stress

II. Critical Thinking Questions and Exercises

DISCUSSION AND ANALYSIS

Discuss the following topics with your classmates.

1. Describe the most common signs and symptoms of coronary vascular disease.
2. For each of the following structures, describe the age-related structural and functional changes in the cardiac system.
3. Compare and contrast the character, duration, aggravating factors, and precipitating events of cardiac and noncardiac chest pain.
4. Draft a detailed assessment guide that the nurse would use to evaluate various symptoms associated with chest pain, shortness of breath, palpitations, fatigue, and syncope.
5. Describe the classic "type A personality" and explain what is meant by "cardiac reactivity."
6. Describe the various characteristics of heart murmurs.
7. Describe the etiology and significance of "gallop sounds."
8. Discuss the value of telemetry to cardiac assessment.

EXAMINING ASSOCIATIONS

Read each analogy. Write the best response in the space provided.

1. The pulmonary artery : lungs :: Aorta: _____system_____.

2. Epicardium : outer layer of cells lining the heart :: _____myocardium_____ : the heart muscle itself.

3. Apical area of the heart : fifth intercostal space : Erb's point: _____3rd ?_____.

4. The first heart sound : closure of the mitral and tricuspid valves :: The second heart sound : closure of _____semilunar_____.

5. Murmurs : malfunctioning valves : Friction rubs: _____abrasion of pericardial surfaces_____

INTERPRETING DATA

Compare the following two figures found in Table 26-2 in the text, depicting the pain pathway of angina pectoris and pericarditis. Answer the associated questions.

Pericarditis

Angina Pectoris

Duration of pain: _____ _____

Precipitating events: _____ _____

And aggravating factors: _____ _____

_____ _____

_____ _____

_____ _____

Alleviating factors: _____ _____

_____ _____

_____ _____

CLINICAL SITUATIONS

Read the following case study. Circle the correct answer.

CASE STUDY: Cardiac Assessment for Chest Pain

Mr. Anderson is a 45-year-old executive with a major oil firm. Lately he has experienced frequent episodes of chest pressure that are relieved with rest. He has requested a complete physical examination. The nurse conducts an initial cardiac assessment.

1. The nurse immediately inspects the patient's skin. She observes a bluish tinge around the patient's lips. She knows that this is an indication of:

a. central cyanosis.

b. pallor.

c. peripheral cyanosis.

d. xanthelasma.

2. The nurse takes a baseline blood pressure measurement after the patient has rested for 10 minutes in a supine position. The reading that reflects a reduced pulse pressure is:
   a. 140/90 mm Hg.
   b. 140/100 mm Hg.
   c. 140/110 mm Hg.
   d. 140/120 mm Hg.

3. Five minutes after the initial blood pressure measurement is taken, the nurse assesses additional readings with the patient in a sitting and then in a standing position. The reading indicative of an abnormal postural response would be:
   a. lying, 140/110; sitting, 130/110; standing, 135/106 mm Hg.
   b. lying, 140/110; sitting, 135/112; standing, 130/115 mm Hg.
   c. lying, 140/110; sitting, 135/100; standing, 120/90 mm Hg.
   d. lying, 140/110; sitting, 130/108; standing, 125/108 mm Hg.

4. The nurse returns Mr. Anderson to the supine position and measures for jugular vein distention. The finding that would initially indicate an abnormal increase in the volume of the venous system would be obvious distention of the veins with the patient at what angle?
   a. 15 degrees
   b. 25 degrees
   c. 35 degrees
   d. 45 degrees

5. The nurse auscultates the apex of the heart by placing a stethoscope over:
   a. Erb's point.
   b. the fifth intercostal space.
   c. the pulmonic area.
   d. the tricuspid area.

CHAPTER 27

Management of Patients With Dysrhythmias and Conduction Problems

I. Interpretation, Completion, and Comparison

MULTIPLE CHOICE

Read each question carefully. Circle your answer.

1. The heart is under the control of the autonomic nervous system. Stimulation of the parasympathetic system results in all of the following *except*:
   a. slowed heart rate.
   b. lowered blood pressure.
   c. reduction in the force of contraction.
   d. positive inotropy.

2. The total time for ventricular depolarization and repolarization is represented on an electrocardiogram (ECG) reading as the:
   a. QRS complex.
   b. QT interval.
   c. ST segment.
   d. TP interval.

3. Ventricular rate and rhythm can be determined by examining what interval on an ECG strip?
   a. PP interval
   b. QT interval
   c. RR interval
   d. TP interval

4. The PR interval on an ECG strip that reflects normal sinus rhythm would be between:
   a. 0.05 and 0.10 seconds.
   b. 0.12 and 0.20 seconds.
   c. 0.15 and 0.30 seconds.
   d. 0.25 and 0.40 seconds.

5. Characteristics of sinus bradycardia include all of the following *except*:
   a. a P wave precedes every QRS complex.
   b. every QRS complex is normal.
   c. the rate is 40 to 60 bpm.
   d. the rhythm is altered.

6. A dysrhythmia common in normal hearts and described by patients as "my heart skipped a beat" is:
   a. premature atrial complex.
   b. atrial flutter.
   c. sinus tachycardia.
   d. ventricular fibrillation.

7. A "sawtooth" P wave is seen on an ECG strip with:
   a. sinus bradycardia.
   b. atrial flutter.
   c. atrioventricular nodal reentry.
   d. premature junctional complex.

8. Atrial fibrillation is associated with a heart rate up to:
   a. 300 bpm.
   b. 400 bpm.
   c. 500 bpm.
   d. 600 bpm.

9. Atrioventricular (AV) nodal reentry tachycardia is characterized by an atrial rate:
   a. of 100 bpm.
   b. between 100 and 150 bpm.
   c. between 150 and 250 bpm.
   d. more than 250 bpm.

10. *Ventricular bigeminy* refers to a conduction defect in which:
   a. conduction is primarily from the AV node.
   b. every other beat is premature.
   c. rhythm is regular but fast.
   d. the rate is between 150 and 250 bpm.

11. With ventricular tachycardia:
   a. conduction originates in the ventricle.
   b. electrical defibrillation is used immediately.
   c. the P wave usually is normal.
   d. the ventricular rate is twice the normal atrial rate.

12. Ventricular fibrillation is associated with an absence of:
   a. heartbeat.
   b. palpable pulse.
   c. respirations.
   d. all of the above.

13. First-degree AV block is characterized by:
   a. a variable heart rate, usually fewer than 60 bpm.
   b. an irregular rhythm.
   c. delayed conduction, producing a prolonged PR interval.
   d. P waves hidden with the QRS complex.

14. A conduction abnormality whereby no atrial impulse travels through the AV node is known as:
   a. first-degree AV block.
   b. second-degree AV block, type 1.
   c. second-degree AV block, type 2.
   d. third-degree AV block.

15. Cardioversion is used to terminate dysrhythmias. With cardioversion, the:
   a. amount of voltage used should exceed 400 W-s.
   b. electrical impulse can be discharged during the T wave.
   c. defibrillator should be set to deliver a shock during the QRS complex.
   d. above statements are all true.

16. When assessing vital signs in a patient with a permanent pacemaker, the nurse needs to know the:
   a. date and time of insertion.
   b. location of the generator.
   c. model number.
   d. pacer rate.

17. Candidates for implantable cardioverter defibrillation (ICD) are patients at high risk who have:
   a. experienced syncope secondary to ventricular tachycardia.
   b. survived sudden cardiac death.
   c. sustained ventricular tachycardia.
   d. experienced one or more of the above.

18. The nurse needs to teach the patient with an automatic ICD that he or she must:
   a. avoid magnetic fields such as metal detection booths.
   b. call for emergency assistance if he or she feels dizzy.
   c. record events that trigger a shock sensation.
   d. be compliant with all of the above.

SHORT ANSWER

Read each statement carefully. Write your response in the space provided.

1. Name the four sites of origin for impulses that are used to name dysrhythmias: _____,
   _____, _____, and _____.

2. Describe the normal electrical conduction through the heart.

   _____

   _____

3. Name five causes of sinus tachycardia: _____, _____, _____,
   _____, and _____.

4. Sinus tachycardia occurs when the ventricular and atrial rate are greater than _____.

5. List a rate and rhythm characteristic that is necessary to diagnose ventricular tachycardia:
   _____ and _____.

6. List three potential collaborative problems that a nurse would choose for a patient with dysrhythmias:
   _____, _____, and _____.

7. Name the one major difference between cardioversion and defibrillation.

   _____

   _____

8. For defibrillation, describe the placement of the electrode paddles on a patient's chest.

   _____

   _____

9. Describe the difference between on-demand and fixed or asynchronous pacemakers.

   _____

   _____

10. Describe the "Maze Procedure" used in cardiac conduction surgery.

   _____

   _____

SCRAMBLEGRAM

Unscramble the letters used to answer each statement, and write the word in the space provided.

1. A term used to describe an irregular or erratic heart rhythm: _____

S H R I C H M D T Y Y

2. The ability of the cardiac muscle to initiate an electrical impulse: _____

T A Y O I T A T I C M U

3. The ability of the cardiac muscle to transmit electrical impulses: _____

O U V T I C N Y I T D C

4. A term used to describe the electrical stimulation of the heart: _____

N O I P T R A D O L Z A E I

5. Stage of conduction in which the ventricles relax: _____

T S L D I A E O

6. Treatment of dysrhythmias by destroying causative cells: _____

N B A I A T L O

II. Critical Thinking Questions and Exercises

EXAMINING ASSOCIATIONS

Read each analogy and fill in the space provided with the best response.

1. The sinus node : right atrium :: Purkinje fibers : _____.

2. Depolarization : systole :: _____ : diastole.

3. The T wave : ventricular repolarization :: The _____ : repolarization of the Purkinje fibers.

4. Normal sinus rhythm : an atrial rate of 60 to 100 bpm :: _____ : an atrial rate less than 60 bpm.

5. Cardizem : atrial flutter :: _____ : atrial fibrillation.

6. First-degree AV block : P:QRS ratio of 1:1 :: Second-degree AV block : P:QRS ratio of

_____ or _____.

CLINICAL SITUATIONS

Graph Analysis

Analyze the following ECG graphs and answer the questions.

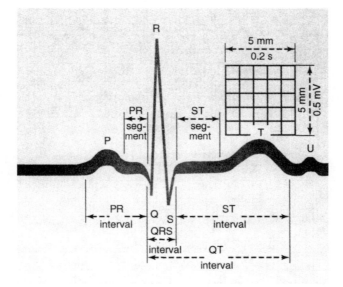

ECG graph and commonly measured complex components. Each small box represents 0.04 seconds on the horizontal axis and 1 mm or 0.1 mV on the vertical axis. The PR interval is measured from the beginning of the P wave to the beginning of the QRS complex; the QRS complex is measured from the beginning of the Q wave to the end of the S wave; the QT interval is measured from the beginning of the Q wave to the end of the T wave.

1. Look at the above graphic recording of cardiac electrical activity. For each action below, choose a wave deflection that corresponds to it, and write the appropriate letter or letters on the line provided.

   a. ____ ventricular muscle repolarization

   b. ____ time required for an impulse to travel through the atria and the conduction system to the Purkinje fibers

   c. ____ atrial muscle depolarization

   d. ____ ventricular muscle depolarization

   e. ____ early ventricular repolarization of the ventricles

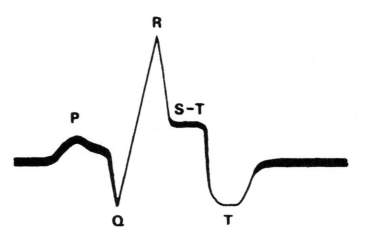

2. Consider the above graphic recording, and identify three alterations that are consistent with myocardial ischemia and infarction hours to days after the attack.

a. _____

b. _____

c. _____

GRAPHIC RECORDINGS

Analyze the graphic recording for each of the following dysrhythmias and describe the altered deflection.

1.

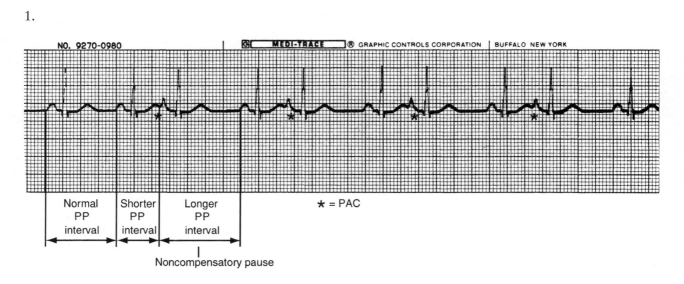

Premature atrial complexes (PACs)

_____

_____

_____

2.

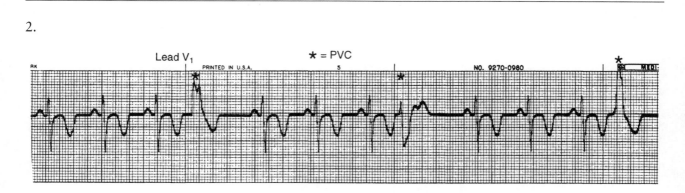

Multifocal PVCs in quadrigeminy

_____

_____

_____

3.

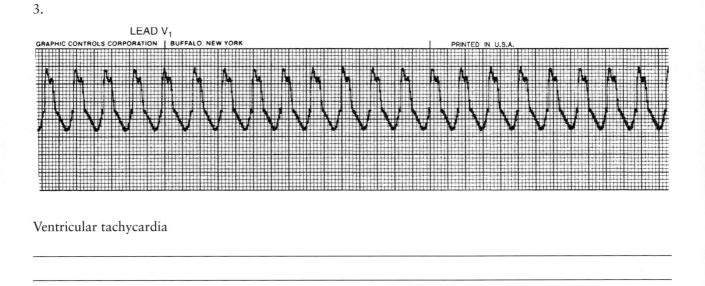

Ventricular tachycardia

_____

_____

_____ .

CLINICAL SITUATIONS

Read the following case studies. Answer the questions in the spaces provided.

CASE STUDY: Permanent Pacemaker

Mr. Woo is a 58-year-old Asian man who is scheduled for permanent pacemaker insertion as treatment for a tachydysrhythmia that does not respond to medication therapy. He is scheduled for an endocardial implant. Answer the following questions related to pacemaker management.

1. Mr. Woo's pacemaker is set at 72 bpm. His heart rate is 76 bpm. Is this expected? _____ (Yes/No). Explain the rationale for your answer. _____

2. Nursing care includes incision site assessment for three potential complications: _____,

   _____, and _____.

3. List four additional complications that Mr. Woo may experience: _____,

   _____, _____, and _____.

4. The most common initial postoperative complication is: _____.

5. List six things about the pacemaker that must be noted on a patient's chart:

   a. _____

   b. _____

   c. _____

   d. _____

   e. _____

   f. _____

6. Describe nursing interventions and expected patient outcomes that should be used to meet the three major goals of patient care:

GOALS

a. _____

b. _____

c. _____

NURSING INTERVENTIONS

a. _____

b. _____

c. _____

EXPECTED OUTCOMES

a. _____

b. _____

c. _____

7. List assessment criteria that should be used to determine whether each of the following expected outcomes of care has been achieved.

a. Freedom from infection _____

b. Adherence to a self-care program _____

c. Maintenance of pacemaker function _____

CHAPTER 28

Management of Patients With Coronary Vascular Disorders

I. Interpretation, Completion, and Comparison

MULTIPLE CHOICE

Read each question carefully. Circle your answer.

1. The most common heart disease for adults in the United States is:
   a. angina pectoris.
   b. coronary artery disease.
   c. myocardial infarction.
   d. valvular heart disease.

2. Lumen narrowing with atherosclerosis is caused by:
   a. atheroma formation on the intima.
   b. scarred endothelium.
   c. thrombus formation.
   d. all of the above.

3. A healthy level of serum cholesterol would be a reading of:
   a. 160 to 190 mg/dL.
   b. 210 to 240 mg/dL.
   c. 250 to 275 mg/dL.
   d. 280 to 300 mg/dL.

4. Which of the following findings is not a significant risk factor for heart disease?
   a. Cholesterol, 280 mg/dL
   b. LDL, 160 mg/dL
   c. High-density lipoproteins (HDL), 80 mg/dL
   d. A ratio of low-density lipoproteins (LDL) to HDL, 4.5 to 1.0

5. Hypertension is repeated blood pressure measurements exceeding:
   a. 110/80 mm Hg.
   b. 120/80 mm Hg.
   c. 130/90 mm Hg.
   d. 140/90 mm Hg.

6. The incidence of coronary artery disease tends to be equal for men and women after the age of:
   a. 45 years.
   b. 50 years.
   c. 55 years.
   d. 65 years.

7. The pain of angina pectoris is produced primarily by:
   a. coronary vasoconstriction.
   b. movement of thromboemboli.
   c. myocardial ischemia.
   d. the presence of atheromas.

8. The nurse advises a patient that sublingual nitroglycerin should alleviate angina pain within:
   a. 3 to 4 minutes.
   b. 10 to 15 minutes.
   c. 30 minutes.
   d. 60 minutes.

9. Patient education includes telling someone who takes nitroglycerin sublingually that he or she should take 1, then go quickly to the nearest emergency department if no relief has been obtained after taking _____ tablet(s) at 5-minute intervals.
   a. 1
   b. 2
   c. 3
   d. 4 to 5

10. The scientific rationale supporting the administration of beta-adrenergic blockers is the drugs' ability to:
    a. block sympathetic impulses to the heart.
    b. elevate blood pressure.
    c. increase myocardial contractility.
    d. induce bradycardia.

11. An antidote for propranolol hydrochloride (a beta-adrenergic blocker) that is used to treat bradycardia is:
    a. digoxin.
    b. atropine.
    c. protamine sulfate.
    d. sodium nitroprusside.

12. Calcium channel blockers act by:
    a. decreasing SA node automaticity.
    b. increasing AV node conduction.
    c. increasing the heart rate.
    d. creating a positive inotropic effect.

13. In the United States, about 1 million people will have an acute myocardial infarction each year. Of these 1 million, what percentage will die?
    a. 10% to 15%
    b. 25%
    c. 30% to 40%
    d. 60%

14. The classic ECG changes that occur with an MI include all of the following *except*:
    a. an absent P wave.
    b. an abnormal Q wave.
    c. T-wave inversion.
    d. ST-segment elevation.

15. The most common site of myocardial infarction is the:
    a. left atrium.
    b. left ventricle.
    c. right atrium.
    d. right ventricle.

16. Which of the following statements about myocardial infarction pain is *incorrect*?
    a. It is relieved by rest and inactivity.
    b. It is substernal in location.
    c. It is sudden in onset and prolonged in duration.
    d. It is viselike and radiates to the shoulders and arms.

17. Myocardial cell damage can be reflected by high levels of cardiac enzymes. The cardiac-specific isoenzyme is:
    a. alkaline phosphatase.
    b. creatine kinase (CK-MB).
    c. myoglobin.
    d. troponin.

18. The most common vasodilator used to treat myocardial pain is:
    a. amyl nitrite.
    b. Inderal.
    c. nitroglycerine.
    d. Pavabid HCl.

19. An intravenous analgesic frequently administered to relieve chest pain associated with myocardial infarction is:
    a. meperidine hydrochloride.
    b. hydromorphone hydrochloride.
    c. morphine sulfate.
    d. codeine sulfate.

20. The need for surgical intervention in coronary artery disease (CAD) is determined by the:
    a. amount of stenosis in the coronary arteries.
    b. myocardial area served by the stenotic artery.
    c. occurrence of previous infarction related to the affected artery.
    d. all of the above.

21. A candidate for percutaneous transluminal coronary angioplasty (PTCA) is a patient with coronary artery disease who:
    a. has compromised left ventricular function.
    b. has had angina longer than 3 years.
    c. has at least 70% occlusion of a major coronary artery.
    d. has questionable left ventricular function.

22. A goal of dilation in PTCA is to increase blood flow through the artery's lumen and achieve a residual stenosis of less than:
    a. 20%.
    b. 35%.
    c. 60%.
    d. 80%.

23. The nurse expects a postoperative PTCA patient to be discharged:
    a. the same day as surgery.
    b. within 24 hours of the procedure.
    c. 3 days later.
    d. after 1 week.

24. The nurse needs to be alert to assess for clinical symptoms of possible postoperative complications of PTCA, which include:
    a. abrupt closure of the artery.
    b. arterial dissection.
    c. coronary artery vasospasm.
    d. all of the above.

25. A candidate for coronary artery bypass grafting (CABG) must meet which of the following criteria?
    a. A blockage that cannot be treated by PTCA
    b. Greater than 60% blockage in the left main coronary artery.
    c. Unstable angina.
    d. All of the above.

26. The most common nursing diagnosis for patients awaiting cardiac surgery is:
    a. activity intolerance.
    b. fear related to the surgical procedure.
    c. decreased cardiac output.
    d. anginal pain.

27. Extremity paresthesia, dysrhythmias (peaked T waves), and mental confusion after cardiac surgery are signs of electrolyte imbalance related to the level of:
    a. calcium.
    b. magnesium.
    c. potassium.
    d. sodium.

28. A complication after cardiac surgery that is associated with an alteration in preload is:
    a. cardiac tamponade.
    b. elevated central venous pressure.
    c. hypertension.
    d. hypothermia.

SHORT ANSWER

Read each statement carefully. Write your response in the space provided.

1. The leading cause of death in the United States for men and women of all ethnic and racial groups is:

   _____.

2. The most common cause of cardiovascular disease is: _____.

3. The most frequently occurring sign of myocardial ischemia is: _____.

4. More than 50% of people with coronary artery disease have the risk factor of:

   _____.

5. List four of seven modifiable risk factors that are considered major causes of coronary artery disease:

   _____, _____, _____, and

   _____.

6. A positive diagnosis of metabolic syndrome occurs when three of the following six conditions are met:

   _____ _____

   _____ _____

   _____ _____

7. Management of coronary heart disease requires a therapeutic range of cholesterol and lipoproteins. An acceptable blood level of total cholesterol is _____ with an LDL/HDL ratio of _____. The desired level of LDL should be _____ mg/dL, and the HDL level should be greater than _____ mg/dL. Triglycerides should be less than _____ mg/dL.

8. The American Heart Association recommends that an average American diet contain about _____% fat.

9. List three of five collaborative problems for a patient with angina: _____,

   _____, and _____.

10. The key, diagnostic indicator for myocardial infarction seen on an electrocardiogram is:

    _____.

11. The vessel most commonly used for CABG is the: _____.

12. List four of seven symptoms seen in postpericardiotomy syndrome. _____,

    _____, _____, and _____.

II. Critical Thinking Questions and Exercises

DISCUSSION AND ANALYSIS

Discuss the following topics with your classmates.

1. Explain why coronary atherosclerosis is such a damaging process.
2. Explain how cigarette smoking contributes to the development of coronary artery disease.
3. Compare and contrast the therapeutic effects and medical/nursing considerations for medications affecting lipoprotein metabolism.
4. Compare and contrast the five types of angina.
5. Describe, in detail, the pain associated with angina pectoris.
6. Discuss the types of questions a nurse would use to assess a patient suspected of experiencing angina.

7. Describe the characteristics of the common presenting symptoms of acute coronary syndrome or acute myocardial infarction.
8. Explain what the phrase "door to balloon time" means.
9. Discuss nursing assessment for the potential complications of cardiac surgery.

EXAMINING ASSOCIATIONS

Examine the association between the items in each cluster and identify the common factor.

1. Abdominal aortic aneurysm, carotid artery disease, diabetes, existing coronary artery disease, and peripheral arterial disease.
2. Abdominal obesity, elevated triglycerides, low level of HDL, hypertension, and impaired function of insulin.
3. Age, cholesterol level, systolic blood pressure, levels of LDL and HDL, and cigarette smoking.
4. Cholesterol abnormalities, cigarette smoking, diabetes mellitus, and hypertension.
5. Total cholesterol, LDL, HDL, and triglycerides.

IDENTIFYING PATTERNS

Review the figure below and answer the following questions.

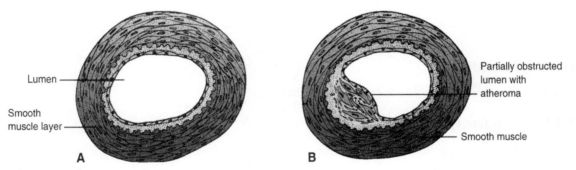

Cross-section of a normal and an atherosclerotic artery. **A,** Cross-section of normal artery in which the lumen is fully patent, open. **B,** Cross-section of artery with diminished patency resulting from atheroma.

1. Describe the underlying pathophysiology that causes a normal artery (**A**) to narrow because of atheroma deposits.

   _____

   _____

   _____

2. An atheroma is described as: _____.

3. A possible complication of rupture or hemorrhage of the lipid core into the plaque is:

   _____

4. A thrombus is a dangerous complication of atherosclerosis because it can lead to: _____ and

   _____.

SUPPORTING ARGUMENTS

Offer a supporting rationale for your response.

1. Explain, supported with a scientific base to your rationale, why cigarette smoking contributes to the severity of coronary heart disease for each of these three factors:

Factor	Scientific Rationale
a. Increased CO levels	a. _____ _____
b. Increased catecholamines	b. _____ _____
c. Increased platelet adhesion	c. _____ _____

2. Argue in support of using calcium channel blockers for the treatment of angina.

   _____

   _____

   _____

CLINICAL SITUATIONS

Read the following case studies. Circle the correct answer.

CASE STUDY: Angina Pectoris

Ermelina, a 64-year-old retired secretary, is admitted to the medical–surgical area for management of chest pain caused by angina pectoris.

1. The nurse knows that the basic cause of angina pectoris is believed to be:
   a. dysrhythmias triggered by stress.
   b. insufficient coronary blood flow.
   c. minute emboli discharged through the narrowed lumens of the coronary vessels.
   d. spasms of the vessel walls owing to excessive secretion of epinephrine (adrenaline).

2. The medical record lists a probable diagnosis of chronic stable angina. The nurse knows that Ermelina's pain:
   a. has increased progressively in frequency and duration.
   b. is incapacitating.
   c. is relieved by rest and is predictable.
   d. usually occurs at night and may be relieved by sitting upright.

3. Ermelina has nitroglycerin at her bedside to take PRN. The nurse knows that nitroglycerin acts in all of the following ways *except*:
   a. causing venous pooling throughout the body.
   b. constricting arterioles to lessen peripheral blood flow.
   c. dilating the coronary arteries to increase the oxygen supply.
   d. lowering systemic blood pressure.

4. Ermelina took a nitroglycerin tablet at 10:00 AM, after her morning care. It did not relieve her pain, so, 5 minutes later, she repeated the dose. Ten minutes later and still in pain, she calls the nurse, who should:

a. administer a PRN dose of diazepam (Valium), try to calm her, and recommend that she rest in a chair with her legs dependent to encourage venous pooling.

b. assist her to the supine position, give her oxygen at 6 L/min, and advise her to rest in bed.

c. help her to a comfortable position, give her oxygen at 2 L/min, and call her physician.

d. suggest that she take double her previous dose after 5 minutes and try to sleep to decrease her body's need for oxygen.

CASE STUDY: Decreased Myocardial Tissue Perfusion

Mr. Lillis, a 46-year-old bricklayer, is brought to the emergency department by ambulance with a suspected diagnosis of myocardial infarction. He appears ashen, is diaphoretic and tachycardiac, and has severe chest pain. The nursing diagnosis is decreased cardiac output, related to decreased myocardial tissue perfusion.

1. The nurse knows that the most critical time period for his diagnosis is:

a. the first hour after symptoms begin.

b. within 24 hours after the onset of symptoms.

c. within the first 48 hours after the attack.

d. between the third and fifth day after the attack.

2. Because the area of infarction develops over minutes to hours, the nurse knows to interpret the following ECG results as indicative of initial myocardial injury:

a. abnormal Q waves.

b. enlarged T wave.

c. inverted T wave.

d. ST segment depression.

3. The nurse evaluates a series of laboratory tests within the first few hours. She knows that a positive indicator of cell damage is:

a. decreased level of troponin.

b. elevated creatine kinase (CK-MB).

c. lower level of myoglobin.

d. all of the above.

4. On the basis of assessment data, the physician diagnoses an acute myocardial infarction. List the drug classification that the nurse knows should be given within 3 to 6 hours of diagnosis: _____. List two common examples: _____ and _____.

5. The nurse needs to look for symptoms associated with one of the major causes of sudden death during the first 48 hours, which is:

a. cardiogenic shock.

b. pulmonary edema.

c. pulmonary embolism.

d. ventricular rupture.

6. The nurse is aware that ischemic tissue remains sensitive to oxygen demands, because scar formation is not seen until the:

a. second week.

b. third week.

c. sixth week.

d. eighth week.

7. Mr. Lillis needs to be advised that myocardial healing will not be complete for about:

a. 2 months.

b. 4 months.

c. 6 months.

d. 8 months.

8. For discharge planning, Mr. Lillis is advised to:

a. avoid large meals.

b. exercise daily.

c. restrict caffeine-containing beverages.

d. do all of the above.

9. The nurse can advise Mr. Lillis that sexual activities can be resumed after what activity tolerance has been achieved?

CHAPTER 29

Management of Patients With Structural, Infectious, and Inflammatory Cardiac Disorders

I. Interpretation, Comparison, and Completion

MULTIPLE CHOICE

Read each question carefully. Circle your answer.

1. Incomplete closure of the tricuspid valve results in a backward flow of blood from the:
   a. aorta to the left ventricle.
   b. left atrium to the left ventricle.
   c. right atrium to the right ventricle.
   d. right ventricle to the right atrium.

2. Backward flow of blood from the left ventricle to the left atrium is through the:
   a. aortic valve.
   b. mitral valve.
   c. pulmonic valve.
   d. tricuspid valve.

3. The pathophysiology of mitral stenosis is consistent with:
   a. aortic stenosis.
   b. left ventricular failure.
   c. left atrial hypertrophy.
   d. all of the above.

4. On auscultation, the nurse suspects a diagnosis of mitral valve regurgitation when which of the following is heard?
   a. Mitral click
   b. High-pitched blowing sound at the apex
   c. Low-pitched diastolic murmur at the apex
   d. Diastolic murmur at the left sternal border

5. The presence of a water-hammer pulse (quick, sharp strokes that suddenly collapse) is diagnostic for:
   a. aortic regurgitation.
   b. mitral insufficiency.
   c. tricuspid insufficiency.
   d. tricuspid stenosis.

6. Severe aortic stenotic disease is consistent with all of the following *except*:
   a. increased cardiac output.
   b. left ventricular hypertrophy.
   c. pulmonary edema.
   d. right-sided heart failure.

7. The most common valvuloplasty procedure is the:
   a. balloon valvuloplasty.
   b. annuloplasty.
   c. chordoplasty.
   d. commissurotomy.

8. Xenographs, used for valve replacement, have a viability of about:
   a. 2 years.
   b. 4 years.
   c. 8 years.
   d. 12 years.

9. The nurse knows that a patient who is to receive a xenograft from a pig or cow will be receiving a (an):
   a. allograft.
   b. autograft.
   c. heterograft.
   d. homograft.

10. The most commonly occurring cardiomyopathy is:
    a. dilated.
    b. hypertrophic.
    c. idiopathic.
    d. restrictive.

11. Probably the most helpful diagnostic test to identify cardiomyopathy is:
    a. serial enzyme studies.
    b. cardiac catheterization.
    c. the echocardiogram.
    d. the phonocardiogram.

12. An immunosuppressant that allowed heart transplantation to become a therapeutic option for end-stage heart disease is:
    a. Procardia.
    b. Cyclosporine.
    c. Calan.
    d. Vancocin.

13. Rheumatic endocarditis is an inflammatory reaction to:
    a. group A, beta-hemolytic streptococcus.
    b. *Pseudomonas aeruginosa*.
    c. *Serratia marcescens*.
    d. *Staphylococcus aureus*.

14. The causative microorganism for rheumatic endocarditis can be accurately identified only by:
    a. a throat culture.
    b. an echocardiogram.
    c. roentgenography.
    d. serum analysis.

15. Clinical manifestations of infective endocarditis may include:
    a. embolization.
    b. focal neurologic lesions.
    c. heart murmurs.
    d. all of the above.

16. The most characteristic symptom of pericarditis is:
    a. dyspnea.
    b. constant chest pain.
    c. fatigue lasting more than 1 month.
    d. uncontrolled restlessness.

17. The characteristic sign of pericarditis is:
    a. a friction rub.
    b. dyspnea.
    c. fever.
    d. hypoxia.

18. Which of the following medications would *not* be used to treat pericarditis because it can decrease blood flow?
    a. Colchicine
    b. Indocin
    c. Motrin
    d. Prednisone

19. A serious consequence of pericarditis is:
    a. cardiac tamponade.
    b. decreased venous pressure.
    c. hypertension.
    d. left ventricular hypertrophy.

SHORT ANSWER

Read each statement carefully. Write your response in the space provided.

1. Describe the basic dysfunction of mitral valve prolapse.

   _____

   _____

2. If dysrhythmias occur with mitral valve prolapsed, the nurse advises the patient to avoid:

   _____, _____, and _____.

3. A nurse, using auscultation to identify aortic regurgitation, would place the stethoscope _____

   and would expect to hear _____.

4. With aortic stenosis, the patient should receive _____ to prevent endocarditis.

5. List four of seven potential complications or collaborative problems for patients with cardiomyopathy:

   _____, _____, _____, and _____.

6. Identify five common indicators for heart transplantation: _____,

   _____, _____, _____,

   and _____.

7. Prompt treatment of streptococcal pharyngitis with _____ can prevent almost all attacks of:

   _____.

8. Briefly describe the pathophysiology of infective endocarditis, beginning with the formation of a vegetation.

   _____

   _____

9. Infective endocarditis is usually caused by the following bacteria: _____,

   _____, _____, and _____.

10. Briefly describe the pathophysiology of myocarditis.

   _____

   _____

   _____

11. Patients with myocarditis may be extremely sensitive to _____ (medication) and should
    therefore be monitored for serum levels to prevent _____.

12. Describe the anatomic landmark for auscultation of a pericardial friction rub.

   _____

   _____

MATCHING

Match the pathophysiology listed in column II with the valvular disorder listed in column I.

Column I

1. _____ Mitral valve prolapse

2. _____ Mitral stenosis

3. _____ Mitral regurgitation

4. _____ Aortic valve stenosis

5. _____ Aortic regurgitation

Column II

a. Leaflet malformation prevents complete closure

b. Can be caused by rheumatic endocarditis

c. Characterized by a significantly widened pulse pressure

d. Blood seeps backward into left atrium

e. Thickening and contracture of mitral valve cusps

II. Critical Thinking Questions and Exercises

DISCUSSION AND ANALYSIS

Discuss the following topics with your classmates.

1. Describe what a nurse would expect to hear when using auscultation to listen to the heart of a patient with mitral valve prolapse.
2. Explain how left ventricular hypertrophy develops from mitral valve insufficiency.
3. Describe the pathophysiology of aortic regurgitation.
4. Describe the characteristic sound of the murmur heard with aortic stenosis.
5. Explain the purpose and process of a balloon valvuloplasty.
6. Explain the purpose and process of valve replacement.
7. Describe the management of a patient who has undergone a valvuloplasty and replacement.
8. Explain the pathophysiology of all cardiomyopathies.
9. Discuss at least five nursing diagnoses and collaborative problems for a patient with cardiomyopathy.
10. Describe the pathophysiology of pericarditis and list at least six underlying causes.

IDENTIFYING PATTERNS

Outline, on the flow chart, the pathophysiologic sequence of events that occurs when mitral valve stenosis leads to right ventricular failure.

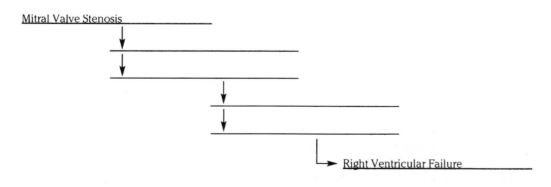

CLINICAL SITUATIONS

Read the following case studies. Fill in the blanks below or circle the correct answer.

CASE STUDY: Infective Endocarditis

Mr. Fontana, a 60-year-old executive, is admitted to the hospital with a diagnosis of infective endocarditis. Pertinent history includes a previous diagnosis of mitral valve prolapse. A physical examination at his physician's office before admission reveals complaints of anorexia, joint pain, intermittent fever, and a 10-lb weight loss in the past 2 months.

1. The nurse knows, prior to assessment, that Mr. Fontana's vague clinical symptoms are characteristic of an insidious disease onset that develops from one of three conditions: _____,

   _____, or _____.

2. While examining Mr. Fontana's eyes during the admission assessment, the nurse notes conjunctival hemorrhages with pale centers caused by emboli in the nerve fiber of the eye. These are known as:
   a. Roth's spots.
   b. Osler's nodes.
   c. Janeway's lesions.
   d. Heberden's nodes.

3. The nurse also assesses for central nervous system manifestations of the infectious disease. She looks for

   symptoms such as: _____, _____, _____, and

   _____.

4. The primary objective of medical management is: _____.

5. Serial blood cultures identified *Streptococcus viridans* as the causative organism, and parenteral antibiotic treatment was initiated. The nurse expects that Mr. Fontana will probably remain on the antibiotic intravenous infusion for:
   a. 5 days.
   b. 1 week.
   c. 2 to 6 weeks.
   d. 8 to 10 weeks.

6. Even with successful treatment, organ damage can occur. Cardiac complications may include:

   _____, _____, _____, and

   _____.

7. Mr. Fontana needs to be advised that prophylactic antibiotic therapy is also recommended for:
   a. tooth extraction.
   b. bronchoscopy.
   c. cystoscopy.
   d. all of the above.

CASE STUDY: Acute Pericarditis

Mrs. Russell is a 46-year-old Caucasian who developed symptoms of acute pericarditis secondary to a viral infection. Diagnosis was based on the characteristic sign of a friction rub and pain over the pericardium.

1. On the basis of knowledge of pericardial pain, the nurse suggests the following body position to relieve the pain symptoms:
   a. flat in bed with feet slightly higher than the head.
   b. Fowler's.
   c. right side-lying.
   d. semi-Fowler's.

2. Based on assessment data, the major nursing diagnosis is: _____.

3. Initial nursing intervention includes maintenance of bed rest until the following symptom disappears:
   a. fever.
   b. friction rub.
   c. pain.
   d. all of the above.

4. Identify three drug classifications that are commonly prescribed for management or treatment:

   _____, _____, and _____.

5. Name the anatomic landmarks used to auscultate for a pericardial friction rub:

   _____

6. List the two major expected patient outcomes for nursing management of a patient with pericarditis:

   _____ and _____.

CHAPTER 30

Management of Patients With Complications From Heart Disease

I. Interpretation, Completion, and Comparison

MULTIPLE CHOICE

Read each question carefully. Circle your answer.

1. The multilumen pulmonary artery catheter allows the nurse to measure hemodynamic pressures at various points in the heart. When the tip enters the small branches of the pulmonary artery, the nurse can assess all of the following measurements *except*:

   a. central venous pressure (CVP).

   b. pulmonary artery capillary pressure (PACP).

   c. pulmonary artery obstructive pressure (PAOP).

   d. pulmonary artery wedge pressure (PAWP).

2. Hemodynamic monitoring by means of a multilumen pulmonary artery catheter can provide detailed information about:

   a. preload.

   b. afterload.

   c. cardiac output.

   d. all of the above.

3. Nursing measures in hemodynamic monitoring include assessing for localized ischemia caused by inadequate arterial flow. The nurse should:

   a. assess the involved extremity for color temperature.

   b. check for capillary filling.

   c. evaluate pulse rate.

   d. do all of the above.

4. The most frequent cause for hospitalization for people older than 75 years of age is:

   a. angina pectoris.

   b. heart failure.

   c. hypertension.

   d. pulmonary edema.

5. The primary cause of heart failure is:

   a. arterial hypertension.

   b. coronary atherosclerosis.

   c. myocardial dysfunction.

   d. valvular dysfunction.

6. The dominant function in cardiac failure is:

   a. ascites.

   b. hepatomegaly.

   c. inadequate tissue perfusion.

   d. nocturia.

7. On assessment, the nurse knows that a patient who reports no symptoms of heart failure at rest but is symptomatic with increased physical activity would have a heart failure classification of:

   a. I.

   b. II.

   c. III.

   d. IV.

8. On assessment, the nurse knows that the presence of pitting edema indicates fluid retention of at least:
   a. 4 lb.
   b. 6 lb.
   c. 8 lb.
   d. 10 lb.

9. The diagnosis of heart failure is usually confirmed by:
   a. a chest x-ray.
   b. an echocardiogram.
   c. an electrocardiogram.
   d. ventriculogram.

10. A key diagnostic laboratory test for heart failure is the:
   a. blood urea nitrogen (BUN).
   b. complete blood cell count.
   c. B-type natriuretic peptide.
   d. serum electrolyte counts.

11. According to the American College of Cardiology and the American Heart Association, a patient presenting with left ventricular dysfunction without symptoms of heart failure would be classified as:
   a. stage A.
   b. stage B.
   c. stage C.
   d. stage D.

12. The treatment for cardiac failure is directed at:
   a. decreasing oxygen needs of the heart.
   b. increasing the cardiac output by strengthening muscle contraction or decreasing peripheral resistance.
   c. reducing the amount of circulating blood volume.
   d. all of the above.

13. A primary classification of medications used in the treatment of systolic heart failure is:
   a. angiotensin-converting enzyme inhibitors.
   b. beta-blockers.
   c. diuretics.
   d. calcium-channel blockers.

14. The nurse knows that this angiotensin-converting enzyme inhibitor ordered by the physician has a rapid onset of action within 15 minutes.
   a. Altace
   b. Capoten
   c. Lotensin
   d. Vasotec

15. An example of a potassium-sparing diuretic that might be prescribed for a person with congestive heart failure is:
   a. Aldactone.
   b. Mykrox.
   c. Zaroxolyn.
   d. Lasix.

16. Digitalis toxicity is a key concern in digitalis therapy. A therapeutic digitalis level should be:
   a. 0.25 to 0.35 mg/mL.
   b. 0.30 to 4.0 mg/mL
   c. 0.5 to 2.0 mg/mL.
   d. 2.5 to 4.0 mg/mL.

17. The primary underlying disorder of pulmonary edema is:
   a. decreased left ventricular pumping.
   b. decreased right ventricular elasticity.
   c. increased left atrial contractility.
   d. increased right atrial resistance.

18. Pulmonary edema is characterized by:
   a. elevated left ventricular end-diastolic pressure.
   b. a rise in pulmonary venous pressure.
   c. increased hydrostatic pressure.
   d. all of the above alterations.

19. With pulmonary edema, there is usually an alteration in:
    a. afterload.
    b. contractility.
    c. preload.
    d. all of the above.

20. A commonly prescribed diuretic that is given intravenously to produce a rapid diuretic effect is:
    a. Bumex.
    b. Lasix.
    c. Mykrox.
    d. Zaroxolyn.

21. Morphine is given in acute pulmonary edema to redistribute the pulmonary circulation to the periphery by decreasing:
    a. peripheral resistance.
    b. pulmonary capillary pressure.
    c. transudation of fluid.
    d. all of the above.

22. A recommended position for a patient in acute pulmonary edema is:
    a. prone, to encourage maximum rest, thereby decreasing respiratory and cardiac rates.
    b. semi-Fowler's, to facilitate breathing and promote pooling of blood in the sacral area.
    c. Trendelenburg, to drain the upper airways of congestion.
    d. upright with the legs down, to decrease venous return.

23. Cardiogenic shock is pump failure that occurs primarily as the result of:
    a. coronary artery stenosis.
    b. left ventricular damage.
    c. myocardial ischemia.
    d. right atrial flutter.

24. Classic signs of cardiogenic shock include all of the following *except*:
    a. bradycardia.
    b. cerebral hypoxia.
    c. hypotension.
    d. oliguria.

25. The nurse expects that positive inotropic medications would be administered to treat cardiogenic shock, with the exception of:
    a. Adrenalin.
    b. Dobutrex.
    c. Intropin.
    d. Levophed.

26. A clinical manifestation of pericardial effusion is:
    a. widening pulse pressure.
    b. a decrease in venous pressure.
    c. shortness of breath.
    d. an increase in blood pressure.

27. The most reliable sign of cardiac arrest is:
    a. absence of a pulse.
    b. cessation of respirations.
    c. dilation of the pupils.
    d. inaudible heart sounds.

28. Brain damage occurs with cessation of circulation after an approximate interval of:
    a. 2 minutes.
    b. 4 minutes.
    c. 6 minutes.
    d. 8 minutes.

29. The drug of choice during cardiopulmonary resuscitation to suppress ventricular dysrhythmias is:
    a. atropine.
    b. epinephrine.
    c. lidocaine.
    d. morphine.

MATCHING

Match the type of ventricular heart failure listed in column II with its associated pathophysiology in column I.

Column I

1. _____ Fatigability

2. _____ Dependent edema

3. _____ Pulmonary congestion predominates

4. _____ Distended neck veins

5. _____ Ascites

6. _____ Dyspnea from fluid in alveoli

7. _____ Orthopnea

8. _____ Hepatomegaly

9. _____ Cough that may be blood-tinged

10. _____ Nocturia

Column II

a. Left-sided heart failure

b. Right-sided heart failure

SHORT ANSWER

Read each statement carefully. Write your response in the space provided.

1. Decipher the formula: CO = HR × SV.

   _____

   _____

2. Distinguish between the terms *preload* and *afterload*.

   Preload: _____

   Afterload: _____

3. Two factors that determine preload are: _____ and _____. Two factors that

   determine afterload are: _____ and _____.

4. Two noninvasive tests are used to assess cardiac hemodynamics: _____ for right ventricular

   preload, _____ for left ventricular afterload, and _____ for left ventricular preload.

5. List four common etiologic factors that cause myocardial dysfunction: _____,

   _____, _____, and _____.

6. Coronary atherosclerosis results in tissue ischemia which causes myocardial dysfunction because

   _____

   _____

7. Name three types of cardiomyopathy: _____, _____,

   and _____; of these, _____ is the most common.

8. The primary clinical manifestations of pulmonary congestion in left-sided heart failure are:

   _____, _____, _____,

   _____, and a probable _____.

9. The primary systemic clinical manifestations of right-sided heart failure are: _____,

   _____, _____, _____,

   _____, _____, and _____.

10. Name four drug classifications normally prescribed for systolic heart failure:

    _____, _____, _____,

    and _____.

11. List four of six common side effects of diuretics: _____, _____,

    _____, and _____.

12. List six symptoms indicative of hypokalemia:

    _____   _____

    _____   _____

    _____   _____

13. Identify six causes of cardiogenic shock:

    _____ _____ _____

    _____ _____ _____

14. The most common thromboembolitic problem among patients with heart failure is:

    _____.

15. For cardiopulmonary resuscitation, the recommended chest compression rate is _____times/min. The

    compression to ventilation ratio of _____ is recommended without stopping for ventilation.

II. Critical Thinking Questions and Exercises

DISCUSSION AND ANALYSIS

Discuss the following topics with your classmates.

1. Explain how the ejection factor, as a test to determine the type of heart failure present, is calculated.
2. Describe in detail the pathophysiologic events that occur in systolic heart failure, especially the fluid dynamic alterations that occur as a result of the conversion of angiotensin I to angiotensin II.
3. Distinguish between the pathophysiology of left-sided and right-sided heart failure.
4. Describe cardiac resynchronization therapy (CRT), a treatment for heart failure.
5. Discuss the key nursing considerations for medications used to treat heart failure.
6. Discuss the nursing assessment, diagnoses, and interventions for a patient with heart failure.
7. Explain the pathophysiology of cardiogenic shock.
8. Explain and demonstrate the process of cardiopulmonary resuscitation (CPR).

IDENTIFYING PATTERNS

Complete the following outline that depicts the pathophysiology of pulmonary edema, beginning with decreased left ventricular pumping ability and ending with hypoxemia and death if not treated.

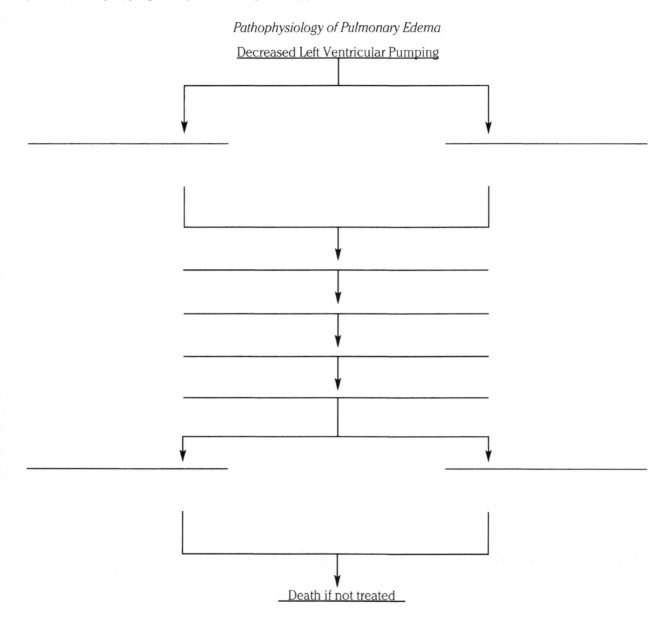

Pathophysiology of Pulmonary Edema

Decreased Left Ventricular Pumping

Death if not treated

CLINICAL SITUATIONS

Read the following case study. Fill in the blanks or circle the correct answer.

CASE STUDY: Pulmonary Edema

Mr. Wolman is to be discharged from the hospital to home. He is 79 years old, lives with his wife, and has just recovered from mild pulmonary edema secondary to congestive heart failure.

1. The most common cause of pulmonary edema is: _____.

2. The sequence of pathophysiologic events is triggered by:
   a. elevated left ventricular end-diastolic pressure.
   b. elevated pulmonary venous pressure.
   c. increased hydrostatic pressure.
   d. impaired lymphatic drainage.

3. The nurse advises Mr. Wolman to rest frequently at home. This advice is based on the knowledge that rest:
   a. decreases blood pressure.
   b. increases the heart reserve.
   c. reduces the work of the heart.
   d. does all of the above.

4. The nurse reminds Mr. Wolman to sleep with two pillows to elevate his head about 10 in. This position is recommended because:
   a. preload can be increased, thus enhancing cardiac output.
   b. pulmonary congestion can be reduced.
   c. venous return to the lungs can be improved, thus reducing peripheral edema.
   d. all of the above can help relieve his symptoms.

5. Mr. Wolman takes 0.25 mg of digoxin once a day. The nurse should tell him about signs of digitalis toxicity, which include:
   a. anorexia.
   b. bradycardia and tachycardia.
   c. nausea and vomiting.
   d. all of the above.

6. Mr. Wolman also takes Lasix (40 mg) twice a day. He is aware of signs related to hypokalemia and supplements his diet with foods high in potassium, such as:
   a. bananas.
   b. raisins.
   c. orange juice.
   d. all of the above.

Assessment and Management of Patients With Vascular Disorders and Problems of Peripheral Circulation

I. Interpretation, Completion, and Comparison

MULTIPLE CHOICE

Read each question carefully. Circle your answer.

1. The most important factor in regulating the caliber of blood vessels, which determines resistance to flow, is:
   a. hormonal secretion.
   b. independent arterial wall activity.
   c. the influence of circulating chemicals.
   d. the sympathetic nervous system.

2. Clinical manifestations of acute venous insufficiency include all of the following *except*:
   a. cool and cyanotic skin.
   b. initial absence of edema.
   c. sharp pain that may be relieved by the elevation of the extremity.
   d. full superficial veins.

3. With peripheral arterial insufficiency, leg pain during rest can be reduced by:
   a. elevating the limb above heart level.
   b. lowering the limb so that it is dependent.
   c. massaging the limb after application of cold compresses.
   d. placing the limb in a plane horizontal to the body.

4. Probably the strongest risk factor for the development of atherosclerotic lesions is:
   a. cigarette smoking.
   b. lack of exercise.
   c. obesity.
   d. stress.

5. Saturated fats are strongly implicated in the causation of atherosclerosis. Saturated fats include all of the following *except*:
   a. corn oil.
   b. eggs and milk.
   c. meat and butter.
   d. solid vegetable oil.

6. The American diet is known to be high in fat. The amount of calories typically supplied by fat in most diets is _____ of the total caloric intake.
   a. 20%
   b. 35%
   c. 60%
   d. 80%

7. Buerger's disease is characterized by all of the following *except*:
   a. arterial thrombus formation and occlusion.
   b. lipid deposits in the arteries.
   c. redness or cyanosis in the limb when it is dependent.
   d. venous inflammation and occlusion.

8. The most outstanding symptom of Buerger's disease is:
   a. a burning sensation.
   b. cramping in the feet.
   c. pain.
   d. paresthesia.

9. The most common cause of all thoracic aortic aneurysms is:
   a. a congenital defect in the vessel wall.
   b. atherosclerosis.
   c. infection.
   d. trauma.

10. Diagnosis of a thoracic aortic aneurysm is done primarily by:
    a. computed tomography.
    b. transesophageal echocardiography.
    c. x-ray.
    d. all of the above.

11. A nurse who suspects the presence of an abdominal aortic aneurysm should look for the presence of:
    a. a pulsatile abdominal mass.
    b. low back pain.
    c. lower abdominal pain.
    d. all of the above.

12. To save a limb that is affected by occlusion of a major artery, surgery must be initiated before necrosis develops, which is usually:
    a. within the first 4 hours.
    b. between 6 and 10 hours.
    c. between 12 and 24 hours.
    d. within 1 to 2 days.

13. Raynaud's disease is a form of:
    a. arterial vessel occlusion caused by multiple emboli that develop in the heart and are transported through the systemic circulation.
    b. arteriolar vasoconstriction, usually on the fingertips, that results in coldness, pain, and pallor.
    c. peripheral venospasm in the lower extremities owing to valve damage resulting from prolonged venous stasis.
    d. phlebothrombosis related to prolonged vasoconstriction resulting from overexposure to the cold.

14. A significant cause of venous thrombosis is:
    a. altered blood coagulation.
    b. stasis of blood.
    c. vessel wall injury.
    d. all of the above.

15. Clinical manifestations of deep vein obstruction include:
    a. edema and limb pain.
    b. ankle engorgement.
    c. leg circumference differences.
    d. all of the above.

16. When administering heparin anticoagulant therapy, the nurse needs to monitor the clotting time to make certain that it is within the therapeutic range of:
    a. one to two times the normal control.
    b. two to three times the normal control.
    c. 3.5 times the normal control.
    d. 4.5 times the normal control.

17. When caring for a patient who has started anticoagulant therapy with warfarin (Coumadin), the nurse knows not to expect therapeutic benefits for:
    a. at least 12 hours.
    b. the first 24 hours.
    c. 2 to 3 days.
    d. 3 to 5 days.

18. Knowing the most serious complication of venous insufficiency, the nurse would assess the patient's lower extremities for signs of:
    a. rudor.
    b. cellulitis.
    c. dermatitis.
    d. ulceration.

19. A nurse should teach a patient with chronic venous insufficiency to do all of the following *except*:
    a. avoid constricting garments.
    b. elevate the legs above the heart level for 30 minutes every 2 hours.
    c. sit as much as possible to rest the valves in the legs.
    d. sleep with the foot of the bed elevated about 6 in.

20. Nursing measures to promote a clean leg ulcer include:
    a. applying wet-to-dry saline solution dressings, which would remove necrotic debris when changed.
    b. flushing out necrotic material with hydrogen peroxide.
    c. using an ointment that would treat the ulcer by enzymatic debridement.
    d. all of the above.

21. The physician prescribed a Tegapore dressing to treat a venous ulcer. The nurse knows that the ankle-brachial index (ABI) must be _____ for the circulatory status to be adequate.
    a. 0.10
    b. 0.25
    c. 0.35
    d. 0.50

22. A varicose vein is caused by:
    a. phlebothrombosis.
    b. an incompetent venous valve.
    c. venospasm.
    d. venous occlusion.

23. Postoperative nursing management for vein ligation and stripping include all of the following *except*:
    a. dangling the legs over the side of the bed for 10 minutes every 4 hours for the first 24 hours.
    b. elevating the foot of the bed to promote venous blood return.
    c. maintaining elastic compression of the leg continuously for about 1 week.
    d. starting the patient ambulating 24 to 48 hours after surgery.

SHORT ANSWER

Read each statement carefully. Write your response in the space provided.

1. Hydrostatic force is defined as _____, whereas osmotic pressure is defined as _____.

2. The hallmark symptom of peripheral arterial occlusive disease is: _____.

3. The clinical picture of a patient presenting with a dissected aorta is: _____.

4. List the six clinical symptoms associated with acute arterial embolism, also known as the six Ps:

_____   _____

_____   _____

_____   _____

5. List the classic triad (Virchow's) of factors associated with the development of venous thromboembolism:

_____, _____, and _____.

6. Venous stasis, postthrombotic syndrome, is characterized by: _____, _____,

_____, and _____.

MATCHING

Match the type of vessel insufficiency listed in column II with its associated symptom listed in column I.

Column I

1. _____ Intermittent claudication

2. _____ Paresthesia

3. _____ Dependent rubor

4. _____ Cold, pale extremity

5. _____ Ulcers of lower legs and ankles

6. _____ Muscle fatigue and cramping

7. _____ Diminished or absent pulses

8. _____ Reddish-blue discoloration with dependency

Column II

a. Arterial insufficiency

b. Venous insufficiency

II. Critical Thinking Questions and Exercises

DISCUSSION AND ANALYSIS

Discuss the following topics with your classmates.

1. Explain what is meant by: flow rate = $\Delta P/R$.
2. Explain the etiology of pain associated with the condition known as "intermittent claudication."
3. Demonstrate the steps required for a nurse to take an accurate ABI calculation.
4. Compare and contrast the various diagnostic tests used to assess abnormalities in the vascular system.
5. Discuss nursing interventions for the nine modifiable risk factors for atherosclerosis.
6. Discuss four nursing diagnoses and related goals for a patient with peripheral vascular problems.
7. Demonstrate the ways that patients with peripheral vascular disease can maintain foot and leg care.
8. Describe the clinical manifestations, assessments, and medical/nursing interventions for patients with peripheral arterial occlusive disease.
9. Compare and contrast the etiology, clinical manifestations, and nursing and medical interventions for a thoracic and abdominal aortic aneurysm.
10. Discuss the four major complications of venous thrombosis and associated nursing interventions.
11. Distinguish between the pathophysiology and clinical manifestations of arterial and venous leg ulcers.
12. Compare and contrast the three treatments used for varicose veins: ligation and stripping, thermal ablation, and sclerotherapy.

EXAMINING ASSOCIATIONS

Read each analogy. Fill in the space provided with the best response.

1. Arteriosclerosis : hardening of the arteries :: _____ : the accumulation of plaque and atheromas.

2. Rudor : reddish-blue discoloration :: _____ : cramplike pain in the extremities with exercise.

3. International normalized ratio (INR) : the measurement of anticoagulant levels :: Ankle-brachial index (ABI) : _____.

4. The intima : inner layer of the arterial wall :: _____ : outer layer of connective tissue.

5. The right lymphatic duct : lymphatic fluid delivery to the right side of the head and neck :: The thoracic duct : _____.

6. Cellulitis : infectious limb swelling :: _____ : lymphatic channel inflammation.

CLINICAL SITUATIONS

Read the following case study. Circle the correct answer.

CASE STUDY: Peripheral Arterial Occlusive Disease

Fred, a 43-year-old construction worker, has a history of hypertension. He smokes two packs of cigarettes a day, is nervous about the possibility of being unemployed, and has difficulty coping with stress. His current concern is calf pain during minimal exercise, which decreases with rest.

1. The nurse assesses Fred's symptoms as being associated with peripheral arterial occlusive disease. The nursing diagnosis is probably:
   a. alteration in tissue perfusion related to compromised circulation.
   b. dysfunctional use of extremities related to muscle spasms.
   c. impaired mobility related to stress associated with pain.
   d. impairment in muscle use associated with pain on exertion.

2. The nurse knows that the hallmark symptom of peripheral arterial occlusion disease is:
   a. intermittent claudication.
   b. phlebothrombosis.
   c. postphlebitis syndrome.
   d. thrombophlebitis.

3. Additional symptoms to support the nurse's diagnosis include all of the following *except*:
   a. blanched skin appearance when the limb is dependent.
   b. diminished distal pulsations.
   c. reddish-blue discoloration of the limb when it is elevated.
   d. warm and rosy coloration of the extremity after exercise.

4. The pain associated with this condition commonly occurs in muscle groups _____.

5. The pain is due to the irritation of nerve endings by the buildup of _____ and

   _____.

6. Pain is experienced when the arterial lumen narrows to about:
   a. 15%.   c. 35%.
   b. 25%.   d. 50%.

7. The nurse notices that several minutes after Jack's leg is dependent, the vessels remain dilated. This is evidenced by the coloring of the skin, which the nurse describes as:
   a. rosy.   c. pallor.
   b. rubor.   d. cyanotic.

8. The nurse is asked to determine ABI. The right posterior tibial reading is 75 mm Hg and the brachial systolic pressure is 150 mm Hg. The ABI would be:
   a. 0.25.   c. 0.65.
   b. 0.50.   d. 0.80.

9. In health teaching, the nurse should suggest methods to increase arterial blood supply, which include:
   a. a planned program involving systematic lowering of the extremity below heart level.   c. graded extremity exercises.
                                                                                             d. all of the above.
   b. Buerger-Allen exercises.

APPLYING CONCEPTS

Examine Figure 31-1 in the text and document the physiologic function of specific components of the vascular system.

1. Superior vena cava _____.

2. Pulmonary circulation _____.

3. Aorta _____.

4. Right and left pulmonary veins _____.

5. Hepatic circulation _____.

6. Systemic circulation _____.

7. Right and left ventricles _____.

8. Right and left atrium _____.

9. Inferior vena cava _____.

10. Renal circulation _____.

CHAPTER 32

Assessment and Management of Patients With Hypertension

I. Interpretation, Completion, and Comparison

MULTIPLE CHOICE

Read each question carefully. Circle your answer.

1. Prehypertension, a precursor to hypertension, can be diagnosed when the diastolic reading is:
   a. between 60 and 70 mm Hg.
   b. at 75 mm Hg.
   c. at 80 mm Hg.
   d. between 85 and 90 mm Hg.

2. Stage 1 hypertension is defined as persistent blood pressure levels in which the systolic pressure is higher than ____ and the diastolic is higher than ____.
   a. 110/60 mm Hg
   b. 120/70 mm Hg
   c. 130/80 mm Hg
   d. 140/90 mm Hg

3. The percentage of adults in the United States who have hypertension is approximately:
   a. 10%.
   b. 15%.
   c. 30%.
   d. 40%.

4. The desired goal for the systolic blood pressure for a person with diabetes mellitus or chronic kidney disease is:
   a. 120 mm Hg.
   b. 130 mm Hg.
   c. 140 mm Hg.
   d. 150 mm Hg.

5. Pharmacologic therapy for patients with uncomplicated hypertension would include the administration of:
   a. Angiotensin-converting enzyme inhibitors.
   b. alpha-blockers.
   c. beta-blockers.
   d. calcium antagonists.

6. A characteristic symptom of damage to the vital organs as a result of hypertension is:
   a. angina.
   b. dyspnea.
   c. epistaxis.
   d. all of the above.

7. An expected nursing diagnosis for a patient with hypertension is:
   a. heart failure.
   b. knowledge deficit.
   c. myocardial infarction.
   d. renal insufficiency.

8. The percentage of patients with hypertension who discontinue their drug therapy, without physician direction, within 1 year after its initiation is estimated to be:
   a. 15%.
   b. 30%.
   c. 50%.
   d. 75%.

9. One of the most significant concerns for medical and nursing management of hypertension is:

   a. complications from medications.

   b. insufficient information.

   c. noncompliance with recommended therapy.

   d. uncontrolled dietary management.

10. Blood pressure control is initially achieved by approximately what percentage of patients when they actively participate in their care?

   a. 10%

   b. 25%

   c. 35%

   d. 70%

SHORT ANSWER

Read each statement carefully. Write your response in the space provided.

1. Blood pressure is the product of _____ multiplied by _____.

2. Cardiac output is the product of _____ multiplied by _____.

3. Approximately _____% of the population has primary hypertension, a class of hypertension with an unidentified cause.

4. Prolonged hypertension can cause significant damage to blood vessels in four "target organs":

_____, _____, _____, and

_____.

5. List six consequences of prolonged, uncontrolled hypertension on the body and its systems.

   _____   _____

   _____   _____

   _____   _____

6. Structural and functional changes in the heart and blood vessels that occur with aging and cause hypertension are: _____, _____,

_____, and _____.

7. Give four examples of conditions that can trigger a hypertensive emergency in which blood pressure must be immediately lowered to at least 180/120 mm Hg: _____, _____,

_____, and _____.

MATCHING

Match the hypertension medication listed in column II with its associated action listed in column I.

Column I

1. _____ Blocks reabsorption of sodium and water in kidneys

2. _____ Stimulates alpha-2 adrenergic receptors

3. _____ Decreases blood volume, renal blood flow, and cardiac output

4. _____ Blocks beta-adrenergic receptors

5. _____ Inhibits aldosterone

6. _____ Impairs synthesis of norepinephrine

Column II

a. Inderal

b. Tenex

c. Aldactone

d. Lasix

e. Serpasil

f. Hygroton

II. Critical Thinking Questions and Exercises

DISCUSSION AND ANALYSIS

Discuss the following topics with your classmates.

1. Discuss in detail several hypotheses about the pathophysiologic basis for elevated blood pressure.
2. Explain how lifestyle changes and medications can control, not cure, hypertension.
3. Compare and contrast the different medications used to treat hypertension and the associated nursing considerations.
4. Discuss the implications for morbidity and mortality for eight risk factors associated with hypertension.
5. Discuss the rationale for and advantages of lifestyle and dietary modifications to prevent/manage hypertension.
6. Compare and contrast a hypertensive crisis with a hypertensive emergency.

IDENTIFYING PATTERNS

Complete the following schematic: "Pathophysiology of Hypertension Secondary to Renal Dysfunction."

Pathophysiology of Essential Hypertension

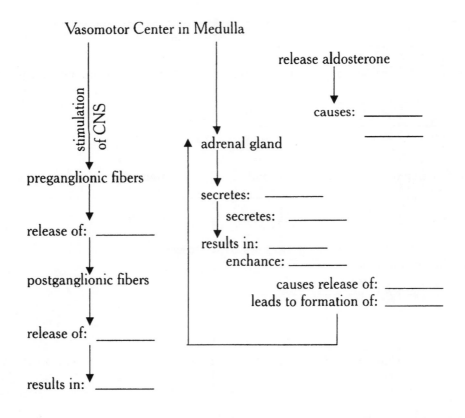

CLINICAL SITUATIONS

Read the following case study. Circle the correct answers.

CASE STUDY: Secondary Hypertension

Georgia, a 30-year-old woman, is diagnosed as having secondary hypertension when serial blood pressure recordings show her average reading to be 170/100 mm Hg. Her hypertension is the result of renal dysfunction.

1. The kidneys help maintain the hypertensive state in essential hypertension by:
   a. increasing their elimination of sodium in response to aldosterone secretion.
   b. releasing renin in response to decreased renal perfusion.
   c. secreting acetylcholine, which stimulates the sympathetic nervous system to constrict major vessels.
   d. doing all of the above.

2. Renal pathology associated with essential hypertension can be identified by:
   a. a urine output greater than 2,000 mL in 24 hours.
   b. a urine specific gravity of 1.005.
   c. hyponatremia and decreased urine osmolality.
   d. increased blood urea nitrogen and creatinine levels.

3. Georgia is prescribed spironolactone (Aldactone), 50 mg once every day. The nurse knows that spironolactone:
   a. blocks the reabsorption of sodium, thereby increasing urinary output.
   b. inhibits renal vasoconstriction, which prevents the release of renin.
   c. interferes with fluid retention by inhibiting aldosterone.
   d. prevents the secretion of epinephrine from the adrenal medulla.

4. Health education for Georgia includes advising her to:
   a. adhere to her dietary regimen.
   b. become involved in a regular program of exercise.
   c. take her medication as prescribed.
   d. do all of the above.

CHAPTER 33

Assessment and Management of Patients With Hematologic Disorders

I. Interpretation, Completion, and Comparison

MULTIPLE CHOICE

Read each question carefully. Circle your answer.

1. The physician expects that the patient has a deficiency in the leukocyte responsible for cell-mediated immunity. The nurse knows to check the white blood cell count for:
   a. basophils.
   b. monocytes.
   c. plasma cells.
   d. T lymphocytes.

2. Myeloid and lymphoid stem cells produce specific types of blood cells. The nurse knows, when evaluating blood tests, that myeloid stem cells differentiate into all of the following types of blood cells *except*:
   a. erythrocytes.
   b. leukocytes.
   c. lymphocytes.
   d. platelets.

3. The nurse notes that a patient, who is a vegetarian, has an abnormal number of megaloblasts. The nurse suspects a deficiency in:
   a. iron.
   b. zinc.
   c. vitamin C.
   d. vitamin B_{12}.

4. An elderly patient presents to the physician's office with a complaint of exhaustion. The nurse, aware of the most common hematologic condition affecting the elderly, knows to check the patient's:
   a. white blood cell count.
   b. red blood cell count.
   c. thrombocyte count.
   d. levels of plasma proteins.

5. A nurse who cares for a patient who has experienced bone marrow aspiration or biopsy should be aware of the most serious hazard of:
   a. hemorrhage.
   b. infection.
   c. shock.
   d. splintering of bone fragments.

6. A person can usually tolerate a gradual reduction in hemoglobin until the level reaches:
   a. 5.0 to 5.5 g/dL.
   b. 4.0 to 4.5 g/dL.
   c. 3.0 to 3.5 g/dL.
   d. 2.0 to 2.5 g/dL.

7. The nurse begins to design a nutritional packet of information for a patient diagnosed with iron deficiency anemia. The nurse would recommend an increased intake of:
   a. fresh citrus fruits.
   b. milk and cheese.
   c. organ meats.
   d. whole-grain breads.

8. A physician prescribes one tablet of ferrous sulfate daily for a 15-year-old girl who experiences heavy flow during her menstrual cycle. The nurse advises the patient and her mother that this over-the-counter preparation must be taken for how many months for iron replenishment to occur?
   a. 1 to 2 months
   b. 3 to 5 months
   c. 6 to 12 months
   d. Longer than 12 months

9. A patient with chronic renal failure is being examined by the nurse practitioner for anemia. The nurse knows to review the laboratory data for a decreased hemoglobin level, red blood cell count, and:
   a. decreased level of erythropoietin.
   b. decreased total iron-binding capacity.
   c. increased mean corpuscular volume.
   d. increased reticulocyte count.

10. The most frequent symptom and complication of anemia is:
    a. bleeding gums.
    b. ecchymosis.
    c. fatigue.
    d. jaundice.

11. The cause of aplastic anemia may:
    a. be related to drugs, chemicals, or radiation damage.
    b. result from the body's T cells attacking the bone marrow.
    c. result from certain infections.
    d. be related to all of the above.

12. During a routine assessment of a patient diagnosed with anemia, the nurse notes the patient's beefy red tongue. The nurse knows that this is a sign of what kind of anemia?
    a. Autoimmune
    b. Folate deficiency
    c. Iron deficiency
    d. Megaloblastic

13. A nurse should know that a diagnosis of hemolytic anemia is associated with all of the following *except*:
    a. abnormality in the circulation of plasma.
    b. decrease in the reticulocyte count.
    c. defect in the erythrocyte.
    d. elevated indirect bilirubin.

14. Absence of intrinsic factor is associated with a vitamin B_{12} deficiency, because the vitamin cannot bind to be transported for absorption in the:
    a. duodenum.
    b. ileum.
    c. jejunum.
    d. stomach.

15. A diagnostic sign of pernicious anemia is:
    a. a smooth, sore, red tongue.
    b. exertional dyspnea.
    c. pale mucous membranes.
    d. weakness.

16. The Schilling test is used to diagnose:
    a. aplastic anemia.
    b. iron deficiency anemia.
    c. megaloblastic anemia.
    d. pernicious anemia.

17. All inherited forms of sickle cell anemia would include all of the following *except*:
    a. autoimmune hemolytic.
    b. G-6-PD deficiency.
    c. thalassemia.
    d. sickle cell anemia.

18. A nurse expects an adult patient with sickle cell anemia to have a hemoglobin value of:
    a. near 3 g/dL.
    b. near 5 g/dL.
    c. between 5 and 7 g/dL.
    d. between 7 and 10 g/dL.

19. Sickle-shaped erythrocytes cause:
    a. cellular blockage in small vessels.
    b. decreased organ perfusion.
    c. tissue ischemia and infarction.
    d. all of the above.

20. A person with sickle cell trait would:
    a. be advised to avoid fluid loss and dehydration.
    b. be protected from crisis under ordinary circumstances.
    c. experience hemolytic jaundice.
    d. have chronic anemia.

21. Polycythemia vera is characterized by bone marrow overactivity, resulting in the clinical manifestations of:
    a. angina.
    b. claudication.
    c. thrombophlebitis.
    d. all of the above.

22. A patient diagnosed with neutropenia resulting from increased destruction of neutrophils would most likely have:
    a. aplastic anemia.
    b. infectious hepatitis.
    c. leukemia.
    d. a lymphoma.

23. The common feature of the leukemias is:
    a. a compensatory polycythemia stimulated by thrombocytopenia.
    b. an unregulated accumulation of white cells in the bone marrow, which replace normal marrow elements.
    c. increased blood viscosity, resulting from an overproduction of white cells.
    d. reduced plasma volume in response to a reduced production of cellular elements.

24. Nursing assessment for a patient with leukemia should include observation for:
    a. fever and infection.
    b. dehydration.
    c. petechiae and ecchymoses.
    d. all of the above.

25. The major cause of death in patients with acute myeloid leukemia is believed to be:
    a. anemia.
    b. dehydration.
    c. embolus.
    d. infection.

26. Multiple myeloma:
    a. can be diagnosed by roentgenograms that show bone lesion destruction.
    b. is a malignant disease of plasma cells that affects bone and soft tissue.
    c. is suspected in any person who evidences albuminuria.
    d. is associated with all of the above.

27. The classic presenting symptom of multiple myeloma is:
    a. debilitating fatigue.
    b. bone pain in the back of the ribs.
    c. gradual muscle paralysis.
    d. severe thrombocytopenia.

28. A patient is admitted with essential thrombocytopenia due to decreased platelet production. The nurse knows that the diagnosis is most likely:
    a. disseminated intravascular coagulation (DIC).
    b. aplastic anemia.
    c. lupus erythematosus.
    d. malignant lymphoma.

29. In the normal blood-clotting cycle, the final formation of a clot will occur:
    a. during the platelet phase.
    b. during the vascular phase.
    c. when fibrin reinforces the platelet plug.
    d. when the plasmin system produces fibrinolysis.

30. Bleeding and petechiae do not usually occur with thrombocytopenia until the platelet count falls below 50,000/mm³. The normal value for blood platelets is:
    a. 50,000 to 100,000/mm³.
    b. 100,000 to 150,000/mm³.
    c. between 150,000 and 350,000/mm³.
    d. greater than 350,000/mm³.

31. Hemophilia is a hereditary bleeding disorder that:
    a. has a higher incidence among males.
    b. is associated with joint bleeding, swelling, and damage.
    c. is related to a genetic deficiency of a specific blood-clotting factor.
    d. is associated with all of the above.

32. Hypoprothrombinemia, in the absence of gastrointestinal or biliary dysfunction, may be caused by a deficiency in vitamin:
    a. A.
    b. B₁₂.
    c. C.
    d. K.

33. A potential blood donor would be rejected if he or she:
    a. had a history of infectious disease exposure within the past 2 to 4 months.
    b. had close contact with a hemodialysis patient within the past 6 months.
    c. had donated blood within the past 3 to 6 months.
    d. had received a blood transfusion 9 to 12 months before the blood donation time.

34. The recommended minimum hemoglobin level for a woman to donate blood is:
    a. 8.0 g/dL.
    b. 10.5 g/dL.
    c. 12.5 g/dL.
    d. 14 g/dL.

SHORT ANSWER

Read each statement carefully. Write your response in the space provided.

1. The volume of blood in humans is about _____5-6_____ L.

2. Blood cell formation (hematopoiesis) occurs in the _____bone marrow_____.

3. Red bone marrow activity is confined in adults to the _____ribs_____, _____sternum_____, _____pelvis_____, and _____vertebral_____.

4. The principal function of the erythrocyte, which is composed primarily of _____hemoglobin_____, is to: _____transport O₂_____.

5. Each 100 mL of blood should normally contain _____15_____ g of hemoglobin.

6. Women of childbearing years need an additional _____2mg,_____ daily of iron to replace that loss during menstruation.

7. The nurse advises a patient who is iron deficient to take extra vitamin _____C_____, which is known for increasing iron absorption.

8. The major function of leukocytes is to: _proted body from bacteria & foreign entities._ ;
the major function of neutrophils is: _phagocytosis_ .

9. Plasma proteins consist primarily of: _albumin_ and _globulins_ .

10. The two most common areas used for bone marrow aspirations in an adult are: _sternum_ and _Iliac crest._

11. The average life expectancy for someone with sickle cell anemia is _42-48_ years.

12. Distinguish between *primary* and *secondary* polycythemia.
proliferate without stopping. _extra production of erythropoietin_

13. Secondary polycythemia is caused by: _erythropoietin_ , which may be in response
to _reduced oxygen_ .

14. The thalassemias (hereditary anemias) are characterized by: _hypochromia_ ,
microcytic , _hemolysis_ , and _anemia_

MATCHING

Match the term listed in column II with its associated definition listed in column I.

Column I

1. __e__ The fluid portion of blood
2. __J__ Another term for platelets
3. __G__ The mature form of white blood cells
4. __O__ The process of continually replacing blood cells
5. __A__ The site of blood cell formation
6. __P__ Makes up 95% of the mass of the red blood cell
7. __f__ The ingestion and digestion of bacteria by neutrophils
8. __B__ The largest classification of leukocytes
9. __q__ A clotting factor present in plasma
10. __h__ A plasma protein primarily responsible for the maintenance of fluid balance
11. __K__ The site of activity for most macrophages
12. __C__ The process of stopping bleeding from a severed blood vessel
13. __R__ A protein that forms the basis of blood clotting
14. __G__ Integral component of the immune system
15. __N__ The term for red blood cell
16. __D__ The letters used for the term reticuloendothelial system
17. __M__ The balance between clot formation and clot dissolution
18. __i__ A term used to describe T lymphocytes

Column II

a. Bone marrow
b. Monocytes
c. Hemostasis
d. RES
e. Plasma
f. Phagocytosis
g. Lymphocytes
h. Albumin
i. T cells
j. Thrombocytes
k. Spleen
l. Neutrophils
m. Hemostasis
n. Erythrocyte
o. Hematopoiesis
p. Hemoglobin
q. Fibrinogen
r. Lymphocytes

II. Critical Thinking Questions and Exercises

DISCUSSION AND ANALYSIS

Discuss the following topics with your classmates.

1. Distinguish between the etiology, clinical manifestations, and nursing interventions for the following anemias: hypoproliferative, bleeding, and hemolytic.
2. Compare the various causes of inherited and acquired hemolytic anemias.
3. Describe the pathophysiology, clinical manifestations, and nursing interventions for a patient with sickle cell anemia. Include a description of sickle cell crisis.
4. Distinguish between the pathophysiology of acute and chronic lymphocytic leukemia and compare nursing interventions for each disease.
5. Compare and contrast the pathophysiology, clinical manifestations, and medical and nursing management for Hodgkin's lymphoma and non-Hodgkin's lymphoma.
6. Discuss the nursing interventions for a patient with thrombocytopenia.
7. Discuss nursing diagnoses and interventions for a patient with DIC.
8. Explain what the "international normalized ratio" (INR) refers to.

CLINICAL SITUATIONS

Read the following case studies. Fill in the blanks or circle the correct answer.

CASE STUDY: Sickle Cell Crises

Tonika, a 15-year-old with sickle cell disease, is admitted to the hospital for treatment of sickle cell crises.

1. On the basis of the knowledge of the inheritance of the sickle cell gene (HBS), the nurse expects the patient to be of _____ descent.
   a. African *(circled)*
   b. Indian
   c. Middle Eastern
   d. Mediterranean

2. The nurse understands that the shape of the red blood cell is altered with this disease. Instead of being round, biconcave, and disclike in appearance, it can be described as _sickle_, _____, _____, and _____; the hemoglobin value is usually _7-10_ g/dL.

3. On assessment, the nurse notes that the patient's face and skull bones are enlarged. She knows this is a compensatory response to: _bone marrow expansion_.

4. The severe pain that occurs during sickle cell crises is the result of: _clotting due to lack of O₂ in capillaries_

5. The nurse understands that Tonika's abdominal pain is probably caused by involvement of the organ most commonly responsible for sequestration crises in young adults, which is the:
   a. kidney.
   b. liver.
   c. pancreas.
   d. spleen. *(circled)*

6. A cardiac response to chronic anemia includes: _fast beating_, _cardiomegaly_, and _heart murmurs_.

7. List three of six possible complications of sickle cell crises: _Pain_, _Sequestration_, and _Aplastic_.

8. Nursing interventions are focused on five goals: _____, _____, _____, _____, and _____.

CASE STUDY: Acute Myeloid Leukemia

John is a 51-year-old accountant recently diagnosed with acute myeloid leukemia.

1. Acute myeloid leukemia results from a defect in the _myeloid stem cell_ and has a peak incidence at _67_ years. The 5-year survival prognosis for those older than 65 is about _4_ %.

2. A bone marrow specimen is diagnostic if it shows an excess of: _immature blast cells_.

3. A characteristic symptom that results from insufficient red blood cell production is:
   a. bleeding tendencies.
   b. fatigue.
   c. susceptibility to infection.
   d. all of the above.

4. The 5-year survival time for those who receive treatment and are younger than 65 years of age averages:
   a. 35%.
   b. 55%.
   c. 75%.
   d. 95%.

5. The major form of therapy that frequently results in remission is:
   a. bone marrow transplantation.
   b. chemotherapy.
   c. radiation.
   d. surgical intervention.

CASE STUDY: Hodgkin's Lymphoma

Ian, a 24-year-old graduate student, was recently diagnosed as having Hodgkin's lymphoma. He sought medical attention because of an annoying pruritus and a small enlargement on the right side of his neck.

1. Ian's disease is classified as Hodgkin's paragranuloma. The nurse knows that this classification is associated with:
   a. a minimal degree of cellular differentiation in the affected nodes.
   b. an excessive production of the Reed–Sternberg cell, the diagnostic atypical cell of Hodgkin's disease.
   c. nodular sclerosis, which reflects advanced malignancy.
   d. replacement of the involved lymph nodes by tumor cells.

2. A positive diagnosis of Hodgkin's lymphoma depends on:
   a. enlarged, firm, and painful lymph nodes.
   b. histologic analysis of an enlarged lymph node.
   c. progressive anemia.
   d. the presence of generalized pruritus.

3. Ian's diagnosis of stage I Hodgkin's lymphoma implies that the disease:
   a. has disseminated diffusely to one or more extrahepatic sites.
   b. involves multiple nodes and is confined to one side of the diaphragm.
   c. is limited to a single node or a single intralymphatic organ or site.
   d. is present above and below the diaphragm and may include spleen involvement.

4. The nurse expects that Ian's course of treatment will involve:
   a. a combination of chemotherapy and radiation.
   b. a drug regimen of nitrogen mustard, vincristine, and a steroid.
   c. chemotherapy with vincristine alone.
   d. radiotherapy to the specific node over a space of 2 to 4 months.

CASE STUDY: Blood Transfusion

Jerry is to receive one unit of packed red cells because he has a hemoglobin level of 8 g/dL and a diagnosis of gastrointestinal bleeding.

1. Before initiating the transfusion, the nurse needs to check:
   a. for the abnormal presence of gas bubbles and cloudiness in the blood bag.
   b. that the blood has been typed and cross-matched.
   c. that the recipient's blood numbers match the donor's blood numbers.
   d. all of the above.

2. Administration technique should include all of the following *except*:
   a. adding 50 to 100 mL of 0.9% NaCl to the packed cells to dilute the solution and speed up delivery of the transfusion.
   b. administering the unit in combination with dextrose in water if the patient needs additional carbohydrates.
   c. administering the unit of blood over 1 to 2 hours.
   d. squeezing the bag of blood every 20 to 30 minutes during administration to mix the cell.

3. The nurse is aware that a transfusion reaction, if it occurs, will probably occur:
   a. 1 to 2 minutes after the infusion begins.
   b. during the first 15 to 30 minutes of the transfusion.
   c. after half the solution has been infused.
   d. several hours after the infusion, when the body has assimilated the new blood components into the general circulation.

4. If a transfusion reaction occurs, the nurse should:
   a. call the physician and wait for directions based on the specific type of reaction.
   b. stop the transfusion immediately and keep the vein patent with a saline or dextrose solution.
   c. slow the infusion rate and observe for an increase in the severity of the reaction.
   d. slow the infusion and request a venipuncture for retyping to start a second transfusion.

CHAPTER 34

Assessment of Digestive and Gastrointestinal Function

I. Interpretation, Completion, and Comparison

MULTIPLE CHOICE

Read each question carefully. Circle your answer.

1. Reflux of food into the esophagus from the stomach is prevented by contraction of the:
   a. ampulla of Vater.
   c. ileocecal valve.
   b. cardiac sphincter.
   d. pyloric sphincter.

2. The digestion of starches begins in the mouth with the secretion of the enzyme:
   a. lipase.
   c. ptyalin.
   b. pepsin.
   d. trypsin.

3. The stomach, which derives its acidity from hydrochloric acid, has a pH of approximately:
   a. 1.0.
   c. 5.0.
   b. 3.5.
   d. 7.5.

4. Intrinsic factor is a gastric secretion necessary for the intestinal absorption of the vitamin that prevents pernicious anemia, that is:
   a. vitamin B_1.
   c. vitamin C.
   b. vitamin B_{12}.
   d. vitamin K.

5. A hormonal regulatory substance that inhibits stomach contraction and gastric secretions is:
   a. acetylcholine.
   c. norepinephrine.
   b. gastrin.
   d. secretin.

6. An enzyme, secreted by the gallbladder, that is responsible for fat emulsification is:
   a. amylase.
   c. maltase.
   b. bile.
   d. steapsin.

7. During the initial assessment of a patient complaining of increased stomach acid related to stress, the nurse knows that the physician will want to consider the influence of the neuroregulator:
   a. gastrin.
   c. norepinephrine.
   b. cholecystokinin.
   d. secretin.

8. Pancreatic secretions into the duodenum:
   a. are stimulated by hormones released in the presence of chyme as it passes through the duodenum.
   b. have an alkaline effect on intestinal contents.
   c. increase the pH of the food contents.
   d. accomplish all of the above.

9. Bile, which emulsifies fat, enters the duodenum through the:
   a. cystic duct.
   b. common bile duct.
   c. common hepatic duct.
   d. pancreatic duct.

10. Secretin is a gastrointestinal hormone that:
    a. causes the gallbladder to contract.
    b. influences contraction of the esophageal and pyloric sphincters.
    c. regulates the secretion of gastric acid.
    d. stimulates the production of bicarbonate in pancreatic juice.

11. The major carbohydrate that tissues use for fuel is:
    a. fructose.
    b. galactose.
    c. glucose.
    d. sucrose.

12. It usually takes how long for food to enter the colon?
    a. 2 to 3 hours after a meal is eaten
    b. 4 to 5 hours after a meal is eaten
    c. 6 to 7 hours after a meal is eaten
    d. 8 to 9 hours after a meal is eaten

13. During a nursing assessment, the nurse knows that the most common symptom of patients with gastrointestinal dysfunction is:
    a. diffuse pain.
    b. dyspepsia.
    c. constipation.
    d. abdominal bloating.

14. When completing a nutritional assessment of a patient who is admitted for a gastrointestinal disorder, the nurse notes a recent history of dietary intake. This is based on the knowledge that a portion of digested waste products can remain in the rectum for how many days after a meal is digested?
    a. 1 day
    b. 2 days
    c. 3 days
    d. 4 days

15. Obstruction of the gastrointestinal tract leads to:
    a. increased force of intestinal contraction.
    b. distention above the point of obstruction.
    c. pain and a sense of bloating.
    d. all of the above.

16. A nurse who is investigating a patient's statement about duodenal pain should assess the:
    a. epigastric area and consider possible radiation of pain to the right subscapular region.
    b. hypogastrium in the right or left lower quadrant.
    c. left lower quadrant.
    d. periumbilical area, followed by the right lower quadrant.

17. Abdominal pain associated with indigestion is usually:
    a. described as crampy or burning.
    b. in the left lower quadrant.
    c. less severe after an intake of fatty foods.
    d. relieved by the intake of coarse vegetables, which stimulate peristalsis.

18. On examination of a patient's stool, the nurse suspects the presence of an upper gastrointestinal bleed when she observes a stool that is:

    a. clay-colored.

    b. greasy and foamy.

    c. tarry and black.

    d. threaded with mucus.

19. Consequences of diarrhea include all of the following *except*:

    a. acidosis.

    b. decreased bicarbonate.

    c. electrolyte imbalance.

    d. hyperkalemia.

20. The nurse has been directed to position a patient for an examination of the abdomen. She knows to place the patient in the:

    a. prone position with pillows positioned to alleviate pressure on the abdomen.

    b. semi-Fowler's position with the left leg bent to minimize pressure on the abdomen.

    c. supine position with the knees flexed to relax the abdominal muscles.

    d. reverse Trendelenburg position to facilitate the natural propulsion of intestinal contents.

21. The nurse auscultates the abdomen to assess bowel sounds. She documents five to six sounds heard in less than 30 seconds. She documents that the patient's bowel sounds are:

    a. normal.

    b. hypoactive.

    c. hyperactive.

    d. none of the above.

22. A gastric analysis with stimulation that results in an excess of gastric acid being secreted could be diagnostic of:

    a. chronic atrophic gastritis.

    b. a duodenal ulcer.

    c. gastric carcinoma.

    d. pernicious anemia.

23. Before a gastroscopy, the nurse should inform the patient that:

    a. he or she must fast for 6 to 12 hours before the examination.

    b. his or her throat will be sprayed with a local anesthetic.

    c. after gastroscopy, he or she cannot eat or drink until the gag reflex returns (1 to 2 hours).

    d. all of the above will be necessary.

24. A flexible sigmoidoscope permits examination of the lower bowel for:

    a. 5 to 10 in.

    b. 10 to 15 in.

    c. 16 to 20 in.

    d. 25 to 35 in.

25. A fiberoptic colonoscopy is most frequently used for a diagnosis of:

    a. bowel disease of unknown origin.

    b. cancer.

    c. inflammatory bowel disease.

    d. occult bleeding.

26. For adults who are older than 50 years of age and at low risk for colorectal cancer, the recommended screening is a:

    a. flexible sigmoidoscopy every 3 years.

    b. colonoscopy every 10 years.

    c. fecal occult blood test annually.

    d. colonoscopy every 2 years.

27. Magnetic resonance imaging (MRI) is contraindicated for patients who have:

    a. permanent pacemakers.

    b. artificial heart valves.

    c. implanted insulin pumps.

    d. all of the above.

28. Patient preparation for esophageal manometry requires the withholding of specific medications such as:
    a. anticholinergics.
    b. calcium-channel blockers.
    c. sedatives.
    d. all of the above.

29. The results of a gastric analysis can be used to diagnose various disease states. An *excess amount of acid* can indicate the presence of:
    a. a duodenal ulcer.
    b. gastric cancer.
    c. a peptic ulcer.
    d. pernicious anemia.

SHORT ANSWER

Read each statement carefully. Write your response in the space provided.

1. Name three pancreatic secretions that contain digestive enzymes: _____, _____, and
   _____.

2. Chyme, partially digested food that is mixed with gastric contents, stimulates segmented contractions, which are _____ and intestinal peristalsis, which is _____.

3. How many hours does it take after eating for food to pass into the terminal ileum? _____ How many hours does it take for food to reach and distend the rectum? _____

4. List three structural changes in the esophagus that occur as the result of aging: _____,
   _____, and _____.

MATCHING

Match the major digestive enzyme in column II with its associated digestive action listed in column I.

Column I

1. _____ Helps convert protein into amino acids
2. _____ Facilitates the production of dextrins and maltose
3. _____ Digests protein and helps form polypeptides
4. _____ Digests carbohydrates and helps form fructose
5. _____ Glucose is a product of this enzyme's action
6. _____ Helps form galactose

Column II

a. Amylase
b. Maltase
c. Sucrase
d. Lactase
e. Pepsin
f. Trypsin

SHORT ANSWER

For each diagnostic test, list one or more patient preparation activities that the nurse must monitor and/or document.

Diagnostic Test	*Patient Preparation*
1. Barium enema	a. _____
	b. _____
	c. _____
	d. _____
	e. _____

Diagnostic Test	*Patient Preparation*
2. Gastric analysis	a. _____
	b. _____
	c. _____
3. Upper gastrointestinal fiberscopic examination	a. _____
	b. _____
	c. _____
4. Fiberoptic colonoscopy	a. _____
	b. _____
	c. _____
	d. _____

II. Critical Thinking Questions and Exercises

IDENTIFYING PATTERNS

Accurate documentation of a pain's location by the nurse is essential to help with a diagnosis. Examine Figure 34-3 in the text and for each site identified, choose the quadrant and the region of the pain's location. Begin clockwise with the first site (referred heart pain) and end with the ninth site (referred liver pain). Use Figure 34-3 as a reference for the names of the quadrants and the regions.

SITE OF REFERRED PAIN

1. Heart (sample)

2. Renal colic

3. Small intestine

4. Ureteral colic

5. Colon

6. Appendicitis

7. Cholecystitis

8. Biliary colic

9. Liver

QUADRANT
Left upper (LUQ)

REGION
Left hypochondriac region

CHAPTER 35

Management of Patients With Oral and Esophageal Disorders

I. Interpretation, Completion, and Comparison

MULTIPLE CHOICE

Read each question carefully. Circle your answer.

1. A nurse knows that adequate nutrition is related to good dental health. As part of health assessment, a nurse also knows that about what percentage of adults 45 to 64 years of age have severe periodontal disease?

   a. 5%

   b. 10%

   c. 15%

   d. 25%

2. Actinic cheilitis is a lip lesion that results from sun exposure and can lead to squamous cell carcinoma. It is evidenced by:

   a. erythema.

   b. fissuring.

   c. white hyperkeratosis.

   d. all of the above.

3. A common disease of oral tissue characterized by painful, inflamed, and swollen gums is:

   a. candidiasis.

   b. gingivitis.

   c. herpes simplex.

   d. periodontitis.

4. A common lesion of the mouth that is also referred to as a "canker sore" is:

   a. aphthous stomatitis.

   b. candidiasis.

   c. leukoplakia buccalis.

   d. lichen planus.

5. The incidence of most dental caries is directly related to an increase in the dietary intake of:

   a. fat.

   b. protein.

   c. salt.

   d. sugar.

6. Postoperative nursing care for drainage of a dentoalveolar or periapical abscess includes all of the following *except*:

   a. soft diet after 24 hours.

   b. fluid restriction for the first 48 hours because the gums are swollen and painful.

   c. external heat by pad or compress to hasten the resolution of the inflammatory swelling.

   d. warm saline mouthwashes every 2 hours while awake.

7. Preventive orthodontics for malocclusion can start as early as age:

   a. 3 years.

   b. 5 years.

   c. 7 years.

   d. 9 years.

8. A patient complains about an inflamed salivary gland below his right ear. The nurse documents probable inflammation of which gland(s)?

   a. Buccal

   b. Parotid

   c. Sublingual

   d. Submandibular

9. Mumps, a viral infection affecting children, is usually an inflammation of which gland(s)?

   a. Buccal

   b. Parotid

   c. Sublingual

   d. Submaxillary

10. Parotitis, frequently seen in the elderly or debilitated patient, is usually caused by:

    a. Methicillin-resistant *Streptococcus aureus* (MRSA).

    b. *Pneumococcus.*

    c. *Staphylococcus aureus.*

    d. *Streptococcus viridans.*

11. A nurse inspects the Stensen duct of the parotid gland to determine inflammation and possible obstruction. The nurse would examine the oral cavity in the area of the:

    a. buccal mucosa next to the upper molars.

    b. dorsum of the tongue.

    c. roof of the mouth next to the incisors.

    d. posterior segment of the tongue near the uvula.

12. Neoplasms of the salivary glands:

    a. are normally malignant and are treated by surgical excision.

    b. commonly recur, and recurrences are more malignant than the original tumor.

    c. are usually always treated with radiation.

    d. are characterized by all of the above.

13. If detected early, prior to lymph node involvement, the 5-year survival rate for oral cancer is about what percent?

    a. 50%

    b. 60%

    c. 70%

    d. 80%

14. The most common site for cancer of the oral cavity is the:

    a. lip.

    b. mouth.

    c. pharynx.

    d. tongue.

15. The typical lesion in oral cancer can be described as:

    a. an indurated ulcer.

    b. a warty growth.

    c. a white or red plaque.

    d. a painful sore.

16. Usually, the first symptom associated with esophageal disease is:

    a. dysphagia.

    b. malnutrition.

    c. pain.

    d. regurgitation of food.

17. The nurse suspects that a patient who presents with the symptom of food "sticking" in the lower portion of the esophagus may have the motility disorder known as:

    a. achalasia.

    b. diffuse spasm.

    c. gastroesophageal reflex.

    d. hiatal hernia.

18. A hiatal hernia involves:

    a. an extension of the esophagus through an opening in the diaphragm.

    b. an involution of the esophagus, which causes a severe stricture.

    c. a protrusion of the upper stomach into the lower portion of the thorax.

    d. a twisting of the duodenum through an opening in the diaphragm.

19. Intervention for a person who has swallowed strong acid includes all of the following *except*:

    a. administering an irritant that will stimulate vomiting.

    b. aspirating secretions from the pharynx if respirations are affected.

    c. neutralizing the chemical.

    d. washing the esophagus with large volumes of water.

20. The most common symptom that patients with gastroesophageal reflux disease (GERD) mention is:

    a. dyspepsia.

    b. odynophagia.

    c. pyrosis.

    d. regurgitation.

21. Cancer of the esophagus occurs primarily in:

    a. black men older than 50 years of age.

    b. black women after menopause.

    c. white men 30 to 40 years old.

    d. white women older than 60 years of age.

22. A common postoperative complication of esophageal surgery for cancer is:

    a. aspiration pneumonia.

    b. hemorrhage.

    c. incompetence of the suture line, resulting in fluid seepage.

    d. the dumping syndrome.

MATCHING

Match the abnormality of the lips, mouth, or gums listed in column II with its associated symptomatology of the lip, mouth, or gums listed in column I.

Column I

1. _____ Ulcerated and painful, white papules

2. _____ Reddened area or rash associated with itching

3. _____ Painful, inflamed, swollen gums

4. _____ White overgrowth of horny layer of epidermis

5. _____ Shallow ulcer with a red border and white or yellow center

6. _____ Hyperkeratotic white patches usually in buccal mucosa

7. _____ Reddened circumscribed lesion that ulcerates and becomes encrusted

8. _____ White patches with rough, hairlike projections usually found on the tongue

Column II

a. Actinic cheilitis

b. Leukoplakia

c. Chancre

d. Canker sore

e. Gingivitis

f. Lichen planus

g. Contact dermatitis

h. Hairy leukoplakia

II. Critical Thinking Questions and Exercises

DISCUSSION AND ANALYSIS

Discuss the following topics with your classmates.

1. Discuss at least eight healthy oral hygiene habits that have been found to promote good dental health.
2. Explain the infectious processes, clinical manifestations, and medical/nursing interventions associated with a periapical abscess.
3. Compare and contrast the clinical manifestations and medical/nursing interventions for sialadenitis and sialolithiasis.
4. Discuss the various nursing interventions for a patient with cancer of the oral cavity.
5. Distinguish between the three types of neck dissection: a classic radical neck, a modified radical neck, and a selective neck.
6. Discuss about nine major nursing diagnoses related to the surgical process of neck dissection.
7. Discuss nursing interventions for the postoperative care of a patient who has had a neck dissection.
8. Compare and contrast the etiology, clinical manifestations, and medical/nursing interventions for achalasia and diffuse esophageal spasm.
9. Discuss the nursing interventions for a patient with cancer of the esophagus.

APPLYING CONCEPTS

Refer to the figure below and answer the following questions related to a neck dissection procedure.

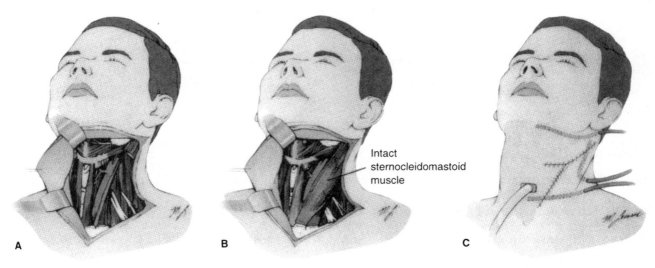

(A) A classic radical neck dissection in which the sternocleidomastoid and smaller muscles are removed. All tissue is removed from the ramus of the jaw to the clavicle. The jugular vein has also been removed. Selective **(B)** is similar but preserves the sternocleidomastoid muscle, internal jugular vein, and the spinal accessory nerve. The wound is closed **(C)**, and portable suction drainage tubes are in place.

Read each question carefully. Either circle the correct answer or write the best response in the space provided.

1. A radical neck dissection (see Figure 35-4) is often performed to help prevent _____, the primary reason for death from neck malignancies.

2. Two common morbidities associated with a radical neck dissection are: _____ and _____.

3. Reconstructive techniques involve grafts that normally use the _____ muscle.

4. List three postoperative complications expected when someone has surgery to the neck area (see A and B):
_____, _____, and _____.

5. Three collaborative, postoperative nursing problems may be: _____, _____, and
_____.

6. After a radical neck dissection, a patient is placed in Fowler's position to:
   a. decrease venous pressure on the skin flaps.
   b. facilitate swallowing.
   c. increase lymphatic drainage.
   d. accomplish all of the above.

7. Postoperatively, a finding that should be immediately reported because it may indicate airway obstruction is:
   a. temperature of 99°F.
   b. pain.
   c. stridor.
   d. localized wound tenderness.

8. A nurse who is caring for a patient who has had radical neck surgery notices an abnormal amount of serosanguineous secretions in the wound suction unit during the first postoperative day. An expected normal amount of drainage is:
   a. between 40 and 80 mL.
   b. approximately 80 to 120 mL.
   c. between 120 and 160 mL.
   d. greater than 160 mL.

9. A major potential complication from graft necrosis or artery damage is hemorrhage from the:
   a. brachial artery.
   b. carotid artery.
   c. innominate artery.
   d. vertebral artery.

10. Postoperatively, the nurse observes excessive drooling. She assesses for damage to the:
    a. facial nerve.
    b. hypoglossal nerve.
    c. spinal accessory nerve.
    d. auditory nerve.

CLINICAL SITUATIONS

Read the following case studies. Fill in the blanks or circle the correct answer.

CASE STUDY: Mandibular Fracture

William, a 17-year-old student, suffered a mandibular fracture while playing football. He is scheduled for jaw repositioning surgery.

1. Preoperatively, the nurse explains the surgical procedure for treatment of a mandibular fracture. Describe the procedure that would be used.

_____

2. Postoperatively, the nurse should immediately position William:
   a. flat on his back to facilitate lung expansion during inspiration.
   b. on his side with his head slightly elevated to prevent aspiration.
   c. supine with his head to the side to promote the drainage of secretions.
   d. with his head lower than his trunk to prevent aspiration of fluids.

3. Postoperatively, the nurse's primary goal is to maintain:
   a. adequate nutrition.
   b. an open airway.
   c. jaw immobilization.
   d. oral hygiene.

4. What would you tell the patient to explain why nasogastric suctioning is needed?

_____

5. For emergency use, which of the following should be available at the head of the bed?
   a. A nasogastric suction tube
   b. A nasopharyngeal suction catheter
   c. A wire cutter or scissors
   d. An oxygen cannula

6. A recommended initial postoperative diet for William would be:
   a. bland pureed.
   b. clear liquid.
   c. full liquid.
   d. semisoft.

7. William must be instructed not to chew food until the ____ postoperative week.
   a. third
   b. fourth
   c. fifth
   d. eighth

8. What essential item must be sent home with William when he is discharged?

_____

CASE STUDY: Cancer of the Mouth

Edith, a 64-year-old mother of two, has been a chain smoker for 20 years. During the past month she noticed a dryness in her mouth and a roughened area that is irritating. She mentioned her symptoms to her dentist, who referred her to a medical internist.

1. On the basis of the patient's health history, the nurse suspects oral cancer. Describe what the nurse would expect the lesion to look like.

_____

2. During the health history, the nurse noted that Edith did not mention a late-occurring symptom of mouth cancer, which is:
   a. drainage.
   b. fever.
   c. odor.
   d. pain.

3. On physical examination, Edith evidenced changes associated with cancer of the mouth, such as:
   a. a sore, roughened area that has not healed in 3 weeks.
   b. minor swelling in an area adjacent to the lesion.
   c. numbness in the affected area of the mouth.
   d. all of the above.

4. To confirm a diagnosis of carcinoma of the mouth, a physician would order:
   a. a biopsy.
   b. a staining procedure.
   c. exfoliative cytology.
   d. roentgenography.

5. A frequent complication of oral surgery when the salivary glands have to be radiated is: _____.

Study Guide for Brunner and Suddarth's Textbook of Medical-Surgical Nursing, 12th edition.

CHAPTER 36

Gastrointestinal Intubation and Special Nutritional Modalities

I. Interpretation, Completion, and Comparison

MULTIPLE CHOICE

Read each question carefully. Circle your answer.

1. The physician ordered a nasoenteric feeding tube with a tungsten-weighted tip. The nurse knows to obtain what kind of tube?
   a. Dobbhoff
   b. Levin
   c. Salem
   d. Sengstaken–Blakemore

2. A nurse prepares a patient for insertion of a nasoenteric tube. The nurse positions the patient:
   a. in high-Fowler's position.
   b. flat in bed.
   c. on his or her right side.
   d. in semi-Fowler's position with his or her head turned to the left.

3. The Levin tube, a commonly used nasogastric tube, has circular markings at specific points. The tube should be inserted to 6 to10 cm beyond what length?
   a. A length of 50 cm (20 in).
   b. A point that equals the distance from the nose to the xiphoid process.
   c. The distance measured from the tip of the nose to the earlobe and from the earlobe to the xiphoid process.
   d. The distance determined by measuring from the tragus of the ear to the xiphoid process.

4. When continuous or intermittent suction is used with a nasogastric tube, the goal is to have the amount of suction in the gastric mucosa reduced to:
   a. 30 to 40 mm Hg.
   b. 60 mm Hg.
   c. 70 to 80 mm Hg.
   d. 100 to 120 mm Hg.

5. One way to confirm placement of a nasogastric tube is to ensure that the nurse tests the pH of the tube aspirate. The nurse knows that the tube placement in the lungs is indicated by what pH?
   a. 1
   b. 2
   c. 4
   d. 6

6. It is essential for the nurse who is managing a gastric sump (Salem) tube to:
   a. maintain intermittent or continuous suction at a rate greater than 120 mm Hg.
   b. keep the vent lumen above the patient's waist to prevent gastric content reflux.
   c. irrigate only through the vent lumen.
   d. do all of the above.

7. A nasoenteric decompression tube can be safely advanced 2 to 3 in every:
   a. 1 hour.
   b. 2 hours.
   c. 4 hours.
   d. 8 hours.

8. Nasoenteric tubes usually remain in place until:
   a. bowel sound is present.
   b. flatus is passed.
   c. peristalsis is resumed.
   d. all of the above mechanisms occur.

9. Symptoms of oliguria, lethargy, and tachycardia in a patient would indicate to the nurse that the patient may be experiencing the initial common potential complication of nasoenteric intubation, which is:
   a. a cardiac dysrhythmia.
   b. fluid volume deficit.
   c. mucous membrane irritation.
   d. pulmonary complications.

10. Osmosis is the process whereby:
    a. particles disperse throughout a liquid medium to achieve an equal concentration throughout.
    b. particles move from an area of greater concentration to an area of lesser concentration to establish equilibrium.
    c. water moves through a membrane from a dilute solution to a more concentrated solution to achieve equal osmolality.
    d. water moves through a membrane from an area of higher osmolality to an area of lesser osmolality to establish equilibrium.

11. Residual content is checked before each intermittent tube feeding. The patient would be reassessed if the residual, on two occasions, was:
    a. about 50 mL.
    b. between 50 and 80 mL.
    c. about 100 mL.
    d. greater than 200 mL.

12. The dumping syndrome occurs when high-carbohydrate foods are administered over a period of less than 20 minutes. A nursing measure to prevent or minimize the dumping syndrome is to administer the feeding:
    a. at a warm temperature to decrease peristalsis.
    b. by bolus to prevent continuous intestinal distention.
    c. with about 100 mL of fluid to dilute the high carbohydrate concentration.
    d. with the patient in semi-Fowler's position to decrease transit time influenced by gravity.

13. Gastrostomy feedings are preferred to nasogastric feedings in the comatose patient, because the:
    a. gastroesophageal sphincter is intact, lessening the possibility of regurgitation.
    b. digestive process occurs more rapidly as a result of the feedings not having to pass through the esophagus.
    c. feedings can be administered with the patient in the recumbent position.
    d. the patient cannot experience the deprivational stress of not swallowing.

14. Initial fluid nourishment after a gastrostomy usually consists of:
    a. distilled water.
    b. 10% glucose and tap water.
    c. milk.
    d. high-calorie liquids.

15. When administering a bolus gastrostomy feeding, the receptacle should be held no higher than:
    a. 9 in.
    b. 18 in.
    c. 27 in.
    d. 36 in.

16. The basic hyperalimentation solution consists of what percentage of glucose?
    a. 10%
    b. 25%
    c. 35%
    d. 50%

17. The preferred route for infusion of parenteral nutrition is the:
   a. brachial vein.
   b. jugular vein.
   c. subclavian vein.
   d. superior vena cava.

18. The most common infectious fungal organism for patients receiving parenteral nutrition is:
   a. *Candida albicans.*
   b. *Klebsiella pneumoniae.*
   c. *Staphylococcus aureus.*
   d. *Staphylococcus epidermidis.*

19. Patients who are receiving total parenteral nutrition should be observed for signs of hyperglycemia, which would include:
   a. diuresis.
   b. lethargy.
   c. stupor.
   d. all of the above.

MATCHING

Match the description of the type of nasogastric, nasoenteric, and regular feeding tube in column II with its appropriate name listed in column I.

Column I

1. _____ Sengstaken–Blakemore

2. _____ Levin

3. _____ Gastric-Sump Salem

4. _____ Moss

5. _____ Dubhoff or Keofeed II

Column II

a. Triple-lumen nasogastric tube that also has a duodenal lumen for postoperative feedings
b. Nasoenteric feeding tube about 6 ft in length
c. Single-lumen, plastic, or rubber nasogastric tube about 4 ft in length
d. Double-lumen, plastic nasogastric tube about 20 cm in length
e. Triple-lumen, rubber nasogastric tube (two lumens are used to inflate the gastric and esophageal balloons)

II. Critical Thinking Questions and Exercises

DISCUSSION AND ANALYSIS

Discuss the following topics with your classmates.

1. Discuss the purposes for gastric intubation.
2. Describe the color of aspirate that distinguishes gastric tube placement versus intestinal placement.
3. Demonstrate, via simulation, the steps a nurse would take to declog an enteral feeding tube.
4. Describe the signs and symptoms that a nurse should assess for a patient experiencing one of three potential complications of enteric tube placement: fluid volume deficit, pulmonary complications, and tube-related irritations.
5. Discuss nursing interventions for four gastrointestinal complications of enteral therapy: diarrhea, nausea and vomiting, gas/bloating/cramping, and constipation.
6. Explain why an infusion pump is always used to administer parenteral nutrition.

CLINICAL SITUATIONS

Read the following case studies. Fill in the blanks or circle the correct answer.

CASE STUDY: Dumping Syndrome

Nancy is 37 years old, 5 ft 7 in tall, and weighs 140 lb. She receives 250 mL of a feeding over a 15-minute period every 4 hours through a nasogastric tube. Nancy has had esophageal surgery for carcinoma.

1. Nancy tells the nurse that she has diarrhea. The nurse suspects Nancy is experiencing the dumping syndrome. The nurse also knows that she needs to eliminate other possible causes, such as: _____, _____, _____, and _____.

2. The nurse reviews Nancy's chart to see what medications she is receiving, because certain drugs increase the frequency of the syndrome in some patients. List three of six medications: _____, _____, and _____.

3. Because of the dumping syndrome, the physician reduces Nancy's current rate of infusion by 50%. The nurse should adjust the rate of the gastrostomy feeding to _____ mL/min.
   a. 8
   b. 10
   c. 12
   d. 16

4. The nurse notes a residual gastric content of 50 mL. She should:
   a. delay the feeding for 2 hours and reassess.
   b. discard the 50 mL and administer the next feeding.
   c. notify the physician.
   d. return the solution through the tube and administer the next feeding.

CASE STUDY: Total Parenteral Nutrition

Penny is 30 years old and single. She is 5 ft 7 in tall, weighs 150 lb, and is receiving parenteral nutrition solution at the rate of 3 L/day. Her postoperative condition warrants receiving nutrients by the intravenous route.

1. The nurse knows that, to spare body protein, Penny's daily calorie intake must be:
   a. about 500 calories per day.
   b. approximately 1,500 calories per day.
   c. around 800 calories per day.
   d. equal to 1,000 calories per day.

2. The nurse estimates Penny's caloric intake for each 1,000 mL of total parenteral nutrition to yield a glucose concentration of _____ calories.
   a. 500
   b. 800
   c. 1,000
   d. 1,500

3. Penny's infusion rate is 120 mL/h. Her rate has slowed because of positional body changes. To compensate, the nurse could safely increase Penny's rate for 8 hours to _____ mL/h.
   a. 100
   b. 125
   c. 138
   d. 146

4. The nurse should observe Penny for signs of rapid fluid intake, which may include:
   a. chills.
   b. fever.
   c. nausea.
   d. all of the above.

5. The nurse weighs Penny daily. After 7 days, Penny's weight gain is abnormal at:
   a. 3.5 lb.
   b. 5.0 lb.
   c. 7.0 lb.
   d. 12 lb.

APPLYING CONCEPTS

Refer to the figure below and answer the following questions.

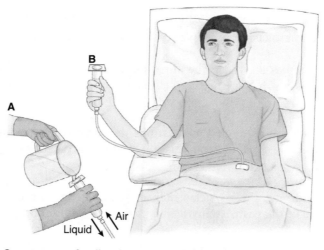

Gastrostomy feeding by gravity. **A,** Feeding is instilled at an angle so that air does not enter the stomach. **B,** Syringe is raised perpendicular to the stomach so that feeding can enter by gravity.

1. List three nursing diagnoses for a postoperative patient that address nursing care for a gastrostomy tube.

   a. _____

   b. _____

   c. _____

2. List three possible collaborative problems for a patient with a gastrostomy tube.

   a. _____

   b. _____

   c. _____

3. When giving an initial tube feeding, the nurse would be looking for _____ around the tube site on the abdomen.

4. A dressing over the tube outlet and the gastrostomy tube protects the skin around the incision from

   _____ and _____ .

5. The syringe, filled with feeding solution, is raised perpendicular to the abdomen so that the solution can enter by gravity. How long should it take for 100 mL to instill?

   _____

6. If the solution fails to instill, the nurse could

_____

_____.

7. The syringe should not be elevated higher than 18 in above the abdominal wall, because:

_____

_____.

8. Explain why the patient in the figure is sitting upright.

_____

_____.

CHAPTER 37

Management of Patients With Gastric and Duodenal Disorders

I. Interpretation, Completion, and Comparison

MULTIPLE CHOICE

Read each question carefully. Circle your answer.

1. Acute gastritis is often caused by:
   a. ingestion of strong acids.
   b. irritating foods.
   c. overuse of aspirin.
   d. all of the above.

2. To promote fluid balance when treating gastritis, the nurse knows that the minimal daily intake of fluids should be:
   a. 1.0 L.
   b. 1.5 L.
   c. 2.0 L.
   d. 2.5 L.

3. The most common site for peptic ulcer formation is the:
   a. duodenum.
   b. esophagus.
   c. pylorus.
   d. stomach.

4. A symptom that distinguishes a chronic gastric ulcer from a chronic duodenal ulcer is the:
   a. absence of any correlation between the presence of the ulcer and a malignancy.
   b. normal to below-normal secretion of acid.
   c. relief of pain after food ingestion.
   d. uncommon incidence of vomiting.

5. Peptic ulcers occur with the most frequency in those between the ages of:
   a. 15 and 25 years.
   b. 20 and 30 years.
   c. 40 and 60 years.
   d. 60 and 80 years.

6. A frequently prescribed proton pump inhibitor of gastric acid is:
   a. Nexium.
   b. Pepcid.
   c. Tagamet.
   d. Zantac.

7. The percentage of patients with peptic ulcers who experience bleeding is:
   a. less than 5%.
   b. 15%.
   c. 25%.
   d. greater than 50%.

8. A characteristic associated with peptic ulcer pain is a:

    a. burning sensation localized in the back or midepigastrium.

    b. feeling of emptiness that precedes meals from 1 to 3 hours.

    c. severe gnawing pain that increases in severity as the day progresses.

    d. combination of all of the above.

9. The best time to administer an antacid is:

    a. with the meal.

    b. 30 minutes before the meal.

    c. 1 to 3 hours after the meal.

    d. immediately after the meal.

10. A Billroth I procedure is a surgical approach to ulcer management whereby:

    a. a partial gastrectomy is performed with anastomosis of the stomach segment to the duodenum.

    b. a sectioned portion of the stomach is joined to the jejunum.

    c. the antral portion of the stomach is removed and a vagotomy is performed.

    d. the vagus nerve is cut and gastric drainage is established.

11. The most common complication of peptic ulcer disease that occurs in 10% to 20% of patients is:

    a. hemorrhage.

    b. intractable ulcer.

    c. perforation.

    d. pyloric obstruction.

12. Nursing interventions associated with peptic ulcers include:

    a. checking the blood pressure and pulse rate every 15 to 20 minutes.

    b. frequently monitoring hemoglobin and hematocrit levels.

    c. observing stools and vomitus for color, consistency, and volume.

    d. all of the above.

13. If peptic ulcer hemorrhage was suspected, an immediate nursing action would be to:

    a. place the patient in a recumbent position with his or her legs elevated.

    b. prepare a peripheral and central line for intravenous infusion.

    c. assess vital signs.

    d. accomplish all of the above.

14. Pyloric (gastric outlet) obstruction can occur when the area distal to the pyloric sphincter becomes stenosed by:

    a. edema.

    b. scar tissue.

    c. spasm.

    d. all of the above.

15. Symptoms associated with pyloric obstruction include all of the following *except*:

    a. anorexia.

    b. diarrhea.

    c. nausea and vomiting.

    d. epigastric fullness.

16. Morbid obesity is a term applied to people who are more than:

    a. 15 kg above their body mass index.

    b. 50 lb above ideal body weight.

    c. 100 lb above ideal body weight.

    d. more than twice their ideal body weight.

17. The average weight loss after bariatric surgery is about what percent of previous body weight?

    a. 25%

    b. 40%

    c. 60%

    d. 80%

18. Pulmonary complications frequently follow upper abdominal incisions, because:

a. aspiration is a common occurrence associated with postoperative injury to the pyloric sphincter or the cardiac sphincter.

b. pneumothorax is a common complication of abdominal surgery when the chest cavity has been entered.

c. the patient tends to have shallow respirations in an attempt to minimize incisional pain.

d. all of the above.

19. Teaching points to help a patient with total gastric resection avoid the dumping syndrome include all of the following *except*:

a. eating small, frequent meals.

b. increasing the carbohydrate content of the diet to supply needed calories for energy.

c. lying down after meals.

d. taking fluids between meals to decrease the total volume in the stomach at one time.

SHORT ANSWER

Read each statement carefully. Write the best response in the space provided.

1. Describe the immediate intervention that should be used to treat the ingestion of a corrosive acid or alkali.

2. Explain why patients with gastritis due to a vitamin deficiency usually have malabsorption of vitamin B_{12}.

3. Name two conditions specifically related to peptic ulcer development: _____ and _____.

4. The bacillus that is commonly associated with gastric and possibly duodenal ulcers: _____.

5. List several findings characteristic of Zollinger–Ellison syndrome.

6. Define the term stress ulcer.

7. Distinguish between Cushing's and Curling's ulcer in terms of cause and location.

8. Explain the current theory about diet modification for peptic ulcer disease.

9. Name four major, potential complications of a peptic ulcer: _____, _____, _____, and _____.

10. Describe the clinical manifestations associated with peptic ulcer perforation.

11. Bariatric surgery works by: _____ and _____.

12. The stomach pouches created by gastric bypass or bonding surgery can hold up to _____ mL of food and fluids.

13. The most common, primary, malignant tumor of the duodenum is: _____. Which portions of the

    duodenum does it involve? The _____ and _____.

SCRAMBLEGRAM

Unscramble the letters used to answer each statement and write the word in the space provided.

1. Lack of hydrochloric acid in digestive secretions of the stomach: _____.

L H O D H I A R C Y R A

2. Inflammation of the stomach: _____.

A R T S G T I I S

3. Vomiting of blood: _____.

M T E S E H S A I M E

4. Term used to describe black and tarry stools: _____.

L N E A M E

5. Opening between the stomach and duodenum: _____.

L R P U S O Y

6. Medical term to describe heartburn: _____.

Y O S P I S R

II. Critical Thinking Questions and Exercises

DISCUSSION AND ANALYSIS

Discuss the following topics with your classmates.

1. Compare and contrast the etiology of chronic and acute gastritis.
2. Describe the pathophysiology of gastritis.
3. Chronic gastritis can be caused by the bacteria *Helicobacter pylori*. Name four diagnostic tests that can be used to determine the presence of the bacteria.
4. Discuss the nursing considerations, including patient teaching, for patients receiving proton pump inhibitors for gastritis.
5. Compare the incidence and symptoms for duodenal versus gastric ulcers.
6. Describe the differences between the three surgical procedures for peptic ulcer disease: vagotomy, pyloroplasty, and antrectomy.
7. Describe the criteria used to select patients for bariatric surgery.
8. Discuss the dietary guidelines for a patient who has had bariatric surgery.
9. Describe the vasomotor and gastrointestinal symptoms found in the dumping syndrome.

EXTRACTING INFERENCES

Examine the figure below. Outline in detail the pathophysiology of peptic ulcer formation. Explain why specific sites are more common and what contributes to common inflammatory sites.

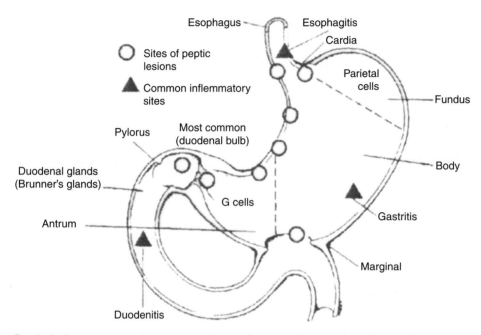

Peptic lesions may occur in the esophagus (esophagitis), stomach (gastritis), or duodenum (duodenitis). Note peptic ulcer sites and common inflammatory sites. Hydrochloric acid is formed by parietal cells in the fundus; gastrin is secreted by G cells in the antrum. The duodenal glands secrete an alkaline mucous solution.

CLINICAL SITUATIONS

Read the following case study. Fill in the blanks or circle the correct answer.

CASE STUDY: Gastric Cancer

Mr. Jackson, a 66-year-old African American, has recently been seen by a physician to confirm a diagnosis of gastric cancer. He has a history of tobacco use and was diagnosed 10 years ago with pernicious anemia. He and his family are shocked about the possibility of this diagnosis because he has been asymptomatic prior to recent complaints of pain and multiple gastrointestinal symptoms.

1. On the basis of her knowledge of disease progression, the nurse assumes that organs adjacent to the
   stomach are also affected such as the_____, _____, _____, and
   _____.

2. On palpitation, the nurse notes two signs that confirm metastasis to the liver: _____ and
   _____.

3. The nurse advises the patient that four diagnostic procedures will be conducted. Two will be used to
   confirm a diagnosis of cancer: _____ and _____; another
   procedure _____ will be performed to assess tumor depth and lymph node
   involvement; and _____ will be used to determine surgical respectability of the probable tumor.

4. The surgical team has decided that a Billroth II would be the best approach to treatment. The nurse explains to the family that this procedure involves a:

a. limited resection in the distal portion of the stomach (removal of about 25% of the stomach).

b. wide resection of the middle and distal portions of the stomach (removal of about 75% of the stomach).

c. proximal subtotal gastrectomy.

d. total gastrectomy and esophagogastrectomy.

5. The nurse explains that combination chemotherapy, more effective than single-agent chemotherapy, frequently follows surgery. The primary agent used would most likely be: _____.

CHAPTER 38

Management of Patients With Intestinal and Rectal Disorders

I. Interpretation, Completion, and Comparison

MULTIPLE CHOICE

Read each question carefully. Circle your answer.

1. The pathophysiology of constipation may be related to interference with:
   a. myoelectric activity of the colon.
   b. mucosal transport.
   c. processes involved in defecation.
   d. all of the above mechanisms.

2. Nursing suggestions to help a person break the constipation habit include all of the following *except*:
   a. a fluid intake of at least 2 L/day.
   b. a low-residue, bland diet.
   c. establishing a regular schedule of exercise.
   d. establishing a regular time for daily elimination.

3. An example of a stimulant laxative that works in 6 to 8 hours is:
   a. Colace.
   b. Colyte.
   c. Dulcolax.
   d. Milk of magnesia.

4. The classification of *moderate diarrhea* refers to the quantity of daily unformed stools described as:
   a. more than two bowel movements a day.
   b. between two and three bowel movements a day.
   c. between three and six bowel movements a day.
   d. more than six bowel movements a day.

5. In assessing stool characteristics associated with diarrhea, the nurse knows that the presence of greasy stools suggests:
   a. disorders of the colon.
   b. inflammatory enteritis.
   c. intestinal malabsorption.
   d. small-bowel disorders.

6. Hypokalemia may occur rapidly in an elderly person who experiences diarrhea. The nurse should immediately report to the physician a critical potassium level of:
   a. 3.5 mEq/L.
   b. 4.5 mEq/L.
   c. 5.5 mEq/L.
   d. 6.5 mEq/L.

7. A disorder of malabsorption that inactivates pancreatic enzymes is:
   a. celiac disease.
   b. cystic fibrosis.
   c. Whipple's disease.
   d. Zollinger–Ellison syndrome.

8. Malabsorption diseases may affect the ability of the digestive system to absorb the major water-soluble:
   a. vitamin A.
   b. vitamin B_{12}.
   c. vitamin D.
   d. vitamin K.

9. A positive Rovsing's sign is indicative of appendicitis. The nurse knows to assess for this indicator by palpating the:
   a. right lower quadrant.
   b. left lower quadrant.
   c. right upper quadrant.
   d. left upper quadrant.

10. The most common site for diverticulitis is the:
    a. duodenum.
    b. ileum.
    c. jejunum.
    d. sigmoid.

11. The incidence of diverticulitis in those older than 80 years of age is about:
    a. 15%.
    b. 35%.
    c. 50%.
    d. 75%.

12. Diverticulitis is clinically manifested by:
    a. a low-grade fever.
    b. a change in bowel habits.
    c. left lower quadrant pain.
    d. all of the above.

13. Common clinical manifestations of Crohn's disease are:
    a. abdominal pain and diarrhea.
    b. edema and weight gain.
    c. nausea and vomiting.
    d. obstruction and ileus.

14. A nurse suspects a diagnosis of regional enteritis when she assesses the symptoms of:
    a. abdominal distention and rebound tenderness.
    b. hyperactive bowel sounds in the right lower quadrant.
    c. intermittent pain associated with diarrhea.
    d. all of the above.

15. Nutritional management for regional enteritis consists of diet therapy that is:
    a. high in fats.
    b. high in fiber.
    c. low in protein.
    d. low in residue.

16. Remission of inflammation in ulcerative colitis is possible with:
    a. antidiarrheal medication.
    b. periods of rest after meals.
    c. steroid therapy.
    d. all of the above.

17. A problem unique to the patient with an ileostomy is that:
    a. regular bowel habits cannot be established.
    b. sexual activity is restricted.
    c. skin excoriation can occur.
    d. the collecting appliance is bulky and large.

18. Postoperative nursing management for a patient with a continent ileostomy includes all of the following *except*:
    a. checking to make certain that the rectal packing is in place.
    b. irrigating the ileostomy catheter every 3 hours.
    c. nasogastric tube feedings, 30 to 50 mL, every 4 to 6 hours.
    d. perineal irrigations after the dressings are removed.

19. Clinical manifestations associated with small-bowel obstruction include all of the following *except*:
    a. dehydration.
    b. pain that is wavelike.
    c. the passage of blood-tinged stool.
    d. vomiting.

20. The 5-year survival rate for cancer of the colon that is detected early is:
    a. less than 20%.
    b. 25% to 35%.
    c. 50% to 60%.
    d. about 90%.

21. Preoperatively, intestinal antibiotics are given for colon surgery to:
    a. decrease the bulk of colon contents.
    b. reduce the bacteria content of the colon.
    c. soften the stool.
    d. do all of the above.

22. For colostomy irrigation, the enema catheter should be inserted into the stoma:
    a. 1 in.
    b. 2 to 3 in.
    c. 4 to 6 in.
    d. 8 in.

23. For colostomy irrigation, the patient should be directed to hold the enema can or bag at shoulder level, approximately how far above the stoma?
    a. 6 in.
    b. 8 to 16 in.
    c. 18 to 24 in.
    d. 30 in.

24. The total quantity of irrigating solution that can be instilled at one session is:
    a. 1,000 mL.
    b. 1,500 mL.
    c. 2,500 mL.
    d. 3,000 mL.

MATCHING

Match the term in column II with its associated definition in column I.

Column I

1. _____ A tubular fibrous tract that extends from an opening beside the anus into the anal canal

2. _____ Dilated and atonic colon caused by a fecal mass

3. _____ A chemotherapeutic agent used to treat colon cancer

4. _____ A food to avoid for a patient with an ileostomy

5. _____ Straining at stool

6. _____ Another name for regional enteritis

7. _____ A highly reliable blood study used to diagnose appendicitis

8. _____ Painful straining at stool

9. _____ The most common bacteria associated with peritonitis

10. _____ Another term for fecal matter

11. _____ An ileal outlet on the abdomen

12. _____ Intestinal rumbling

13. _____ Another food to avoid for a patient with an ileostomy

Column II

a. Valsalva maneuver
b. Tenesmus
c. Stoma
d. Corn
e. Fistula
f. Peritonitis
g. Crohn's disease
h. TPN
i. 5-FU
j. Effluent
k. CEA
l. Laxatives
m. Megacolon
n. Borborygmus
o. Celery
p. *E. coli*

14. _____ The most popular "over-the-counter" medication purchased in the United States

15. _____ Intravenous nutrition used for inflammatory bowel disease

16. _____ The most common complication of colon cancer

Match the type of laxative listed in column III with its classification in column II. Then match the classification in column II with its action listed in column I.

Column I	Column II	Column III
1. _____ Magnesium ions alter stool consistency	a. _____ Bulk forming	I. Mineral oil
2. _____ Surfactant action hydrates stool	b. _____ Stimulant	II. Metamucil
3. _____ Electrolytes induce diarrhea	c. _____ Fecal softener	III. Milk of magnesia
4. _____ Polysaccharides and cellulose mix with intestinal contents	d. _____ Lubricant	IV. Dulcolax
5. _____ Colon is irritated and sensory nerve endings stimulated	e. _____ Saline agent	V. Colace
6. _____ Hydrocarbons soften fecal matter	f. _____ Osmotic agent	VI. Colyte

SHORT ANSWER

Read each statement carefully. Write your response in the space provided.

1. The three most common changes in the gastrointestinal tract that are symptoms of functional disorders or diseases are: _____, _____, and _____.

2. Name two diseases of the colon commonly associated with constipation: _____ and _____.

3. The pathophysiology of constipation is associated with interference with three major functions of the colon: _____, _____, and _____.

4. The recommended dietary intake of fiber is how many grams per day? _____. This intake, along with 1.5 to 2 L of fluids daily, should prevent constipation that occurs with fewer than how many bowel movements per week? _____.

5. The most common bacteria found in antibiotic-associated diarrhea is: _____.

6. The four most common complications of diverticulitis are: _____, _____, _____, and _____.

7. List four common bacteria found in peritonitis: _____, _____, _____, and _____.

8. The three most common causes of small-bowel obstruction are: _____ followed by _____ and _____.

9. The majority of large-bowel obstructions are caused by: _____.

10. List the six risk factors for colorectal cancer:

_____   _____

_____   _____

_____   _____

II. Critical Thinking Questions and Exercises

DISCUSSION AND ANALYSIS

Discuss the following topics with your classmates.

1. Discuss the physiologic processes that result in the urge to defecate.
2. Explain the Valsalva maneuver that can occur as a complication of constipation.
3. Discuss the patient education implications for laxatives: bulk forming, lubricant, fecal softeners, and osmotic agents.
4. Discuss the pathophysiology, clinical manifestations, and medical/nursing interventions for irritable bowel syndrome (IBS).

5. For each of these three diseases, explain the pathophysiology of malabsorption:

Pancreatic insufficiency: _____

Zollinger–Ellison syndrome: _____

Celiac disease: _____

6. Describe the nursing care management for a patient with inflammatory bowel disease (IBD).
7. Discuss the nursing interventions for patients undergoing ostomy surgery.
8. Explain the steps involved in changing an ostomy appliance.
9. Compare and contrast the five different surgical procedures used in colorectal cancer surgery.
10. Explain the differences between the etiology and clinical manifestations of five mechanical causes of intestinal obstruction: adhesions, intussusception, a volvulus, hernia, and tumor.
11. Compare and contrast the clinical manifestations and nursing interventions for eight potential complications of intestinal surgery.
12. Describe the steps for irrigating a colostomy.
13. Compare the etiology, clinical manifestations, and medical and nursing interventions for patients with diseases of the anorectum: anorectal abscess, anal fistula and fissure, hemorrhoids, pilonidal sinus or cyst, and sexually transmitted diseases.

RECOGNIZING CONTRADICTIONS

Rewrite each statement correctly. Underline the key concepts.

1. Diarrhea is a condition in which there is an increased frequency of bowel movements (more than six per day) associated with increased amount and consistency.
2. The most serious complication of appendicitis is strangulation of adjacent bowel tissue, which occurs in 5% of the cases.
3. Peritonitis, the most common reason for emergency abdominal surgery, occurs in about 10% of the population.
4. The major cause of death from peritonitis is hypovolemia.
5. The most common areas affected in Crohn's disease are the sigmoid colon and the cecum.
6. Surgery is rarely necessary for the treatment of regional enteritis.
7. Rectal bleeding is the most common symptom of colon cancer.

CLINICAL SITUATIONS

Read the following case studies. Fill in the blanks or circle the correct answer.

CASE STUDY: Appendicitis

Rory, an 18-year-old girl, is admitted to the hospital with a possible diagnosis of appendicitis. She had been symptomatic for several days before admission.

1. During assessment, the nurse is looking for positive indicators of appendicitis, which include all of the following *except*:
   a. a low-grade fever.
   b. abdominal tenderness on palpation.
   c. thrombocytopenia.
   d. vomiting.

2. On physical examination, the nurse should be looking for tenderness on palpation at McBurney's point, which is located in the:
   a. left lower quadrant.
   b. left upper quadrant.
   c. right lower quadrant.
   d. right upper quadrant.

3. Symptoms suggestive of acute appendicitis include:
   a. a positive Rovsing's sign.
   b. increased abdominal pain with coughing.
   c. tenderness around the umbilicus.
   d. all of the above.

4. Preparation for an appendectomy includes:
   a. an intravenous infusion.
   b. prophylactic antibiotic therapy.
   c. salicylates to lower an elevated temperature.
   d. all of the above.

CASE STUDY: Peritonitis

Sharon has peritonitis subsequent to ambulatory peritoneal dialysis. Her presenting symptoms are pain, abdominal tenderness, and nausea.

1. On assessment, the nurse should be looking for additional symptoms diagnostic of peritonitis, which include:
   a. abdominal rigidity.
   b. diminished peristalsis.
   c. leukocytosis.
   d. all of the above.

2. A central venous pressure (CVP) catheter is inserted to monitor fluid balance. The nurse's readings indicate low circulatory volume. The reading is probably between:
   a. 2 and 4 cm H_2O.
   b. 6 and 8 cm H_2O.
   c. 10 and 12 cm H_2O.
   d. 14 and 16 cm H_2O.

3. Given Sharon's CVP reading indicating hypovolemia, the nurse should assess for all of the following *except*:
   a. bradycardia.
   b. hypotension.
   c. oliguria.
   d. tachypnea.

4. With treatment, Sharon's peritonitis subsides. However, the nurse continues to assess for the common complication of:
   a. abscess formation.
   b. respiratory arrest owing to excessive pressure on the diaphragm.
   c. umbilical hernia.
   d. urinary tract infection.

IDENTIFYING PATTERNS

Review Figure 38-2 in the text and answer the following questions about IBS.

1. List at least five etiological factors associated with the change in intestinal motility in IBS:

   _____, _____, _____,

   _____, and _____.

2. The primary symptom in IBS is: _____.

3. Based on the figure above, describe the pathophysiologic changes that result in IBS:

   _____.

4. Five standard diagnostic tests used in IBS are: _____,

   _____, _____, _____,

   and _____.

5. Goals of medical management include: _____, _____,

   _____, and _____.

6. Describe the nurses' role in providing patient and family education.

   _____

CHAPTER 39

Assessment and Management of Patients With Hepatic Disorders

I. Interpretation, Completion, and Comparison

MULTIPLE CHOICE

Read each question carefully. Circle your answer.

1. The majority of blood supply to the liver, which is rich in nutrients from the gastrointestinal tract, comes from the:
   a. hepatic artery.
   b. hepatic vein.
   c. portal artery.
   d. portal vein.

2. The liver plays a major role in glucose metabolism by:
   a. producing ketone bodies.
   b. synthesizing albumin.
   c. participating in gluconeogenesis.
   d. doing all of the above.

3. The liver synthesizes prothrombin only if there is enough:
   a. vitamin A.
   b. vitamin B_{12}.
   c. vitamin D.
   d. vitamin K.

4. The substance necessary for the manufacture of bile salts by hepatocytes is:
   a. albumin.
   b. bilirubin.
   c. cholesterol.
   d. vitamin D.

5. The main function of bile salts is:
   a. albumin synthesis.
   b. fat emulsification in the intestines.
   c. lipid manufacture for the transport of proteins.
   d. urea synthesis from ammonia.

6. Hepatocellular dysfunction results in all of the following *except*:
   a. decreased serum albumin.
   b. elevated serum bilirubin.
   c. increased blood ammonia levels.
   d. increased levels of urea.

7. Jaundice becomes evident when serum bilirubin levels exceed:
   a. 0.5 mg/dL.
   b. 1.0 mg/dL.
   c. 1.5 mg/dL.
   d. 2.5 mg/dL.

8. The liver converts ammonia to urea. What level of ammonia would suggest liver failure?
   a. 40 µg/dL
   b. 100 mg/dL
   c. 200 µg/dL
   d. 300 mg/dL

9. The most common cause of parenchymal cell damage and hepatocellular dysfunction is:
   a. infectious agents.
   b. malnutrition.
   c. metabolic disorders.
   d. toxins.

10. Negative sodium balance is important for a patient with ascites. An example of food permitted on a low-sodium diet is:
   a. one-forth cup of peanut butter.
   b. one cup of powdered milk.
   c. one frankfurter.
   d. two slices of cold cuts.

11. The nurse expects that the diuretic of choice for a patient with ascites would be:
   a. Aldactone.
   b. ammonium chloride.
   c. Diamox.
   d. Lasix.

12. An indicator of probable esophageal varices is:
   a. hematemesis.
   b. a positive guaiac test.
   c. melena.
   d. all of the above.

13. The mortality rate from the first bleeding episode for esophageal varices is about:
   a. 10% to 15%.
   b. 15% to 25%.
   c. 30% to 50%.
   d. 80% or higher.

14. Bleeding esophageal varices result in a decrease in:
   a. nitrogen load from bleeding.
   b. renal perfusion.
   c. serum ammonia.
   d. all of the above.

15. The initial model of therapy to treat variceal hemorrhage that decreases portal pressure and produces constriction is:
   a. Corgard.
   b. Isordil.
   c. Pitressin.
   d. Somatostatin.

16. A person who consumes contaminated shellfish would probably develop:
   a. hepatitis B.
   b. hepatitis C.
   c. hepatitis D.
   d. hepatitis E.

17. The hepatitis virus that is transmitted via the fecal-oral route is:
   a. hepatitis A virus.
   b. hepatitis B virus.
   c. hepatitis C virus.
   d. hepatitis D virus.

18. Immune serum globulin provides passive immunity against type A hepatitis in those not vaccinated if it is administered within 2 weeks of exposure. Immunity is effective for about:
   a. 1 month.
   b. 2 months.
   c. 3 months.
   d. 4 months.

19. Choose the correct statement about hepatitis B vaccine.
   a. All persons at risk should receive active immunization.
   b. Evidence suggests that the human immunodeficiency virus (HIV) may be harbored in the vaccine.
   c. Booster doses are recommended every 5 years.
   d. One dose in the dorsogluteal muscle is recommended.

20. Indications for postexposure vaccination with hepatitis B immune globulin include:

    a. accidental exposure to HbAg-positive blood.

    b. perinatal exposure.

    c. sexual contact with those who are positive for HbAg.

    d. all of the above exposures.

21. This hepatitis virus caused by contaminated needles shared by drug users is expected to increase fourfold by 2015. This type of hepatitis, which is also the most common cause for liver transplantation, is:

    a. hepatitis A.

    b. hepatitis B.

    c. hepatitis C.

    d. hepatitis D.

22. The chemical most commonly implicated in toxic hepatitis is:

    a. chloroform.

    b. gold compounds.

    c. phosphorus.

    d. all of the above hepatotoxins.

23. Acetaminophen, found in over-the-counter (OTC) drugs, is the leading cause of acute liver failure. A popular drug containing acetaminophen is:

    a. Advil.

    b. Aleve.

    c. Motrin.

    d. Tylenol.

24. Fulminant hepatic failure may progress to hepatic encephalopathy about how many weeks after disease onset?

    a. 2 weeks

    b. 4 weeks

    c. 6 weeks

    d. 8 weeks

25. The major causative factor in the etiology of cirrhosis is:

    a. acute viral hepatitis.

    b. chronic alcoholism.

    c. chronic biliary obstruction.

    d. infection (cholangitis).

26. Late symptoms of hepatic cirrhosis include all of the following *except*:

    a. edema.

    b. hypoalbuminemia.

    c. hypokalemia.

    d. hyponatremia.

27. Cirrhosis results in shunting of portal system blood into collateral blood vessels in the gastrointestinal tract. The most common site is:

    a. the esophagus.

    b. the lower rectum.

    c. the stomach.

    d. a combination of all of the above.

28. Signs of advanced liver disease include:

    a. ascites.

    b. jaundice.

    c. portal hypertension.

    d. all of the above.

29. The most common single cause of death in patients with cirrhosis is:

    a. congestive heart failure.

    b. hepatic encephalopathy.

    c. hypovolemic shock.

    d. ruptured esophageal varices.

30. Hepatic lobectomy for cancer can be successful when the primary site is localized. Because of the regenerative capacity of the liver, a surgeon can remove up to what percentage of liver tissue?

    a. 25%

    b. 50%

    c. 75%

    d. 90%

SHORT ANSWER

Read each statement carefully. Write your answer in the space provided.

1. What percentage of the liver needs to be damaged before liver function tests are abnormal?

   _____.

2. The two major complications of a liver biopsy are: _____ and _____.

3. The mortality rate for hepatitis B can be as high as what percent? _____.

4. The most common reason for liver transplantation is exposure to _____.

5. Hepatocellular carcinoma is caused by: _____, _____, _____, and

   _____.

6. The leading cause of death after liver transplantation is: _____.

MATCHING

Match the vitamin listed in column II with the signs of deficiency due to severe chronic liver disease listed in column I.

Column I

1. _____ Hypoprothrombinemia
2. _____ Beriberi and polyneuritis
3. _____ Hemorrhagic lesions of scurvy
4. _____ Night blindness
5. _____ Macrocytic anemia
6. _____ Skin and neurologic changes
7. _____ Mucous membrane lesions

Column II

a. Vitamin A
b. Vitamin C
c. Vitamin K
d. Folic acid
e. Thiamine
f. Riboflavin
g. Pyridoxine

II. Critical Thinking Questions and Exercises

DISCUSSION AND ANALYSIS

Discuss the following topics with your classmates.

1. Discuss the age-related changes of the hepatobiliary system.
2. Demonstrate on a classmate how to palpate the abdomen to assess the liver.
3. Distinguish between hemolytic, hepatocellular, and obstructive jaundice in regard to etiology.
4. Describe the pathophysiology of ascites.
5. Review with your classmates the nursing interventions for a patient having a paracentesis.
6. Describe how balloon tamponade works.
7. Distinguish between three types of portal system shunts used to surgically bypass variceal bleeding sites.
8. Explain the pathophysiology of hepatic encephalopathy.
9. Explain the pathophysiology of alcoholic cirrhosis.
10. Compare and contrast the five types of viral hepatitis (A, B, C, D, and E) according to mode of transmission, etiology, and outcome.

CLINICAL SITUATIONS

Read the following case studies. Circle the correct answer.

CASE STUDY: Liver Biopsy

Veronica is scheduled for a liver biopsy. The staff nurse assigned to care for Veronica is to accompany her to the treatment room.

1. Before a liver biopsy, the nurse should check to see that:
   a. a compatible donor blood is available.
   b. coagulation studies have been completed.
   c. vital signs have been assessed.
   d. all of the above have been done.

2. The nurse begins preparing Veronica for the biopsy by assisting her to the correct position, which is:
   a. jackknife, with her entire back exposed.
   b. recumbent, with her right upper abdomen exposed.
   c. lying on her right side, with the left upper thoracic area exposed.
   d. supine, with the left lateral chest wall exposed.

3. The nurse knows that the biopsy needle will be inserted into the liver between the:
   a. third and fourth ribs.
   b. fourth and fifth ribs.
   c. sixth and seventh ribs.
   d. eighth and ninth ribs.

4. Immediately before needle insertion, Veronica needs to be instructed to:
   a. breathe slowly and deeply so that rib cage expansion will be minimized during needle insertion.
   b. inhale and exhale deeply several times, then exhale and hold her breath at the end of expiration until the needle is inserted.
   c. pant deeply and continue panting during needle insertion so pain perception will be minimized.
   d. take a deep inspiration and not breathe for 30 to 40 seconds so that the area for needle insertion can be determined; she should then resume normal breathing for the remainder of the procedure.

5. After the biopsy, the nurse assists Veronica to:
   a. high-Fowler's position, in which she can effectively take deep breaths and cough.
   b. ambulate while splinting her incision.
   c. assume the Trendelenburg position to prevent postbiopsy shock.
   d. the right side-lying position with a pillow placed under the right costal margin.

CASE STUDY: Paracentesis

Wendy is scheduled for a paracentesis because of ascites formation subsequent to cirrhosis of the liver.

1. Before the procedure, the nurse obtains several drainage bottles. She knows that the maximum amount of fluid to be aspirated at one time is:
   a. 1 L.
   b. 2 L.
   c. 3 L.
   d. 4 L.

2. The nurse helps Wendy to assume the proper position for a paracentesis, which is:
   a. recumbent so that the fluid will pool to the lower abdomen.
   b. lying on her left side so that fluid will not exert pressure on the liver.
   c. semi-Fowler's to avoid shock and provide the most comfort.
   d. upright with her feet resting on a support so that the puncture site will be readily visible.

3. After the paracentesis, Wendy should be observed for signs of vascular collapse, which include all of the following *except*:
   a. bradycardia.
   b. hypotension.
   c. oliguria.
   d. pallor.

CASE STUDY: Alcoholic or Nutritional Cirrhosis

Nathan, a 50-year-old physically disabled veteran, has lived alone for 30 years. He has maintained his independence despite chronic back pain resulting from a war injury. He has a long history of depression and limited food intake. He drinks 6 to 10 bottles of beer daily. He was recently admitted to a veteran's hospital with a diagnosis of alcoholic or nutritional cirrhosis. He was asymptomatic for ascites.

1. On assessment, the nurse notes early clinical manifestations of alcoholic or nutritional cirrhosis, which include all of the following *except*:
   a. pain caused by liver enlargement.
   b. a sharp edge to the periphery of the liver.
   c. a liver decreased in size and nodular.
   d. a firm liver.

2. An abnormal laboratory finding for Nathan is a:
   a. blood ammonia level of 35 mg/dL.
   b. serum albumin concentration of 4.0 g/dL.
   c. total serum bilirubin level of 0.9 mg/dL.
   d. total serum protein level of 5.5 g/dL.

3. Nathan is 5 ft 8 in tall and weighs 154 lb. The physician recommends 50 cal/kg for weight gain. Nathan's daily caloric intake would be approximately:
   a. 2,200 calories.
   b. 2,800 calories.
   c. 3,500 calories.
   d. 3,800 calories.

4. A recommended daily protein intake for Nathan to gain weight is:
   a. 31 to 44 g.
   b. 41 to 54 g.
   c. 51 to 64 g.
   d. 61 to 74 g.

5. The physician recommends a sodium-restricted diet. The nurse expects the suggested sodium intake to be approximately:
   a. 250 to 500 mg/24 h.
   b. 500 to 1,000 mg/24 h.
   c. 2,000 to 2,500 mg/24 h.
   d. 3,000 to 3,500 mg/24 h.

CASE STUDY: Liver Transplantation

Denise, a 54-year-old mother of three, is scheduled for a liver transplantation subsequent to an extensive hepatic malignancy with multifocal tumors greater than 8 cm in diameter.

1. Denise is hopeful that her surgery will be successful. She is aware, however, that her chance of survival at 5 years is about:
   a. 10%.
   b. 30%.
   c. 50%.
   d. 70%.

2. Denise knows that a successful outcome to transplantation will be compromised by:
   a. fluid and electrolyte disturbances.
   b. malnutrition.
   c. immunosuppressive therapy.
   d. all of the above.

3. The nurse is aware that postoperatively the most common complication after liver transplantation is:

   a. bleeding.   c. infection.

   b. hypotension.   d. portal hypertension.

4. The nurse knows that a patient receiving cyclosporine to prevent rejection of a transplanted liver may develop a drug side effect of:

   a. nephrotoxicity.   c. thrombocytopenia.

   b. septicemia.   d. all of the above reactions.

CHAPTER 40

Assessment and Management of Patients With Biliary Disorders

I. Interpretation, Completion, and Comparison

MULTIPLE CHOICE

Read each question carefully. Circle your answer.

1. Bile is stored in the:
   a. cystic duct.
   b. duodenum.
   c. gallbladder.
   d. common bile duct.

2. A patient is diagnosed with gallstones in the bile ducts. The nurse knows to review the results of blood work for a:
   a. serum ammonia concentration of 90 mg/dL.
   b. serum albumin concentration of 4.0 g/dL.
   c. serum bilirubin level greater than 1.0 mg/dL.
   d. serum globulin concentration of 2.0 g/dL.

3. The major stimulus for increased bicarbonate secretion from the pancreas is:
   a. amylase.
   b. lipase.
   c. secretin.
   d. trypsin.

4. An action not associated with insulin is the:
   a. conversion of glycogen to glucose in the liver.
   b. lowering of blood glucose.
   c. promotion of fat storage.
   d. synthesis of proteins.

5. The nurse knows that a patient with low blood sugar would have a blood glucose level of:
   a. 55 to 75 mg/dL.
   b. 80 to 120 mg/dL.
   c. 130 to 150 mg/dL.
   d. 160 to 180 mg/dL.

6. A patient with calculi in the gallbladder is said to have:
   a. cholecystitis.
   b. cholelithiasis.
   c. choledocholithiasis.
   d. choledochotomy.

7. Statistics show that there is a greater incidence of gallbladder disease for women who are:
   a. multiparous.
   b. obese.
   c. older than 40 years of age.
   d. characterized by all of the above.

8. The obstruction of bile flow due to cholelithiasis can interfere with the absorption of:
   a. vitamin A.
   b. vitamin B_6.
   c. vitamin B_{12}.
   d. vitamin C.

9. Clinical manifestations of common bile duct obstruction include all of the following *except*:
   a. amber-colored urine.
   b. clay-colored feces.
   c. pruritus.
   d. jaundice.

10. The diagnostic procedure of choice for cholelithiasis is:
    a. x-ray.
    b. oral cholecystography.
    c. cholecystography.
    d. ultrasonography.

11. Pharmacologic therapy is frequently used to dissolve small gallstones. It takes about how many months of medication with UDCA or CDCA for stones to dissolve?
    a. 1 to 2 months
    b. 3 to 5 months
    c. 6 to 8 months
    d. 6 to 12 months

12. Chronic pancreatitis, commonly described as autodigestion of the pancreas, is often not detected until what percentage of the exocrine and endocrine tissue is destroyed?
    a. 10% to 25%
    b. 30% to 50%
    c. 60% to 75%
    d. 80% to 90%

13. Mild acute pancreatitis is characterized by:
    a. edema and inflammation.
    b. pleural effusion.
    c. sepsis.
    d. disseminated intravascular coagulopathy.

14. A major symptom of pancreatitis that brings the patient to medical care is:
    a. severe abdominal pain.
    b. fever.
    c. jaundice.
    d. mental agitation.

15. The nurse should assess for an important early indicator of acute pancreatitis, which is a prolonged and elevated level of:
    a. serum calcium.
    b. serum lipase.
    c. serum bilirubin.
    d. serum amylase.

16. Nursing measures for pain relief for acute pancreatitis include:
    a. encouraging bed rest to decrease the metabolic rate.
    b. teaching the patient about the correlation between alcohol intake and pain.
    c. withholding oral feedings to limit the release of secretin.
    d. all of the above.

17. The risk for pancreatic cancer is directly proportional to:
    a. age.
    b. dietary intake of fat.
    c. cigarette smoking.
    d. presence of diabetes mellitus.

18. With pancreatic carcinoma, insulin deficiency is suspected when the patient evidences:
    a. an abnormal glucose tolerance.
    b. glucosuria.
    c. hyperglycemia.
    d. all of the above.

19. Clinical manifestations associated with a tumor of the head of the pancreas include:
    a. clay-colored stools.
    b. dark urine.
    c. jaundice.
    d. all of the above.

20. A nurse should monitor blood glucose levels for a patient who is diagnosed as having hyperinsulinism. A value inadequate to sustain normal brain function is:
   a. 30 mg/dL.
   b. 50 mg/dL.
   c. 70 mg/dL.
   d. 90 mg/dL.

21. Zollinger–Ellison tumors are associated with hypersecretion of:
   a. aldosterone.
   b. gastric acid.
   c. insulin.
   d. vasopressin.

SHORT ANSWER

Read each statement carefully. Write your response in the space provided.

1. The capacity of the gallbladder for bile storage is: _____mL.

2. The endocrine secretions of the pancreas are: _____, _____, and _____.

3. Digestive enzymes are secreted by the pancreas; _____ aids in the digestion of carbohydrates, _____ aids protein digestion, and _____ aids the digestion of fats.

4. The primary cause of acute cholecystitis is: _____.

5. The most serious complication after a laparoscopic cholecystectomy is: _____.

6. The criteria for predicting the severity of pancreatitis and associated mortality is evidenced by some of these clinical signs: _____, _____, _____, and _____.

7. A major cause of morbidity and mortality in patients with acute pancreatitis is: _____.

8. What percentage of patients have advanced pancreatic cancer when it is first detected? _____. What is the 5-year survival rate? _____.

II. Critical Thinking Questions and Exercises

CLINICAL SITUATIONS

Read the following case studies. Circle the correct answer or fill in the blank space.

CASE STUDY: Cholecystectomy

Brenda, a 33-year-old obese mother of four, is diagnosed as having acute gallbladder inflammation. She is 5 ft 4 in tall and weighs 190 lb. The physician decides to delay surgical intervention until Brenda's acute symptoms subside.

1. Brenda's initial course of treatment would probably consist of:
   a. analgesics and antibiotics.
   b. intravenous fluids.
   c. nasogastric suctioning.
   d. all of the above.

2. After her acute attack, Brenda was limited to low-fat liquids. As foods are added to her diet, she needs to know that she should avoid:

   a. cooked fruits.

   b. eggs and cheese.

   c. lean meats.

   d. rice and tapioca.

3. Brenda is being medicated with chenodeoxycholic acid. The nurse needs to tell Brenda that the drug may not be effective if it is taken in conjunction with:

   a. dietary cholesterol.

   b. estrogens.

   c. oral contraceptives.

   d. any of the above.

Because Brenda's symptoms continue to recur, she is scheduled for gallbladder surgery.

1. Brenda has signed a consent form for removal of her gallbladder and ligation of the cystic duct and artery. She is scheduled to undergo a:

   a. cholecystectomy.

   b. cholecystostomy.

   c. choledochostomy.

   d. choledocholithotomy.

2. Postoperative nursing observation includes assessing for:

   a. indicators of infection.

   b. leakage of bile into the peritoneal cavity.

   c. obstruction of bile drainage.

   d. all of the above.

3. Brenda needs to know that fat restriction is usually lifted after the biliary ducts dilate to accommodate bile once held by the gallbladder. This takes about:

   a. 1 week.

   b. 2 to 3 weeks.

   c. 4 to 6 weeks.

   d. 2 months.

CASE STUDY: Chronic Pancreatitis

Carl, a 56-year-old traveling salesman, has recently been diagnosed with chronic pancreatitis.

1. Describe the pathophysiologic sequence of the inflammatory process.

   _____

2. The nurse knows that the major cause of chronic pancreatitis is _____ with a median age of _____ years at diagnosis.

3. A characteristic clinical symptom of chronic pancreatitis is: _____.

4. Dysfunction of the pancreatic islet cells leads to a diagnosis of: _____.

5. A recommended surgical procedure that allows drainage of pancreatic secretions into the jejunum is:

   _____

6. Long-term management requires two dietary modifications: _____ and _____.

CHAPTER 41

Assessment and Management of Patients With Diabetes Mellitus

I. Interpretation, Completion, and Comparison

MULTIPLE CHOICE

Read each question carefully. Circle your answer.

1. Glucose intolerance increases with age. The incidence in those older than 65 years is:
   - a. 20%
   - b. 50%
   - c. 65%
   - d. 80%

2. The ethnic group with the *lowest* incidence of diabetes mellitus in the United States is:
   - a. African Americans.
   - b. Caucasians.
   - c. Hispanics.
   - d. Native Americans.

3. As a cause of death by disease in the United States, diabetes mellitus ranks:
   - a. first.
   - b. second.
   - c. third.
   - d. fourth.

4. A patient is diagnosed with type 1 diabetes. The nurse knows that all of the following are probable clinical characteristics *except*:
   - a. ketosis-prone.
   - b. little endogenous insulin.
   - c. obesity at diagnoses.
   - d. younger than 30 years.

5. A patient who is diagnosed with type 1 diabetes mellitus would be expected to:
   - a. be restricted to an American Diabetic Association diet.
   - b. have no damage to the islet cells of the pancreas.
   - c. need exogenous insulin.
   - d. need to receive daily doses of a hypoglycemic agent.

6. Possible risk factors associated with type 1 diabetes mellitus include:
   - a. an autoimmune susceptibility to diabetogenic viruses.
   - b. environmental factors.
   - c. the presence of human leukocyte antigen (HLA).
   - d. all of the above.

7. Clinical manifestations associated with a diagnosis of type 1 diabetes mellitus include all of the following *except*:
   - a. hypoglycemia.
   - b. hyponatremia.
   - c. ketonuria.
   - d. polyphagia.

8. The nurse is asked to assess a patient for glucosuria. The nurse would secure a specimen of:
   a. blood.
   b. sputum.
   c. stool.
   d. urine.

9. Knowing that gluconeogenesis helps to maintain blood levels, a nurse should:
   a. document weight changes because of fatty acid mobilization.
   b. evaluate the patient's sensitivity to low room temperatures because of decreased adipose tissue insulation.
   c. protect the patient from sources of infection because of decreased cellular protein deposits.
   d. do all of the above.

10. A nurse is assigned to care for a patient who is suspected of having type 2 diabetes mellitus. Clinical manifestations for which the nurse should assess include:
   a. blurred or deteriorating vision.
   b. fatigue and muscle cramping.
   c. wounds that heal slowly or respond poorly to treatment.
   d. all of the above.

11. There seems to be a strong positive correlation between type 2 diabetes mellitus and:
   a. hypotension.
   b. kidney dysfunction.
   c. obesity.
   d. sex.

12. The lowest fasting plasma glucose level suggestive of a diagnosis of diabetes is:
   a. 90 mg/dL.
   b. 115 mg/dL.
   c. 126 mg/dL.
   d. 180 mg/dL.

13. The most sensitive test for diabetes mellitus is the:
   a. fasting plasma glucose.
   b. 2-hour postload glucose.
   c. intravenous glucose.
   d. urine glucose.

14. A female diabetic patient who weighs 130 lb has an ideal body weight of 116 lb. For weight reduction of 2 lb/week, her daily caloric intake should be approximately:
   a. 1,000 calories.
   b. 1,200 calories.
   c. 1,500 calories.
   d. 1,800 calories.

15. The nurse should encourage exercise in the management of diabetes, because it:
   a. decreases total triglyceride levels.
   b. improves insulin utilization.
   c. lowers blood glucose.
   d. accomplishes all of the above.

16. Self-monitoring of blood glucose is recommended for patients with:
   a. abnormal renal glucose thresholds.
   b. hypoglycemia without warning symptoms.
   c. unstable diabetes.
   d. all of the above conditions.

17. An example of a commonly administered intermediate-acting insulin is:
   a. NHP.
   b. Iletin II.
   c. Humalog.
   d. Humulin U.

18. The nurse knows that an intermediate-acting insulin should reach its "peak" in:
   a. 1 to 2 hours.
   b. 3 to 4 hours.
   c. 4 to 12 hours.
   d. 16 to 20 hours.

19. Insulin pumps in use today:
    a. can deliver a premeal dose (bolus) of insulin before each meal.
    b. deliver a continuous basal rate of insulin at 0.5 to 2.0 units/h.
    c. prevent unexpected savings in blood glucose measurements.
    d. are capable of doing all of the above.

20. A probable candidate for diabetic management with oral antidiabetic agents is the patient who is:
    a. non–insulin-dependent.
    b. stable and not prone to ketosis.
    c. unable to be managed by diet alone.
    d. characterized by all of the above.

21. An example of a first-generation sulfonylurea used in type 2 diabetes is:
    a. Dia-Beta
    b. Glyset
    c. Starlix
    d. Tolinase

22. The nurse should expect that insulin therapy will be temporarily substituted for oral antidiabetic therapy if the diabetic patient:
    a. develops an infection with fever.
    b. suffers trauma.
    c. undergoes major surgery.
    d. develops any or all of the above.

23. The tissue area that provides the fastest absorption rate for regular insulin is believed to be the:
    a. abdominal area.
    b. anterior thigh.
    c. deltoid area.
    d. gluteal site.

24. Rotation sites for insulin injection should be separated from one another by 2.5 cm (1 in) and should be used only once every:
    a. third day.
    b. week.
    c. 2 to 3 weeks.
    d. 2 to 4 weeks.

25. Hypoglycemia, an abnormally low blood glucose concentration, occurs with a glucose level that is:
    a. lower than 50 to 60 mg/dL.
    b. between 60 and 80 mg/dL.
    c. between 75 and 90 mg/dL.
    d. 95 mg/dL.

26. A clinical feature that distinguishes a hypoglycemic reaction from a ketoacidosis reaction is:
    a. blurred vision.
    b. diaphoresis.
    c. nausea.
    d. weakness.

27. The nurse knows that treatment modalities for diabetic ketoacidosis should focus on management of:
    a. acidosis.
    b. dehydration.
    c. hyperglycemia.
    d. all of the above.

28. The major electrolyte of concern in the treatment of diabetic ketoacidosis is:
    a. calcium.
    b. magnesium.
    c. potassium.
    d. sodium.

29. Mortality rates for patients with diabetes are positively correlated with atherosclerotic complications, especially in the coronary arteries, which account for about what percentage of all deaths in these patients?
    a. 10%
    b. 30%
    c. 40%
    d. 60%

30. Macrovascular disease has a direct link with:
    a. hypertension.
    b. increased triglyceride levels.
    c. obesity.
    d. all of the above.

31. Clinical nursing assessment for a patient with microangiopathy who has manifested impaired peripheral arterial circulation includes all of the following *except*:
    a. integumentary inspection for the presence of brown spots on the lower extremities.
    b. observation for paleness of the lower extremities.
    c. observation for blanching of the feet after the legs are elevated for 60 seconds.
    d. palpation for increased pulse volume in the arteries of the lower extremities.

32. With nonproliferative (background) retinopathy, examination of the retina may reveal:
    a. leakage of fluid or serum (exudates).
    b. microaneurysms.
    c. focal capillary single closure.
    d. all of the above pathologic changes.

33. A diagnostic manifestation of proliferative retinopathy is:
    a. decreased capillary permeability.
    b. microaneurysm formation.
    c. neovascularization into the vitreous humor.
    d. the leakage of capillary wall fragments into surrounding areas.

34. A nurse caring for a diabetic patient with a diagnosis of nephropathy would expect the urinalysis report to indicate:
    a. albumin.
    b. bacteria.
    c. red blood cells.
    d. white blood cells.

35. With peripheral neuropathy, a diabetic patient has limited sensitivity to:
    a. heat.
    b. pain.
    c. pressure.
    d. all of the above.

36. Nursing care for a diabetic patient with peripheral neuropathy includes:
    a. assessing pain patterns to rule out peripheral vascular insufficiency.
    b. inspecting the feet for breaks in skin integrity.
    c. palpating the lower extremities for temperature variations.
    d. all of the above.

37. During surgery, glucose levels will rise, because there is an increased secretion of:
    a. cortisol.
    b. epinephrine.
    c. glucagon.
    d. all of the above.

38. The nurse expects that a type 1 diabetic patient may receive what percentage of his or her usual morning dose of insulin preoperatively?
    a. 10% to 20%
    b. 25% to 40%
    c. 50% to 60%
    d. 85% to 90%

MATCHING

Match the physiologic change listed in column II with its associated term listed in column I.

Column I

1. _____ Gluconeogenesis
2. _____ Glucosuria
3. _____ Glycogenolysis
4. _____ Nephropathy
5. _____ Retinopathy

Column II

a. Filtered glucose that the kidney cannot absorb spills over into urine
b. Glycogen breaks down in the liver through the action of glucagon
c. New glucose is produced from amino acids
d. Microvascular changes develop in the eyes
e. Small vessel disease affects the kidneys

SHORT ANSWER

Read each statement carefully. Write your response in the space provided.

1. In the United States, diabetes mellitus is the leading cause of three pathologic conditions: _____, _____, and _____.

2. The renal threshold for glucose is: _____.

3. Gestational diabetes occurs in _____% of pregnant women.

4. The main goal of diabetes treatment is to: _____.

5. List the five major components of management for diabetes: _____, _____, _____, _____, and _____.

6. A person is overweight when the body mass index (BMI) is: _____; obesity is diagnosed with a BMI of _____.

7. The current recommended distribution of calories for a diabetic patient's meal plan is _____% carbohydrates, _____% fat, and _____% protein.

8. The recommended amount of daily fiber intake is: _____ g.

9. Two examples of rapid-acting insulin are: _____ and _____.

10. The most common risk of insulin pump therapy is: _____.

11. The sulfonylureas act by: _____.

12. List the four main areas for insulin injection: _____, _____, _____, and _____.

13. List three major acute complications of diabetes: _____, _____, and _____.

14. Clinical manifestations characteristic of hyperglycemic, hyperosmolar, nonketotic syndrome would include: _____, _____, _____, and _____.

15. Identify five possible collaborative problems that a nurse should be aware of for a patient newly diagnosed with hyperglycemia, hyperosmolar, and nonketotic syndrome: _____, _____, _____, _____, and _____.

16. The leading cause of blindness in the United States among those between the ages of 20 and 74 years of age is: _____.

II. Critical Thinking Questions and Exercises

DISCUSSION AND ANALYSIS

Discuss the following topics with your classmates.

1. Discuss the eight risk factors associated with diabetes mellitus and the nurse's role in health education.
2. Compare the clinical characteristics and clinical implications for the four major classifications of diabetes: type 1, type 2, gestational, and diabetes mellitus associated with other conditions or syndromes.
3. Describe the six major activities of insulin.
4. Explain how insulin regulation is altered in the diabetic state.
5. Describe the pathophysiologic difference between type 1 and type 2 diabetes.
6. Explain the primary cause of gestational diabetes mellitus.
7. Explain the term *glycemic index*.
8. Describe the major complications of insulin therapy.
9. Demonstrate how to mix rapid-acting and longer-acting insulin in the same syringe.
10. Demonstrate the proper technique for self-injection of insulin and disposal of the syringes.
11. Distinguish between the *dawn phenomenon* and the *Somogyi* effect.
12. Discuss a patient education plan for diabetic patients to follow when they are sick (sick day rules).

EXAMINING ASSOCIATIONS

For each of the clinical characteristics listed below, choose the associated classification of diabetes mellitus. Enter "1" for type 1 diabetes mellitus or "2" for type 2 diabetes mellitus.

1. _____ Etiology includes obesity
2. _____ Ketosis is rare
3. _____ Patient usually thin at diagnosis
4. _____ Patient needs insulin to preserve life
5. _____ Patient often has islet cell antibodies
6. _____ Patient has no islet cell antibodies
7. _____ Onset can occur at any age
8. _____ Usually is diagnosed after age 30 years
9. _____ Hyperosmolar nonketotic syndrome is a complication
10. _____ There is little or no endogenous insulin

IDENTIFYING PATTERNS

In diagram format, illustrate the pathophysiologic sequence of changes that occur with type 1 diabetes, from "decreased insulin production by beta cells" to "ketoacidosis." Any outline format is acceptable as long as a cause-and-effect sequence can be seen.

APPLYING CONCEPTS

Examine the figure below and answer the following questions.

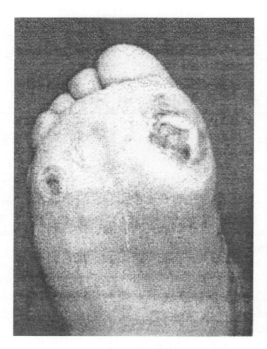

Neuropathic ulcers occur on pressure points in areas with diminished sensation in diabetic polyneuropathy. Pain is absent (and therefore the ulcer may go unnoticed).

1. Explain how each of the following diabetic complications leads to the formation of neuropathic ulcers and foot infections.

   a. Sensory neuropathy causes: _____

   b. Autonomic neuropathy causes: _____

   c. Motor neuropathy causes: _____

2. Appropriate foot care could prevent up to _____% of lower extremity amputations as a result of foot infections and complications.

3. Explain how peripheral vascular disease affects the progression of a foot infection and ulcer formation.

4. Explain how hyperglycemia affects the spread of a foot infection.

5. The three events that typically occur in sequence and lead to the development of a diabetic foot ulcer are:

   _____, _____, and _____.

6. List five daily activities related to foot care that a nurse should instruct a diabetic patient to complete:

_____, _____,

_____, _____, and

_____.

7. Foot infections and ulcers may progress to the point that amputation is necessary, because:

_____.

CLINICAL SITUATIONS

Read the following case studies. Circle the correct answer.

CASE STUDY: Type 1 Diabetes

Albert, a 35-year-old insulin-dependent diabetic patient, is admitted to the hospital with a diagnosis of pneumonia. He has been febrile since admission. His daily insulin requirement is 24 units of NPH.

1. Every morning Albert is given NPH insulin at 7:30 AM. Meals are served at 8:30 AM, 12:30 PM, and 6:30 PM. The nurse expects that the NPH insulin will reach its maximum effect (peak) between the hours of:
   a. 11:30 AM and 1:30 PM.
   b. 11:30 AM and 7:30 PM.
   c. 3:30 PM and 9:30 PM.
   d. 5:30 PM and 11:30 PM.

2. A bedtime snack is provided for Albert. This is based on the knowledge that intermediate-acting insulins are effective for an approximate duration of:
   a. 6 to 8 hours.
   b. 10 to 14 hours.
   c. 16 to 20 hours.
   d. 24 to 28 hours.

3. Albert refuses his bedtime snack. This should alert the nurse to assess for:
   a. an elevated serum bicarbonate and a decreased blood pH.
   b. signs of hypoglycemia earlier than expected.
   c. symptoms of hyperglycemia during the peak time of NPH insulin.
   d. sugar in the urine.

CASE STUDY: Hypoglycemia

Betty, an 18-year-old type 1 diabetic patient, is unconscious when admitted to the hospital. Her daily dose of insulin has been 32 units of NPH each morning.

1. On the basis of the knowledge of hypoglycemia, the nurse would expect that Betty's serum glucose level on admission is approximately:
   a. 50 mg/dL.
   b. 70 mg/dL.
   c. 90 mg/dL.
   d. 110 mg/dL.

2. Betty is given 1 mg of glucagon hydrochloride, subcutaneously, in the emergency department. Knowledge about the action of this drug alerts the nurse to observe for latent symptoms associated with:
   a. glucosuria.
   b. hyperglycemia.
   c. ketoacidosis.
   d. rebound hypoglycemia.

3. After Betty is medically stabilized, she is admitted to the clinical area for observation and health teaching. The nurse should make sure that Betty is aware of warning symptoms associated with hypoglycemia, such as:

    a. emotional changes.

    b. slurred speech and double vision.

    c. staggering gait and incoordination.

    d. all of the above.

4. Betty should also be taught that hypoglycemia may be prevented by:

    a. eating regularly scheduled meals.

    b. eating snacks to cover the peak time of insulin.

    c. increasing food intake when engaging in increased levels of physical exercise.

    d. doing all of the above.

CASE STUDY: Diabetic Ketoacidosis

Christine, a 64-year-old woman, is admitted to the clinical area with a diagnosis of diabetic ketoacidosis. On admission, she is drowsy yet responsive.

1. Nursing actions for a diagnosis of ketoacidosis include:

    a. monitoring urinary output by means of an indwelling catheter.

    b. evaluating serum electrolytes.

    c. testing for glucosuria and acetonuria.

    d. all of the above.

2. The nurse should expect that the rehydrating intravenous solution used will be:

    a. 0.9% saline solution.

    b. 5% dextrose in water.

    c. 10% dextrose in water.

    d. sterile water.

3. In evaluating the laboratory results, the nurse expects all of the following to indicate ketoacidosis *except*:

    a. a decreased serum bicarbonate level.

    b. an elevated blood glucose.

    c. an increased blood urea.

    d. an increased blood pH.

4. The physician notes a change in Christine's respirations. Her breathing is described as Kussmaul respirations. The nurse knows that these respirations are:

    a. deep.

    b. labored.

    c. rapid.

    d. shallow.

5. Christine is started on low-dose intravenous insulin therapy. Nursing assessment includes all of the following *except* frequent:

    a. blood pressure measurements to monitor the degree of hypotension.

    b. estimates of serum potassium, because increased blood glucose levels are correlated with elevated potassium levels.

    c. evaluation of blood glucose levels, because glucose levels should decline as insulin levels increase.

    d. elevation of serum ketones to monitor the course of ketosis.

6. As blood glucose levels approach normal, the nurse should assess for signs of electrolyte imbalance associated with:

    a. hypernatremia.

    b. hypercapnia.

    c. hypocalcemia.

    d. hypokalemia.

CHAPTER 42

Assessment and Management of Patients With Endocrine Disorders

I. Interpretation, Completion, and Comparison

MULTIPLE CHOICE

Read each question carefully. Circle your answer.

1. An example of exocrine glands are the:
   a. adrenals.
   b. ovaries.
   c. parathyroids.
   d. sweat glands.

2. The nurse knows that the anterior pituitary gland is responsible for secreting all of the following *except* the:
   a. adrenocorticotropic hormone (ACTH).
   b. antidiuretic hormone (ADH).
   c. follicle-stimulating hormone (FSH).
   d. thyroid-stimulating hormone (TSH).

3. The major structure balancing the rapid action of the nervous system with slower hormonal action is the:
   a. hypothalamus.
   b. pineal gland.
   c. hypophysis.
   d. thyroid gland.

4. Diabetes insipidus is a disorder related to a deficiency of:
   a. growth hormone.
   b. prolactin.
   c. oxytocin.
   d. vasopressin.

5. When thyroid hormone is administered for prolonged hypothyroidism, the nurse knows to monitor the patient for:
   a. angina.
   b. depression.
   c. mental confusion.
   d. hypoglycemia.

6. The preferred medication for treating hypothyroidism is:
   a. lithium.
   b. Proprandol.
   c. propylthiouracil.
   d. Synthroid.

7. A clinical manifestation *not* usually associated with hyperthyroidism is:
   a. a pulse rate slower than 90 bpm.
   b. an elevated systolic blood pressure.
   c. muscular fatigability.
   d. weight loss.

8. Patients with hyperthyroidism are characteristically:
   a. apathetic and anorexic.
   b. calm.
   c. emotionally stable.
   d. sensitive to heat.

9. Iodine or iodide compounds are used for hyperthyroidism because they do all of the following *except*:
   a. decrease the basal metabolic rate.
   b. increase the vascularity of the gland.
   c. lessen the release of thyroid hormones.
   d. reduce the size of the gland.

10. The objectives of pharmacotherapy for hyperthyroidism include:
    a. destroying overreactive thyroid cells.
    b. preventing thyroid hormonal synthesis.
    c. increasing the amount of thyroid tissue.
    d. all of the above.

11. Signs of thyroid storm include all of the following *except*:
    a. bradycardia.
    b. delirium or somnolence.
    c. dyspnea and chest pain.
    d. hyperpyrexia.

12. Medical management for thyroid crisis includes:
    a. intravenous dextrose fluids.
    b. hypothermia measures.
    c. oxygen therapy.
    d. all of the above.

13. Pharmacotherapy for thyroid storm would *not* include the administration of:
    a. acetaminophen.
    b. iodine.
    c. propylthiouracil.
    d. synthetic levothyroxine.

14. The most common type of goiter is etiologically related to a deficiency of:
    a. thyrotropin.
    b. iodine.
    c. thyroxine.
    d. calcitonin.

15. The nurse knows that the most common and least aggressive type of cancer is:
    a. anaplastic.
    b. follicular adenocarcinoma.
    c. medullary.
    d. papillary adenocarcinoma.

16. A diagnosis of hyperparathyroidism can be established by all of the following signs *except*:
    a. a negative reading on a Sulkowitch test.
    b. a serum calcium level of 12 mg/dL.
    c. an elevated level of parathyroid hormone.
    d. bone demineralization seen on an x-ray film.

17. A recommended breakfast for a hyperparathyroid patient would be:
    a. cereal with milk and bananas.
    b. fried eggs and bacon.
    c. orange juice and toast.
    d. pork sausage and cranberry juice.

18. One of the most important and frequently occurring complications of hyperparathyroidism is:
    a. kidney stones.
    b. pancreatitis.
    c. pathologic fractures.
    d. peptic ulcer.

19. The pathophysiology of hypoparathyroidism is associated with all of the following *except*:
    a. a decrease in serum calcium.
    b. an elevation of blood phosphate.
    c. an increase in the renal excretion of phosphate.
    d. a lowered renal excretion of calcium.

20. The goal of medical management for hypoparathyroidism is to:
    a. achieve a serum calcium level of 9 to 10 mg/dL.
    b. eliminate clinical symptoms.
    c. reverse the symptoms of hypocalcemia.
    d. accomplish all of the above.

21. Nursing management for a hypoparathyroid patient would not include:
    a. maintaining a quiet, subdued environment.
    b. making certain that calcium gluconate is kept at the bedside.
    c. observing the patient for signs of tetany.
    d. supplementing the diet with milk and milk products.

22. A pheochromocytoma is an adrenal medulla tumor that causes arterial hypertension by increasing the level of circulating:
    a. catecholamines.
    b. enzymes.
    c. hormones.
    d. glucocorticoids.

23. A positive test for overactivity of the adrenal medulla is an epinephrine value of:
    a. 50 pg/mL.
    b. 100 pg/mL.
    c. 100 to 300 pg/mL.
    d. 450 pg/mL.

24. Laboratory findings suggestive of Addison's disease include all of the following *except*:
    a. a relative lymphocytosis.
    b. hyperkalemia and hyponatremia.
    c. hypertension.
    d. hypoglycemia.

25. A positive diagnosis of Cushing's syndrome is associated with:
    a. the disappearance of lymphoid tissue.
    b. a reduction in circulating eosinophils.
    c. an elevated cortisol level.
    d. all of the above.

26. Clinical manifestations of Cushing's syndrome may be modified with a diet that is:
    a. high in protein.
    b. low in carbohydrates.
    c. low in sodium.
    d. all of the above.

27. A patient with aldosteronism would be expected to exhibit all of the following symptoms *except*:
    a. alkalosis.
    b. hypokalemia.
    c. hyponatremia.
    d. an increased pH.

28. The nurse needs to be aware that large-dose corticosteroid therapy is most effective when administered:
    a. at 8:00 AM.
    b. at 8:00 PM.
    c. between 4:00 AM and 5:00 AM.
    d. between 4:00 PM and 6:00 PM.

29. Nursing assessment for a patient who is receiving corticosteroid therapy includes observation for the unacceptable side effect of:
    a. glaucoma.
    b. facial mooning.
    c. potassium loss.
    d. weight gain.

MATCHING

Match the hormonal function listed in column II with its corresponding hormone listed in column I.

Column I

1. _____ Glucagon
2. _____ Aldosterone
3. _____ Oxytocin
4. _____ Somatotropin
5. _____ Vasopressin
6. _____ Calcitonin
7. _____ Prolactin
8. _____ Melatonin
9. _____ Parathormone
10. _____ Insulin

Column II

a. Controls excretion of water by the kidneys

b. Lowers blood sugar

c. Inhibits bone resorption

d. Influences metabolism that is essential for normal growth

e. Supports sexual maturation

f. Promotes the secretion of milk

g. Stimulates the reabsorption of sodium and the elimination of potassium

h. Promotes glycogenolysis

i. Increases the force of uterine contractions during parturition

j. Regulates serum calcium

SHORT ANSWER

Read each statement carefully. Write your response in the space provided.

1. The term used to describe the regulation of hormone concentration in the bloodstream is: _____.

2. Hormones are classified four ways: _____, _____, _____, and _____.

3. The two major hormones secreted by the posterior lobe of the pituitary gland are: _____, which controls _____ and _____, which facilitates _____.

4. Oversecretion of adrenocorticotropic hormone (ACTH) or the growth hormone results in _____ disease.

5. A deficiency of ADH or vasopressin can result in the disorder known as _____, which is characterized by _____ and _____.

6. The thyroid gland produces three hormones: _____, _____, and _____.

7. The most common cause of hypothyroidism is: _____.

8. Hyperthyroidism is second only to _____ as a common endocrine disorder.

9. The most common type of hyperthyroidism is: _____.

10. The two most common medications used to treat hyperthyroidism are: _____ and _____.

11. Tetany is suspected when either of these signs are positive: _____ or

    _____.

12. Name the three types of steroid hormones produced by the adrenal cortex: _____,

    _____, and _____.

SCRAMBLEGRAM

Unscramble the letters to answer each statement.

1. The master gland of the endocrine system is the: _____.

I U I Y T P R T A

2. The pituitary gland is controlled by the: _____.

O A T M P U A S H H L Y

3. Another name for the growth hormone is: _____.

P O T T I A S N R O O M

4. Excessive secretion of ADH results in a syndrome that causes fluid retention, which is identified by the five

    letters: _____.

H D A I S

5. The thyroid gland depends on the uptake of _____ to synthesize its hormones.

E O N I D I

6. The term used to describe "bulging eyes" found in patients with hyperthyroidism is: _____.

H M P L O S E A X O H T

7. The term used to describe hyperirritability of the nerves and excessive muscular twitching secondary to

    hypocalcemia is: _____.

Y T N A E T

II. Critical Thinking Questions and Exercises

DISCUSSION AND ANALYSIS

Discuss the following topics with your classmates.

1. Describe the clinical manifestations, nursing interventions, and medical management for diabetes insipidus.
2. Distinguish between four diagnostic thyroid tests: serum thyroid-stimulating hormone, serum free T4, serum T3 and T4, and the T3 resin uptake test.

3. Draft six nursing diagnoses and related goals for a patient with hypothyroidism.
4. Explain how radiation can induce thyroid cancer.
5. Compare and contrast the etiology and clinical manifestations of Addison's disease and Cushing's syndrome.

CLINICAL SITUATIONS

Read the following case studies. Circle the correct answer.

CASE STUDY: Primary Hypothyroidism

Connie had been hospitalized for 1 week for studies to confirm a diagnosis of primary hypothyroidism.

1. Several tests were used in Connie's assessment. All of the following results are consistent with her diagnosis of hypothyroidism *except* for:

   a. an increased level of thyrotropin (TSH).

   b. a low uptake of radioactive iodine (^{131}I).

   c. a protein-bound iodine reading of 3 mg/dL.

   d. a T_3 uptake value of 45%.

2. Nursing care for Connie includes assessing for clinical manifestations associated with hypothyroidism. A manifestation not consistent with her diagnosis is a:

   a. change in her menstrual pattern.

   b. pulse rate of 58 bpm.

   c. temperature of 95.88°F.

   d. weight loss of 10 lb over a 2-week period.

3. The principal objective of medical management is to:

   a. irradiate the gland in an attempt to stimulate hormonal secretion.

   b. replace the missing hormone.

   c. remove the diseased gland.

   d. withhold exogenous iodine to create a negative feedback response, which will force the gland to secrete hormones.

4. Nursing comfort measures for Connie should include:

   a. encouraging frequent periods of rest throughout the day.

   b. offering her additional blankets to help prevent chilling.

   c. using a cleansing lotion instead of soap for her skin.

   d. all of the above.

5. Health teaching for Connie includes making sure that she knows that iodine-based chemotherapy is:

   a. administered intravenously for 1 week so that her symptoms may be rapidly put into remission.

   b. needed for life.

   c. recommended for 1 to 3 months.

   d. used until her symptoms disappear.

CASE STUDY: Hyperparathyroidism

Emily is a 65-year-old woman and has been complaining of continued emotional irritability. Her family described her as always being "on edge" and neurotic. After several months of exacerbated symptoms, Emily underwent a complete physical examination and was diagnosed with hyperparathyroidism.

1. Emily's clinical symptoms are all related to an increase in serum:

   a. calcium.

   b. magnesium.

   c. potassium.

   d. sodium.

2. As a nurse, you know that the normal level of the mineral identified in the previous question is:
   a. 8.8 to 10 mg/dL.
   b. 1.3 to 2.1 mEq/L.
   c. 3.5 to 5.0 mEq/L.
   d. 135 to 148 mmol/L.

3. Describe eight symptoms usually seen when hyperparathyroidism involves several body systems:

   _____, _____, _____, _____,

   _____, _____, _____, and _____.

4. Name one of the most important organ complications of hyperparathyroidism: _____.

5. A musculoskeletal symptom found with hyperparathyroidism is:
   a. deformities due to demineralization.
   b. pain on weight bearing.
   c. pathologic fractures due to osteoclast growth.
   d. all of the above.

6. The recommended treatment for primary hyperparathyroidism is:
   a. pharmacotherapy until the elevated serum levels return to normal.
   b. surgical removal of the abnormal parathyroid tissue.
   c. adrenalectomy.
   d. all of the above treatments.

7. Acute hypercalcemic crises can occur in hyperparathyroidism. The treatment would involve immediate:
   a. administration of diuretic agents to promote renal excretion of calcium.
   b. phosphate therapy to correct hypophosphatemia.
   c. dehydration with large volumes of intravenous fluids.
   d. management with all of the above modalities.

CASE STUDY: Subtotal Thyroidectomy

Darrell, a 37-year-old father of two, has just returned to the clinical area from the recovery room. Darrell has had a subtotal thyroidectomy.

1. Postoperatively, Darrell is assisted from the stretcher to the bed. The most comfortable position for him to assume would be:
   a. high-Fowler's position with his neck supported by a soft collar.
   b. recumbent position with his neck hyperextended and supported by a neck pillow.
   c. recumbent position with sandbags preventing his neck from rotating.
   d. semi-Fowler's position with his head supported by pillows.

2. Postoperative bleeding when the patient is in the dorsal position would probably be evidenced:
   a. anteriorly.
   b. laterally.
   c. posteriorly.
   d. in any of the above areas.

3. Indicators of internal bleeding include:
   a. a sensation of fullness at the incision site.
   b. hypotension.
   c. tachycardia.
   d. all of the above.

4. The nurse should assess for the common manifestation of recurrent laryngeal nerve damage, which is:
   a. any voice change.
   b. the inability to speak.
   c. pain while speaking.
   d. pain while swallowing.

5. The nurse expects Darrell's postoperative diet to be:
   a. clear liquids, such as tea and carbonated beverages.
   b. high in calories.
   c. low in fat and protein.
   d. low in minerals, especially calcium.

6. The nurse should monitor serum calcium levels for hypocalcemia, which will occur with a serum calcium level of:
   a. 5 mg/dL.
   b. 9 mg/dL.
   c. 13 mg/dL.
   d. 17 mg/dL.

CHAPTER 43

Assessment of Renal and Urinary Tract Function

I. Interpretation, Completion, and Comparison

MULTIPLE CHOICE

Read each question carefully. Circle your answer.

1. An abnormal constituent of urine is:
   a. creatinine.
   b. glucose.
   c. potassium.
   d. urea.

2. The normal quantity of water ingested and excreted in the urine is approximately:
   a. 0.5 L/day.
   b. 1.5 L/day.
   c. 2.5 L/day.
   d. 4.0 L/day.

3. The normal amount of sodium ingested and excreted in the urine is approximately:
   a. 2 to 3 g/day.
   b. 4 to 5 g/day.
   c. 6 to 8 g/day.
   d. 9 to 10 g/day.

4. Increased blood osmolality will result in:
   a. antidiuretic hormone (ADH) stimulation.
   b. an increase in urine volume.
   c. diuresis.
   d. less reabsorption of water.

5. A major sensitive indicator of kidney disease is the:
   a. blood urea nitrogen level.
   b. creatinine clearance level.
   c. serum potassium level.
   d. uric acid level.

6. A major manifestation of uremia is:
   a. a decreased serum phosphorus level.
   b. hyperparathyroidism.
   c. hypocalcemia with bone changes.
   d. increased secretion of parathormone.

7. Significant nursing assessment data relevant to renal function should include information about:
   a. any voiding disorders.
   b. the patient's occupation.
   c. the presence of hypertension or diabetes mellitus.
   d. all of the above.

8. Oliguria is said to be present when urinary output is:
   a. less than 30 mL/h.
   b. about 100 mL/h.
   c. between 300 and 500 mL/h.
   d. between 500 and 1,000 mL/h.

9. A 24-hour urine collection is scheduled to begin at 8:00 AM. The nurse should begin the procedure:
   a. after discarding the 8:00 AM specimen.
   b. at 8:00 AM, with or without a specimen.
   c. 6 hours after the urine is discarded.
   d. with the first specimen voided after 8:00 AM.

10. The nurse should inform a patient that preparation for intravenous urography includes:
    a. a liquid restriction for 8 to 10 hours before the test.
    b. liquids before the test.
    c. enemas until clear.
    d. remaining NPO from midnight before the test.

11. Nursing responsibilities after renal angiography include:
    a. assessment of peripheral pulses.
    b. color and temperature comparisons between the involved and uninvolved extremities.
    c. examination of the puncture site for swelling and hematoma formation.
    d. all of the above.

12. A cystoscope allows visualization of the:
    a. bladder.
    b. ureteral orifices.
    c. urethra.
    d. above areas.

13. Nursing management after a renal brush biopsy includes:
    a. assessing for the clinical manifestations of hemorrhage.
    b. encouraging a fluid intake of 3 L every 24 hours.
    c. obtaining a sample of each voided urine to compare it with a prebiopsy specimen.
    d. all of the above.

SHORT ANSWER

Read each statement carefully. Write the best response in the space provided.

1. The functional unit of each kidney is the _____, located in the _____ of the kidney.

2. Normal adult bladder capacity is _____ mL of urine.

3. The urine osmolality that indicates an early sign of kidney disease is: _____.

4. The regulation of the amount of sodium excreted depends on the hormone _____.

5. When a person is dehydrated, the urine osmolality is: _____.

6. Water is reabsorbed, rather than excreted, under the control of the _____.

7. The normal serum pH is: _____; urine pH is: _____.

8. The major waste product of protein metabolism is: _____. Approximately how many grams are produced and excreted daily? _____.

9. The test that most accurately reflects glomerular filtration and renal excretory function is the:

   _____.

II. Critical Thinking Questions and Exercises

DISCUSSION AND ANALYSIS

Discuss the following topics with your classmates.

1. Describe the blood circulation through the kidneys and the filtration role of the glomerulus.
2. Compare the filtration functions of the cortical and juxtamedullary nephrons.
3. Explain the three-step process of urine formation that involves glomerular filtration, tubular reabsorption, and tubular secretion.
4. Explain why renal glycosuria may occur.
5. Describe the role of the ADH in maintaining the blood osmolality.
6. Explain the role of the kidneys in maintaining acid–base balance.
7. Discuss the etiology and nursing assessments for problems associated with changes in voiding; for example, dysuria, nocturia, proteinuria, urgency, enuresis, and incontinence.
8. Demonstrate how to percuss the bladder to check for residual urine.

IDENTIFYING PATTERNS

Draw the sequence of pathophysiologic events that are triggered when the blood pressure decreases and the hormone renin is released from the cells in the kidneys.

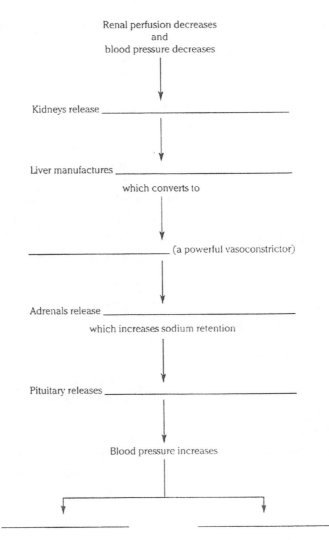

Renal perfusion decreases
and
blood pressure decreases

Kidneys release _____

Liver manufactures _____

which converts to

_____ (a powerful vasoconstrictor)

Adrenals release _____

which increases sodium retention

Pituitary releases _____

Blood pressure increases

_____   _____

CHAPTER 44

Management of Patients With Renal Disorders

I. Interpretation, Completion, and Comparison

MULTIPLE CHOICE

Read each question carefully. Circle your answer.

1. The most accurate indicator of fluid loss or gain in an acutely ill patient is:
   a. blood pressure.
   b. capillary refill.
   c. serum sodium levels.
   d. weight.

2. The nurse notes that a patient who is retaining fluid had a 1-kg weight gain. The nurse knows that this is equivalent to about:
   a. 250 mL.
   b. 500 mL.
   c. 750 mL.
   d. 1,000 mL.

3. A patient is admitted with electrolyte imbalance. He has carpopedal spasm, ECG changes, and a positive Chvostek's sign. The nurse suspects a deficit of:
   a. calcium.
   b. magnesium.
   c. phosphorus.
   d. sodium.

4. Acute glomerulonephritis refers to a group of kidney diseases in which there is:
   a. an inflammatory reaction.
   b. an antigen–antibody reaction to streptococci that results in circulating molecular complexes.
   c. cellular complexes that lodge in the glomeruli and injure the kidney.
   d. a combination of all of the above.

5. In most cases, the major stimulus to acute glomerulonephritis is:
   a. *Escherichia coli.*
   b. group A streptococcal infection of the throat.
   c. *Staphylococcus aureus.*
   d. *Neisseria gonorrhoeae.*

6. Laboratory findings consistent with acute glomerulonephritis include all of the following *except*:
   a. hematuria.
   b. polyuria.
   c. proteinuria.
   d. white cell casts.

7. Chronic glomerulonephritis is manifested by:
   a. anemia secondary to erythropoiesis.
   b. hypercalcemia and decreased serum phosphorus.
   c. hypokalemia and elevated bicarbonate.
   d. metabolic alkalosis.

8. The major manifestation of nephrotic syndrome is:
   a. hematuria.
   b. hyperalbuminemia.
   c. edema.
   d. anemia.

9. A clinical diagnosis of nephrotic syndrome is consistent with an exceedingly high level of:
   a. albumin.
   b. low-density lipoproteins.
   c. protein in the urine.
   d. serum cholesterol.

10. Acute renal failure (ARF) caused by parenchymal damage to the glomeruli or kidney tubules results in all of the following *except*:
    a. decreased GFR.
    b. increased urine's specific gravity.
    c. impaired electrolyte balance.
    d. progressive azotemia.

11. Oliguria is a clinical sign of ARF that refers to a daily urine output of:
    a. 1.5 L.
    b. 1.0 L.
    c. less than 400 mL.
    d. less than 50 mL.

12. A fall in CO_2-combining power and blood pH indicates what state accompanying renal function?
    a. Metabolic acidosis
    b. Metabolic alkalosis
    c. Respiratory acidosis
    d. Respiratory alkalosis

13. Hyperkalemia is a serious electrolyte imbalance that occurs in ARF and results from:
    a. protein catabolism.
    b. electrolyte shifts in response to metabolic acidosis.
    c. tissue breakdown.
    d. all of the above.

14. Potassium intake can be restricted by eliminating high-potassium foods such as:
    a. butter.
    b. citrus fruits.
    c. cooked white rice.
    d. salad oils.

15. A patient with ARF and negative nitrogen balance is expected to lose about:
    a. 0.5 kg/day.
    b. 1.0 kg/day.
    c. 1.5 kg/day.
    d. 2.0 kg/day.

16. The leading cause of end-stage renal disease is:
    a. diabetes mellitus.
    b. hypertension.
    c. glomerulonephritis.
    d. toxic agents.

17. A patient with stage 3, chronic renal failure would be expected to have:
    a. a GFR of >90 mL/min/1.73 m^2.
    b. a GFR = 30 to 59 mL/min/1.73 m^2.
    c. severe decreases in GFR.
    d. kidney failure.

18. In chronic renal failure (end-stage renal disease), decreased glomerular filtration leads to:
    a. increased pH.
    b. decreased creatinine clearance.
    c. increased blood urea nitrogen (BUN).
    d. all of the above.

19. Decreased levels of erythropoietin, a substance normally secreted by the kidneys, leads to which serious complication of chronic renal failure?
    a. Anemia
    c. Hyperkalemia
    b. Acidosis
    d. Pericarditis

20. Recent research about the long-term toxicity of aluminum products has led physicians to recommend antacids that lower serum phosphorus, such as:
    a. calcium carbonate.
    c. magaldrate.
    b. sodium bicarbonate.
    d. milk of magnesia.

21. Dietary intervention for renal deterioration includes limiting the intake of:
    a. fluid.
    c. sodium and potassium.
    b. protein.
    d. all of the above.

22. The process that underlies and supports the procedure of hemodialysis is:
    a. diffusion.
    c. ultrafiltration.
    b. osmosis.
    d. all of the above processes.

23. An incomplete protein *not* recommended for the diet of a patient managed by long-term hemodialysis is that found in:
    a. eggs.
    c. milk.
    b. fish.
    d. nuts.

24. With peritoneal dialysis, urea and creatinine pass through the peritoneum by:
    a. active transport.
    c. filtration.
    b. diffusion and osmosis.
    d. ultrafiltration.

25. At the end of five peritoneal exchanges, the patient's fluid loss was 500 mL. This loss is equal to approximately:
    a. 0.5 lb.
    c. 1.5 lb.
    b. 1.0 lb.
    d. 2 lb.

26. The major danger after renal surgery is:
    a. abdominal distention owing to reflex cessation of intestinal peristalsis.
    c. paralytic ileus caused by manipulation of the colon during surgery.
    b. hypovolemic shock caused by hemorrhage.
    d. pneumonia caused by shallow breathing because of severe incisional pain.

27. Preoperative management for a patient who is to undergo kidney transportation includes:
    a. bringing the metabolic state to as normal a level as possible.
    c. suppressing immunologic defense mechanisms.
    d. all of the above.
    b. making certain that the patient is free of infection.

28. Postoperative management for a recipient of a transplanted kidney includes:
    a. aseptic technique to avoid infection.
    c. protective isolation while immunosuppressive drug therapy is at its maximum dosage.
    b. hourly urinary output measurements to estimate the degree of kidney function.
    d. all of the above.

MATCHING

Match the symptom listed in column II with its associated fluid or electrolyte imbalance listed in column I.

Column I

1. _____ Calcium deficit
2. _____ Calcium excess
3. _____ Fluid volume deficit
4. _____ Fluid volume excess
5. _____ Magnesium deficit
6. _____ Potassium deficit
7. _____ Potassium excess
8. _____ Protein deficit
9. _____ Sodium deficit
10. _____ Sodium excess

Column II

a. Carpopedal spasm and tetany
b. Muscle hypotonicity and flank pain
c. Oliguria and weight loss
d. Positive Chvostek's sign
e. Crackles and dyspnea
f. Chronic weight loss and fatigability
g. Fingerprinting on the sternum
h. Irritability and intestinal colic
i. Rough, dry tongue and thirst
j. Soft, flabby muscles and weakness

SHORT ANSWER

Read each statement carefully. Write your response in the space provided.

1. The primary cause of chronic kidney disease is: _____.

2. Nephrosclerosis is primarily caused by: _____ and _____.

3. List the six major clinical manifestations of glomerular injury:

_____   _____

_____   _____

_____   _____

4. Describe the physical appearance of the urine early in the stage of acute glomerulonephritis.

_____.

5. Two blood levels that are significantly increased in ARF are: _____ and _____.

6. Name five physiologic disorders that characterize the nephrotic syndrome: _____, _____, _____, _____, and _____.

7. List the six risk factors for renal cancer:

_____   _____

_____   _____

_____   _____

8. List three major conditions that cause ARF. For each category, give one to two examples.

   a. _____   Examples: _____

   b. _____   Examples: _____

   c. _____   Examples: _____

9. In ARF, name two clinical signs of hyperkalemia: _____ and _____.

10. List at least six clinical manifestations seen in chronic renal failure.

11. List six potential complications of dialysis treatment.

   _____   _____

   _____   _____

   _____   _____

12. The leading cause of death for patients undergoing chronic hemodialysis is: _____.

13. The most common and serious complication of continuous ambulatory peritoneal dialysis (CAPD) is:

   _____.

14. Two complications of renal surgery that are believed to be caused by reflex paralysis of intestinal peristalsis and manipulation of the colon or duodenum during surgery are: _____ and

   _____.

II. Critical Thinking Questions and Exercises

DISCUSSION AND ANALYSIS

1. Describe the general management strategies for electrolyte imbalances for the following: sodium, potassium, calcium, magnesium, and phosphorus.
2. Describe the pathophysiology of acute glomerulonephritis.
3. Describe the pathophysiology, clinical manifestations, and medical management for a patient with polycystic kidney disease.
4. Describe nursing measures to prevent acute renal failure (ARF).
5. Describe the signs and symptoms of chronic renal failure, per system, i.e., neurological, cardiovascular, gastrointestinal, etc.
6. Compare the indications for acute versus chronic dialysis.
7. Describe the major complications of hemodialysis.
8. Explain the hemodynamics behind and the procedure for peritoneal dialysis.
9. Describe the medical and nursing management for patients who have experienced renal trauma.

APPLYING CONCEPTS

Examine Figure 44-5 in the text and answer the following questions.

1. A needle is inserted into the arterial segment of the fistula to: _____.

2. A needle is inserted into the venous segment of the fistula to: _____.

3. A new fistula requires _____ months to mature. This time is necessary because:

   _____.

4. Describe the exercise the patient should perform to help increase the vessel size.

   _____.

5. The most commonly used synthetic graft material is: _____.

   Grafts allow access in as little as _____ days.

CLINICAL SITUATIONS

Read the following case study. Circle the correct answer.

CASE STUDY: Continuous Ambulatory Peritoneal Dialysis

Edward, a 29-year-old diabetic patient, chose CAPD as a way of managing his end-stage renal disease.

1. Edward chose CAPD because it helped him:
   a. avoid severe dietary restrictions.
   b. control his blood pressure.
   c. have control over his daily activities.
   d. do all of the above.

2. Using CAPD, Edward needs to dialyze himself:
   a. approximately four to five times a day with no night changes.
   b. every 3 hours while awake.
   c. every 4 hours around the clock.
   d. once in the morning and once in the evening every day.

3. Edward needs to be aware that toxic wastes are exchanged during the equilibration or dwell time, which usually lasts for:
   a. 10 to 15 minutes.
   b. 30 minutes.
   c. 1 hour.
   d. 2 to 3 hours.

4. Edward needs to be taught how to detect signs of the most serious and most common complication of CAPD, which is:
   a. an abdominal hernia.
   b. anorexia.
   c. edema.
   d. peritonitis.

5. Edward's diet should be modified to be:
   a. high in carbohydrates.
   b. high in fats.
   c. high in protein.
   d. low in bran and fiber.

CASE STUDY: Acute Renal Failure

Fran is hospitalized with a diagnosis of ARF. She had been taking gentamicin sulfate for a pseudomonal infection.

1. The nurse knows that the kidney is susceptible to damage by nephrotoxic antibiotic agents, because it functions as a major excretory pathway and receives ____ of cardiac output at rest.
   a. 5%
   b. 15%
   c. 25%
   d. 45%

2. The nurse needs to assess for symptoms consistent with pathology secondary to reduced renal blood flow. Symptoms would include:
   a. reduced glomerular filtration.
   b. renal ischemia.
   c. tubular damage.
   d. all of the above.

3. During the oliguric phase of ARF, Fran's protein intake for her 156-lb body weight should be approximately:
   a. 35 g/24 h.
   b. 70 g/24 h.
   c. 120 g/24 h.
   d. 156 g/24 h.

4. While evaluating laboratory studies, the nurse expects that Fran's oliguric phase will be marked by all of the following *except*:
   a. blood urea nitrogen of 10 mg/dL.
   b. serum creatinine of 0.8 mg/dL.
   c. serum potassium of 6 mEq/L.
   d. urinary volume less than 600 mL/24 h.

5. After the diuretic phase, the nurse should recommend a:
   a. high-potassium diet.
   b. high-protein diet.
   c. low-carbohydrate diet.
   d. low-fat diet.

6. The nurse expects the period of recovery to follow a period of oliguria and to last approximately:
   a. 2 weeks.
   b. 6 weeks.
   c. 2 months.
   d. 6 to 12 months.

CHAPTER 45

Management of Patients With Urinary Disorders

I. Interpretation, Completion, and Comparison

MULTIPLE CHOICE

Read each question carefully. Circle your answer.

1. An example of an upper urinary tract infection (UTI) is:
   a. acute pyelonephritis.
   b. cystitis.
   c. prostatitis.
   d. urethritis.

2. A sign of possible UTI is:
   a. a negative urine culture.
   b. an output of 200 to 900 mL with each voiding.
   c. cloudy urine.
   d. urine with a specific gravity of 1.005 to 1.022.

3. The most common site of a lower UTI is the:
   a. bladder.
   b. kidney.
   c. prostate.
   d. urethra.

4. There is an increased risk of UTIs in the presence of:
   a. altered metabolic states.
   b. immunosuppression.
   c. urethral mucosa abrasion.
   d. all of the above.

5. The most common organism responsible for UTIs in women and the elderly is:
   a. *Klebsiella.*
   b. *Escherichia coli.*
   c. *Proteus.*
   d. *Pseudomonas.*

6. A first-line fluoroquinolone antibacterial agent for UTIs that has been found to be significantly effective is:
   a. Bactrim.
   b. Cipro.
   c. Macrodantin.
   d. Septra.

7. Frequently, a urinary analgesic is prescribed for relief of burning, pain, and other symptoms of a UTI. An example would be:
   a. Bactrim.
   b. Levaquin.
   c. Pyridium.
   d. Septra.

8. Health information for a female patient diagnosed as having cystitis includes all of the following *except*:
   a. cleanse around the perineum and urethral meatus (from front to back) after each bowel movement.
   b. drink liberal amounts of fluid.
   c. shower rather than bathe in a tub.
   d. void no more frequently than every 6 hours to allow urine to dilute the bacteria in the bladder.

9. Complications of chronic pyelonephritis include:
   a. end-stage renal disease.
   b. hypertension.
   c. kidney stone formation.
   d. all of the above.

10. The type of incontinence that results from a sudden increase in intra-abdominal pressure is:
    a. reflex incontinence.
    b. stress incontinence.
    c. overflow incontinence.
    d. urge incontinence.

11. Incontinence or dyssynergia is a voiding dysfunction found in the following neurogenic disorder:
    a. cerebellar ataxia.
    b. diabetes.
    c. multiple sclerosis.
    d. Parkinson's disease.

12. Fluid management as a method of behavioral therapy for incontinence requires a daily liquid intake of:
    a. 0.5 mL.
    b. 1.0 mL.
    c. 1.5 mL.
    d. 2.0 mL.

13. Spastic neurogenic bladder is associated with all of the following *except*:
    a. a loss of conscious sensation and cerebral motor control.
    b. a lower motor neuron lesion.
    c. hypertrophy of the bladder walls.
    d. reduced bladder capacity.

14. The major complication of neurogenic bladder is:
    a. hypertrophy.
    b. infection.
    c. pain.
    d. spasm.

15. The major cause of death for patients with neurologic impairment of the bladder is:
    a. myocardial infection.
    b. pulmonary edema.
    c. septicemia.
    d. renal failure.

16. Nursing measures for the patient with neurogenic bladder include:
    a. encouraging a liberal fluid intake.
    b. keeping the patient as mobile as possible.
    c. offering a diet low in calcium.
    d. all of the above.

17. When managing a closed urinary drainage system, the nurse needs to remember not to:
    a. allow the drainage bag to touch the floor.
    b. disconnect the bag.
    c. raise the drainage bag above the level of the patient's bladder.
    d. do any of the above.

18. A woman is taught to catheterize herself by inserting the catheter into the urethra:
    a. 0.5 to 1 in.
    b. 2 in.
    c. 3 in.
    d. 5 in.

19. A major clinical manifestation of renal stones is:
    a. dysuria.
    b. hematuria.
    c. infection.
    d. pain.

20. Patients with urolithiasis need to be encouraged to:
    a. increase their fluid intake so that they can excrete 2,500 mL to 4,000 mL every day, which will help prevent additional stone formation.
    b. participate in strenuous exercises so that the tone of smooth muscle in the urinary tract can be strengthened to help propel calculi.
    c. supplement their diet with calcium needed to replace losses to renal calculi.
    d. limit their voiding to every 6 to 8 hours so that increased volume can increase hydrostatic pressure, which will help push stones along the urinary system.

21. A patient being prescribed a diet moderately reduced in calcium and phosphorus should be taught to avoid:
    a. citrus fruits.
    b. milk.
    c. pasta.
    d. whole grain breads.

22. The most common symptom of cancer of the bladder is:
    a. back pain.
    b. dysuria.
    c. visible, painless hematuria.
    d. infection.

23. The predominant cause of bladder cancer is:
    a. chronic renal failure.
    b. cigarette smoking.
    c. environmental pollution.
    d. metastasis from another primary site.

24. The most effective intravesical agent for transurethral resection or fulguration for bladder cancer is:
    a. bacille Calmette-Guerin (BCG).
    b. doxorubicin.
    c. ethoglucid.
    d. thiotepa.

25. The urinary diversion whereby the patient will void from his rectum for the rest of his life is known as a:
    a. cutaneous ureterostomy.
    b. nephrostomy.
    c. suprapubic cystotomy.
    d. ureterosigmoidostomy.

SHORT ANSWER

Read each statement carefully. Write your response in the space provided.

1. There are three natural defenses to bacterial invasion of the urinary tract: _____ (protein), _____ (immunoglobulin), and _____, which interferes with the adherence of *Escherichia coli.*

2. The three organisms most frequently found in UTIs are: _____, _____, and _____.

3. Name common signs and symptoms associated with an uncomplicated lower UTI (cystitis).

4. The most common cause of recurrent UTIs in elderly males is: _____.

5. Patients with indwelling catheters are most likely to be infected by one of the following four organisms: _____, _____, _____, and _____.

6. List five reasons for catheterization: _____,

_____, _____, _____, and

_____.

7. List six signs and/or symptoms associated with catheter-induced UTIs:

_____   _____

_____   _____

_____   _____

8. List three crystalline substances known to form calcium-based stones in the urinary tract:

_____, _____, and _____.

II. Critical Thinking Questions and Exercises

RECOGNIZING CONTRADICTIONS

Rewrite each statement correctly. Underline the key concepts.

1. The majority of hospital-acquired (nosocomial) urinary tract infections are uncomplicated and community-acquired.
2. Urethrovesical reflux refers to the backward flow of urine from the bladder into the kidney.
3. Urinary tract anti-infectives are considered first-line medications for the treatment of urge incontinence.
4. Patients diagnosed with calcium-based renal stones are advised to avoid foods such as shellfish and organ meats.

DISCUSSION AND ANALYSIS

Discuss the following topics with your classmates.

1. Describe six categories of risk factors for UTIs.
2. Discuss why the elderly are more prone to UTI and name seven factors that contribute to UTIs in the elderly.
3. Compare the clinical symptoms and nursing interventions for acute versus chronic pyelonephritis.
4. Discuss at least 10 of the 14 common risk factors for urinary incontinence.
5. Describe the various causes of transient incontinence (reversible if condition is treated).
6. Explain the various teaching points that a nurse should cover to help patients promote urinary continence.
7. Explain general principles/guidelines that a nurse should follow to prevent infection in a patient with an indwelling urinary catheter.
8. Describe the eight risks factors for bladder cancer.

CHAPTER 46

Assessment and Management of Female Physiologic Processes

I. Interpretation, Completion, and Comparison

MULTIPLE CHOICE

Read each question carefully. Circle your answer.

1. The menstrual cycle is dependent on hormone production. The hormone responsible for stimulating progesterone is:

    a. androgens.

    b. estradiol.

    c. the follicle-stimulating hormone.

    d. the luteinizing hormone.

2. A neighbor tells you that she has had vaginal bleeding for the past several days. She is postmenopausal and has not had a menstrual period for the past 4 years. You recommend that she:

    a. should see her gynecologist or physician as soon as possible.

    b. should mention the bleeding episode to her physician at her next appointment.

    c. should disregard this bleeding episode, because it is probably normal.

    d. should use a birth control method, because she may be fertile with her next ovulation.

3. An annual pelvic examination should begin at age:

    a. 14 years.

    b. 18 years.

    c. 21 years.

    d. 25 years.

4. During an internal vaginal examination, the nurse practitioner notes a frothy and malodorous discharge. She suspects it is caused by the bacteria:

    a. *Candida.*

    b. *Eschar.*

    c. *Trichomonas.*

    d. *Escherichia coli.*

5. The results of a patient's cytologic test for cancer (Pap test) were interpreted as class II. The nurse explains that a class II finding indicates:

    a. squamous cell abnormalities.

    b. malignancy.

    c. suggestive but not conclusive malignancy.

    d. the absence of atypical or abnormal cells.

6. Newer classifications are being used to describe the findings of the cytologic smear. For example, a high-grade, squamous, intraepithelial lesion corresponds to all of the following *except*:

    a. CIN grade 1.

    b. CIN grade 2.

    c. CIS.

    d. CIN grade 3.

7. After a cervical cone biopsy, the patient needs to be instructed to:

    a. leave the packing in place for 18 to 24 hours.

    b. report any excessive bleeding.

    c. delay sexual intercourse until healing occurs.

    d. do all of the above.

8. The normal menstrual cycle usually lasts 4 to 5 days with a loss of about how much blood?

    a. 30 mL

    b. 60 mL

    c. 90 mL

    d. 120 mL

9. To prevent toxic shock syndrome (TSS), the nurse advises the 15-year-old girl to change tampons every:

    a. 2 to 3 hours.

    b. 4 to 6 hours.

    c. 8 hours.

    d. 12 hours.

10. A middle-aged woman experiencing dyspareunia can use what medication to diminish the discomfort?

    a. Ibuprofen

    b. Petroleum jelly

    c. K-Y jelly

    d. Aspirin

11. A nutritional recommendation for postmenopausal women would be a dietary increase in:

    a. calcium.

    b. iron.

    c. salt.

    d. vitamin K.

12. Premenstrual syndrome (PMS) may be caused by estrogen rising and progesterone decreasing during the phase of the menstrual cycle known as:

    a. follicular.

    b. luteal.

    c. ovulation.

    d. premenstrual.

13. In educating a patient with PMS about changing her dietary practices, the nurse would recommend that she increase her intake of:

    a. magnesium.

    b. vitamin D.

    c. iron.

    d. zinc.

14. Pain at the time of the regular menstrual flow is referred to as:

    a. dysmenorrhea.

    b. amenorrhea.

    c. menorrhagia.

    d. metrorrhagia.

15. In the United States, the percentage of pregnancies that are unplanned is about:

    a. 20%.

    b. 30%.

    c. 50%.

    d. 80%.

16. The most common side effect of transdermal contraceptives is:

    a. breast cancer.

    b. withdrawal bleeding.

    c. thrombophlebitis.

    d. application site allergic reactions.

17. Statistically, use of the calendar rhythm method as a means of contraception yields a pregnancy rate of:

    a. less than 10%.

    b. between 10% and 20%.

    c. about 40%.

    d. about 80%.

18. Spontaneous abortion occurs in 10% to 20% of pregnancies. Spontaneous abortion occurs most commonly at:

    a. 4 weeks.

    b. 4 to 6 weeks.

    c. 8 to 12 weeks.

    d. 16 weeks.

19. The highest incidence of ectopic pregnancy occurs in the:

    a. cervix.

    b. interstitial tissue.

    c. fallopian tube.

    d. abdominal area.

20. Rupture of the fallopian tube in an ectopic pregnancy usually occurs:
    a. within the first 2 weeks.   c. at 2 months.
    b. at 4 to 6 weeks.   d. at 3 months.

SHORT ANSWER

Read each statement carefully. Write your response in the space provided.

1. Puberty usually begins at ages _____ to _____ but may occur as early as age

   _____.

2. The pituitary gland releases two essential hormones: _____ hormone causes

   the ovaries to secrete estrogen and _____ hormone stimulates the production of
   progesterone.

3. Menopause usually begins at age _____ to _____ years with a

   median age of _____. Perimenopause can begin as early as

   _____.

4. List at least seven danger signals that any woman should report to a health care professional:

   _____   _____

   _____   _____

   _____   _____

   _____

5. The number of women who experience domestic violence each year is about:

   _____.

6. Approximately, _____% of women are victims of childhood incest.

7. The most accurate outpatient procedure for evaluating a woman for endometrial cancer is:

   _____.

8. List four of eight major symptoms a woman with PMS may experience: _____,

   _____, _____, and _____.

9. Menopause puts a woman at risk for four serious conditions: _____,

   _____, _____, and _____.

10. Explain why amenorrhea occurs with anorexia and bulimia.

    _____

    _____

11. Describe the physiologic basis for "the pill" as a contraceptive.

    _____

    _____

12. Identify at least six risk factors that would absolutely contraindicate the use of oral contraceptives:

_____, _____, _____, _____, _____, and _____.

13. Explain how the injectable contraceptive of Depo-Provera works.

_____

_____

14. Explain how the emergency use of estrogen or estrogen and a progestin can prevent pregnancy within 5 days of an episode of unprotected sexual intercourse (e.g., rape, torn condom).

_____

_____

15. Describe in vitro fertilization (IVF).

_____

_____

MATCHING

Match the term in column II with its corresponding definition in column I.

Column I

1. _____ Painful sexual intercourse
2. _____ Bladder protruding into the vagina
3. _____ Beginning of menstruation
4. _____ Description of ovaries and fallopian tubes
5. _____ Painful menstruation
6. _____ Implantation of endometrial tissue in other areas of the pelvis
7. _____ Pain on movement of the cervix
8. _____ Absence of menstrual flow

Column II

a. Adnexa
b. Amenorrhea
c. Chandelier sign
d. Cystocele
e. Dysmenorrhea
f. Dyspareunia
g. Endometriosis
h. Menarche

II. Critical Thinking Questions and Exercises

DISCUSSION AND ANALYSIS

Discuss the following topics with your classmates.

1. Discuss the information that should be obtained during a nursing health assessment, including essential data like health-related behaviors, annual examinations, and prior immunizations.
2. Describe the practice of female genital mutilation (FGM), common in Africa and the Middle East, and the nurse's role in assessment.
3. Discuss the risks and benefits of hormone replacement for the medical management of menopause.
4. Outline the health history questions and physical assessment modifications necessary for a woman with a disability.
5. Compare the benefits and risks of combined hormonal contraceptives.
6. Explain the postexposure prophylaxis recommended by the CDC (2002) for rape victims, including HIV testing.

RECOGNIZING CONTRADICTIONS

Rewrite each statement correctly. Underline the key concepts.

1. The Women's Health Initiative (WHI) study (2002) found that hormone replacement therapy, postmenopause, greatly reduced the presence of heart disease.
2. Women born to mothers who took diethylstilbestrol (DES) during their pregnancy have a higher than average chance of suffering miscarriage.
3. A cervical cone biopsy may be performed without anesthesia because the cervix is less sensitive to pain.
4. Magnetic resonance imaging (MRI) exposes the patient to radiation and is more expensive than other pelvic diagnostic aids.
5. Estrogen prepares the uterus for implantation of the fertilized ovum.
6. Progesterone can cause painful cramps during ovulation because it causes myometrial contractility and arteriolar vasospasm.
7. The leading cause of a pregnancy-related death in the woman's first trimester is hemorrhage, post spontaneous abortion.

EXTRACTING INFERENCES

Refer to the figure below when answering the following questions about ectopic pregnancies.

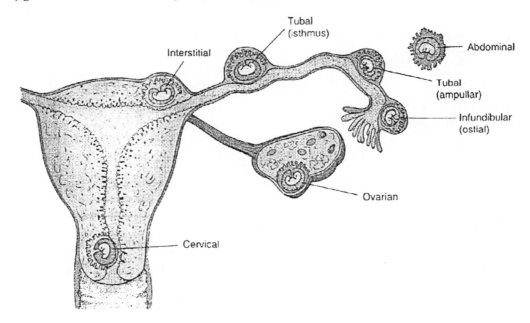

1. Explain what occurs after the ovum is fertilized to cause an ectopic pregnancy.

   _____

   _____

2. List several possible causes of ectopic implantation.

   _____

   _____

3. Look at the ovum implanted in the tubal (isthmus) area. What symptoms would you expect the woman to exhibit before tubal rupture occurs?

   _____

   _____

4. Name three possible surgical options to treat ectopic pregnancies: _____,
_____, and _____.

5. Postoperative medical management would include assessing the level of beta-HCG to: _____.

6. Potential maternal complications for ectopic pregnancies are: _____ and _____.

CLINICAL SITUATIONS

CASE STUDY: Toxic Shock Syndrome

Irene, a 23-year-old woman, is admitted to the emergency department in shock with an elevated temperature. She is diagnosed as having TSS.

1. The nurse knows that TSS is a bacterial infection associated with the use of tampons. The bacterial toxin is believed to be:
   a. *Escherichia coli.*
   b. *Haemophilus influenzae.*
   c. *Staphylococcus aureus.*
   d. *Pseudomonas aeruginosa.*

2. The onset of TSS is characterized by the sudden appearance of:
   a. an elevated temperature (up to 102°F).
   b. a red, macular rash.
   c. myalgia and dizziness.
   d. uncontrolled hypotension.

3. Signs associated with TSS include all of the following *except*:
   a. an elevated blood urea nitrogen level.
   b. a decreased bilirubin level.
   c. leukocytosis.
   d. oliguria.

4. Diagnostic evaluation is made from examination of cultures from:
   a. the blood and urine.
   b. the cervix.
   c. the vagina.
   d. all of the above areas.

5. A priority of medical management is:
   a. alleviating respiratory distress.
   b. treating the shock.
   c. controlling the infection.
   d. managing the emotional distress.

CHAPTER 47

Management of Patients With Female Reproductive Disorders

I. Interpretation, Completion, and Comparison

MULTIPLE CHOICE

Read each question carefully. Circle your answer.

1. Conditions that increase a woman's chances of developing candidiasis, caused by *Candida albicans*, include:
   - a. corticosteroids.
   - b. diabetes mellitus.
   - c. antibiotic therapy.
   - d. all of the above.

2. Metronidazole (Flagyl) is the recommended treatment for a vaginal infection caused by:
   - a. *Candida albicans*.
   - b. *Escherichia coli*.
   - c. *Streptococcus*.
   - d. *Trichomonas vaginalis*.

3. The nurse knows that a patient diagnosed with Bartholinitis would most likely be infected with:
   - a. *Candida albicans*.
   - b. *Chlamydia*.
   - c. *Gardnerella vaginalis*.
   - d. *Trichomonas vaginalis*.

4. Nursing interventions for the relief of pain and discomfort for a woman with a vulvovaginal infection include:
   - a. warm perineal irrigations.
   - b. sitz baths.
   - c. cornstarch for chafed inner thighs.
   - d. all of the above.

5. The *most common* sexually transmitted disease among young, sexually active people is:
   - a. candidiasis.
   - b. human papillomavirus.
   - c. endocervicitis.
   - d. salpingitis.

6. The bacterium responsible for mucopurulent cervicitis is:
   - a. *Chlamydia*.
   - b. *Gardnerella*.
   - c. *Staphylococcus*.
   - d. *Pseudomonas*.

7. The incidence of chlamydia and gonorrhea infections in young females in the United States is:
   - a. 1 in 100.
   - b. 1 in 50.
   - c. 1:20.
   - d. 1:10.

8. The percentage of women who have both chlamydia and gonorrhea is:
   - a. 15%.
   - b. 25%.
   - c. 50%.
   - d. 80%.

9. A risk factor(s) for women diagnosed with pelvic inflammatory disease (PID) annually in the United States is (are):

   a. early age of first intercourse.

   b. multiple sex partners.

   c. previous pelvic infection.

   d. all of the above.

10. The leading cause of new HIV infection in women is:

    a. heterosexual transmission.

    b. homosexual transmission.

    c. blood transfusions.

    d. intravenous drug use.

11. The percentage of women in their 20s who acquire HIV is:

    a. 20%.

    b. 30%.

    c. 50%.

    d. 80%.

12. Mrs. Jakes has had a pessary inserted for long-term treatment of a prolapsed uterus. As part of your teaching plan, you would advise Mrs. Jakes to:

    a. see her gynecologist to remove and clean the pessary at regular intervals.

    b. keep the insertion site clean and dry.

    c. avoid sexual intercourse.

    d. avoid climbing stairs as much as possible.

13. The most common vulvar tumor is known as:

    a. Bartholin's cyst.

    b. Skene's duct cyst.

    c. vulvodynia.

    d. vestibular cyst.

14. Fibroid tumors occur in what percentage of women during their reproductive years?

    a. 5% to 10%

    b. 10% to 15%

    c. 20% to 40%

    d. 50% to 60%

15. Mrs. Schurman, who has been diagnosed as having endometriosis, asks for an explanation of the disease. The best response for the nurse is to explain that:

    a. she has developed an infection in the lining of her uterus.

    b. tissue from the lining of the uterus has implanted in areas outside the uterus.

    c. the lining of the uterus is thicker than usual, causing heavy bleeding and cramping.

    d. the lining of the uterus is too thin because endometrial tissue has implanted outside the uterus.

16. The highest frequency of endometriosis is found in the:

    a. cervix.

    b. cul-de-sac.

    c. ovaries.

    d. ureterovesical peritoneum.

17. Mrs. Schurman's treatment involves taking oral danazol (Danocrine), 800 mg/day, for 9 months. Danazol is:

    a. a gonadotropin that decreases ovarian and pituitary stimulations.

    b. an antigonadotropin that increases pituitary stimulation and decreases ovarian stimulation.

    c. a gonadotropin that decreases pituitary stimulation and increases ovarian stimulation.

    d. an antigonadotropin that decreases pituitary and ovarian stimulations.

18. Risk factors commonly associated with cancer of the cervix include:

    a. chronic cervical infections.

    b. exposure to diethylstilbestrol (DES) in utero.

    c. multiple sexual partners.

    d. all of the above.

19. By incidence, where does cervical cancer rank among the most common female reproductive cancers?
    a. First
    b. Second
    c. Third
    d. Fourth

20. The two chief symptoms of early carcinoma of the cervix are:
    a. leukoplakia and metrorrhagia.
    b. dyspareunia and foul-smelling vaginal discharge.
    c. "strawberry" spots and menorrhagia.
    d. leukorrhea and irregular vaginal bleeding or spotting.

21. Using the International Classification of Carcinoma of the Uterine Cervix, a stage II Pap smear result indicates:
    a. cancer in situ.
    b. vaginal invasion.
    c. pelvic wall invasion.
    d. bladder extension.

22. A postmenopausal woman who has irregular uterine or vaginal bleeding should be encouraged by a nurse to:
    a. stop taking her Premarin (hormonal therapy).
    b. see her gynecologist as soon as possible.
    c. disregard this phenomenon because it is common during this life stage.
    d. mention it to her physician during her next annual examination.

23. Cancer of the uterus is the most common pelvic neoplasm in women; among cancers for women, it ranks:
    a. first.
    b. second.
    c. third.
    d. fourth.

24. Women who experience postmenopausal bleeding have what percentage of a chance of developing cancer of the uterus?
    a. 10%
    b. 20%
    c. 35%
    d. 75%

25. The most common symptom of cancer of the vulva is:
    a. a foul-smelling discharge.
    b. bleeding.
    c. pain.
    d. pruritus.

26. The primary treatment for vulvar malignancy is:
    a. chemotherapy creams.
    b. laser vaporization.
    c. radiation.
    d. wide excision.

27. Postoperative nursing care for a simple vulvectomy should include:
    a. cleansing the wound daily.
    b. offering a low-residue diet.
    c. positioning the patient with pillows.
    d. all of the above.

28. As a cause of cancer deaths related to the female reproductive system, ovarian cancer ranks:
    a. first.
    b. second.
    c. third.
    d. fourth.

29. The risk of ovarian cancer for women over their lifetime is:
    a. 1 in 20.
    b. 1 in 30.
    c. 1 in 50.
    d. 1 in 70.

30. Women who have the BRCA1 and BRCA2 genes have a lifetime risk of developing ovarian cancer as high as:
    a. 20%.
    c. 60%.
    b. 40%.
    d. 80%.

31. A diagnosis of stage III ovarian cancer indicates that growth involves:
    a. only the ovaries.
    c. metastases outside the pelvis.
    b. the ovaries with pelvic extension.
    d. distant metastases.

MATCHING

Match the word in column II with its associated definition in column I.

Column I

Column II

1. _____ Intense burning and inflammation of the vulva
2. _____ A preferred treatment for candidiasis
3. _____ The recommended treatment for trichomoniasis
4. _____ The drug of choice for herpes genitalis
5. _____ A potential complication of toxic shock syndrome
6. _____ The downward displacement of the bladder toward the vaginal orifice
7. _____ This test is used for diagnosis of cervical cancer
8. _____ Term used to describe the surgical procedure in which the uterus, cervix, and ovaries are removed
9. _____ A term used to describe vaginal bleeding
10. _____ Another name for benign tumors of the uterus
11. _____ In utero exposure to this drug increases the incidence of vaginal cancer
12. _____ A risk factor for uterine cancer
13. _____ Exercises that strengthen the pelvic muscles
14. _____ An opening between two hollow organs
15. _____ Displacement of the uterus into the vaginal canal
16. _____ Cysts that arise from parts of the ovum

a. Fibroids
b. Fistula
c. Cystocele
d. Mycostatin
e. Acyclovir
f. Vulvodynia
g. Dermoid
h. Septic shock
i. Menorrhagia
j. DES
k. Kegal
l. Prolapse
m. HRT
n. Pap smear
o. Hysterectomy
p. Flagyl

II. Critical Thinking Questions and Exercises

DISCUSSION AND ANALYSIS

Discuss the following topics with your classmates.

1. Discuss patient-teaching points to decrease/minimize the 10 common risk factors for vulvovaginal infections.
2. Explain why a decrease in estrogen can lead to vaginal infections.
3. Describe the pathophysiology and latest treatment for human papillomavirus infections.
4. Explain the extent of organ involvement with PID.
5. Discuss the nursing management, preoperative, postoperative, and community-based care, for patients who have had surgery for pelvic organ prolapsed.
6. Compare the risk factors for cervical and uterine cancer.

CLINICAL SITUATIONS

CASE STUDY: Bacterial Vaginosis

Read the following case studies. Fill in the blanks or circle the correct answer.

Maryanne, a 19-year-old college student, has recently noticed increased vaginal discharge that is grey to yellowish white in color.

1. After examination, the nurse prepares a wet mount (vaginal smear). When potassium hydroxide solution is added to the smear, a fishy odor is noted. Maryanne probably has a nonspecific vaginitis known as:
   a. bacterial vaginosis.
   b. candidiasis.
   c. trichomonas vaginalis.
   d. atopic vaginitis.

2. A diagnostic sign of bacterial vaginosis is:
   a. a scanty to minimal discharge.
   b. a vaginal pH of >4.7.
   c. painful menstruation.
   d. a greenish discharge between periods.

3. Metronidazole (Flagyl) is prescribed to be taken twice a day for 1 week. While taking this medication, Maryanne should be instructed to:
   a. avoid dairy products.
   b. avoid sunlight.
   c. avoid alcohol.
   d. lie down flat for at least 30 minutes after inserting the medication.

4. If Maryanne's vaginal infection recurs, the nurse should recommend that:
   a. her sexual partner be tested and treated.
   b. she refrain from sexual intercourse.
   c. she avoid the use of tampons.
   d. she take only showers and no tub baths for awhile.

5. An appropriate nursing diagnosis for Maryanne is:
   a. Altered Comfort—pain and discomfort related to burning or itching from the infectious process.
   b. Self-care Deficit related to inability to perform activities of daily living.
   c. Altered Comfort related to *Gardnerella*-associated vaginitis.
   d. Altered Comfort related to candidiasis.

CASE STUDY: Herpes Genitalis

Paige, a 37-year-old mother of one, has just been recently diagnosed with herpes genitalis, a recurrent, lifelong viral infection.

1. Herpes genitalis, a sexually transmitted disease, causes blisters on the:
   a. cervix.
   b. external genitalia.
   c. vagina.
   d. all of the above areas.

2. The initial painful infection usually lasts:
   a. 1 week.
   b. 2 weeks.
   c. 4 weeks.
   d. 6 weeks.

3. The herpes virus that is accountable for about 80% of genital and perineal lesions is:
   a. Epstein-Barr virus.
   b. cytomegalovirus.
   c. herpes simplex, type 2.
   d. varicella zoster.

4. At least _____ people, mostly young Caucasian adolescents and young adults, are infected.

5. To acquire the infection, one must have had close human contact with one of five sites on the body:

_____, _____, _____, _____,

and _____.

6. Since there is no cure for HSV-2 infection, list three antiviral agents that manage symptoms:

_____, _____, and _____.

7. List four probable nursing diagnoses for Paige: _____, _____,

_____, and _____.

CASE STUDY: Pelvic Inflammatory Disease

Donna is a 26-year-old graduate student who has been sexually active with multiple partners for 5 years. Last year she experienced several incidences of cervicitis. She now believes she has PID.

1. On the basis of your knowledge of PID, you know that the inflammatory condition of the pelvic cavity may involve the following five areas: _____, _____, _____,

_____, and _____.

2. Choose six words to describe the characteristics of the infection: _____, _____,

_____, _____, _____, and _____.

3. Name the two most common causative organisms for PID:

_____ and _____.

4. List five disorders that can result from the PID infection: _____,

_____, _____, _____, and _____.

5. Name four localized symptoms and six generalized symptoms of PID.

Localized	*Generalized*
1. _____	1. _____
2. _____	2. _____
3. _____	3. _____
4. _____	4. _____
	5. _____
	6. _____

CHAPTER 48

Assessment and Management of Patients With Breast Disorders

I. Interpretation, Completion, and Comparison

MULTIPLE CHOICE

Read each question carefully. Circle your answer.

1. The optimal time for breast self-examination is usually beginning at which day(s) after menses begins?
   a. Third to fourth
   b. Fifth to seventh
   c. Eighth to ninth
   d. After tenth day

2. The average percentage of women who perform breast self-examination is believed to be about:
   a. 15%.
   b. 25%.
   c. 40%.
   d. 80%.

3. Mammography can diagnose breast cancer before it is clinically palpable, meaning that the lump can be detected by x-ray when it is approximately of what size?
   a. 1 cm
   b. 1 mm
   c. 2 cm
   d. 2 mm

4. As part of health teaching, the nurse needs to alert patients that mammography can yield a false-negative result in how many instances out of 100?
   a. 5 to 10
   b. 10 to 15
   c. 15 to 20
   d. 20 to 25

5. Mammography should be used to annually screen women every year, beginning at age:
   a. 25 years.
   b. 30 years.
   c. 35 years.
   d. 40 years.

6. Characteristics of the lumps present in cystic disease of the breasts include all of the following *except*:
   a. a rapid increase and decrease in size.
   b. increased tenderness before menstruation.
   c. a painless or tender lump.
   d. skin dimpling and nipple retraction.

7. The risk of developing breast cancer for women is now 1 in:
   a. 8.
   b. 15.
   c. 25.
   d. 40.

8. Over 80% of breast cancers are diagnosed after age:
   a. 40 years.
   b. 50 years.
   c. 65 years.
   d. 75 years.

9. The current 5-year survival rate for stage I breast cancer is about:
   a. 60%.
   b. 75%.
   c. 88%.
   d. 98%.

10. Carcinoma in situ, a noninvasive form of cancer, has what percentage cure rate with surgical treatment?
    a. 75%
    b. 85%
    c. 90 to 95%
    d. About 98%

11. A 1998 clinical study yielded significant reduction in the incidence of breast cancer for those participants who took the chemopreventive agent:
    a. doxorubicin.
    b. methotrexate.
    c. raloxifene.
    d. tamoxifen.

12. The strongest factor (80% correlation) that influences the incidence of breast cancer is:
    a. chemical elements.
    b. environmental pollution.
    c. genetic predisposition.
    d. the number of menstrual cycles.

13. The chance of developing breast cancer doubles if:
    a. the woman had her first child after 30 years of age.
    b. the woman's mother had breast cancer.
    c. the woman was exposed to radiation after puberty.
    d. all of the above are true.

14. The majority of breast cancers occur in the:
    a. upper, inner quadrant.
    b. lower, inner quadrant.
    c. upper, outer quadrant.
    d. lower, outer quadrant.

15. Early clinical manifestations of breast carcinoma include all of the following *except*:
    a. a nontender lump.
    b. asymmetry of the breasts.
    c. nipple retraction.
    d. pain in the breast tissue.

16. A noninvasive breast tumor that is 2 cm or less in size is classified as:
    a. stage I.
    b. stage II.
    c. stage III.
    d. stage IV.

17. Carcinoma of the breast results from cell doubling. A cell that doubles every 60 days for 30 doublings would become palpable after (1 cm or larger) in:
    a. 3 years.
    b. 5 years.
    c. 10 years.
    d. 15 years.

18. At diagnosis of breast carcinoma, the risk for the presence of metastasis is about:
    a. 25%.
    b. 38%.
    c. 55%.
    d. 73%.

19. The most common site for regional metastasis for breast carcinoma is(are) the:
    a. adrenals.
    b. axillary lymph node.
    c. lungs.
    d. liver.

20. If the number of positive axillary lymph nodes is between five and six on biopsy, the risk for breast cancer recurrence is:

    a. less than 10%.

    b. 15%.

    c. 30%.

    d. greater than 50%.

21. A patient is scheduled for removal of her left breast and the axillary lymph nodes; the pectoralis minor muscle is to be left in place. This surgical intervention is called:

    a. an extended radical mastectomy.

    b. a modified radical mastectomy.

    c. a quadrantectomy.

    d. a simple mastectomy.

22. Suggested postoperative positioning of the affected arm after surgical intervention (mastectomy) is:

    a. abduction to promote incisional healing.

    b. adduction to minimize trauma to sensitive tissue.

    c. elevation to promote lymphatic drainage.

    d. extension to facilitate isometric exercises.

23. Postmastectomy arm exercises facilitate the development of collateral circulation, which decreases lymphedema. Collateral circulation is usually developed within:

    a. 1 month.

    b. 3 months.

    c. 5 months.

    d. 8 to 10 months.

24. A patient with lymphedema in an arm should be advised to avoid:

    a. blood pressure assessments in that arm.

    b. injections or needles in that arm.

    c. prolonged exposure of that arm to sunlight.

    d. all of the above.

25. The most common hormonal method of intervention is the use of:

    a. Cytadren.

    b. diethylstilbestrol.

    c. Megace.

    d. tamoxifen.

26. A monoclonal antibody that is used for targeted chemotherapy is:

    a. Aranesp.

    b. Epogen.

    c. Herceptin.

    d. Arimidex.

27. The most commonly encountered breast condition in the male is:

    a. breast cancer.

    b. mastitis.

    c. gynecomastia.

    d. cystic breast disease.

MATCHING

Match the term in column II with its corresponding definition in column I.

Column I

1. _____ Overdeveloped breast tissue usually seen in boys

2. _____ Breast augmentation

3. _____ Mammography after injection of dye

4. _____ Breast cancer in the ductal system

5. _____ Breast pain, usually hormonal in nature

6. _____ Infection of breast tissue

7. _____ Partial breast radiation

Column II

a. Galactography

b. Mastalgia

c. Paget's disease

d. Mastitis

e. Gynecomastia

f. Brachytherapy

g. Mammoplasty

II. Critical Thinking Questions and Exercises

DISCUSSION AND ANALYSIS

Discuss the following topics with your classmates.

1. Describe some abnormal clinical signs and symptoms that may be observed during inspection of the breasts.
2. Demonstrate the procedure to use for breast palpation.
3. Discuss the differences among the various types of breast biopsies.
4. Discuss the various causes of nipple discharge.
5. Discuss the pre- and postoperative nursing interventions for a patient having a total mastectomy.
6. Demonstrate the usual regimen of arm and shoulder exercises after breast surgery.
7. Explain the self-care instructions for patients receiving radiation therapy.

CLINICAL SITUATIONS

Read the following case study. Circle the correct answer.

CASE STUDY: Simple Mastectomy

Louise is 53 years old and single. The biopsy findings indicate that she has a malignancy in her breast. She is scheduled for a simple mastectomy.

1. On the basis of the knowledge about the cause of breast cancer, the nurse knows that the highest incidence of this type of cancer is found:
   a. among those who give birth to their first child after 35 years of age.
   b. among those who have had multiple pregnancies.
   c. in the unmarried woman who has not had children.
   d. in the woman who has menopause after 50 years of age.

2. On examination, Louise's tumor is found in the anatomic area where tumors usually develop, the:
   a. medial half of the breast.
   b. nipple area.
   c. posterior segment, inferior to the nipple.
   d. upper, outer quadrant.

3. Louise is advised that if she chooses not to seek treatment, her life expectancy will be:
   a. less than 1 year.
   b. between 2 and 3 years.
   c. about 5 years.
   d. as long as 10 years.

4. The nurse can advise Louise that surgical management for her stage I cancer has a cure rate of:
   a. 30%.
   b. 50%.
   c. 90%.
   d. 100%.

5. Postoperative care of the incision includes all of the following *except*:
   a. applying cocoa butter to increase elasticity.
   b. drying the area with slight friction to stimulate the circulation.
   c. gently bathing the area with a nonabrasive soap.
   d. massaging the area.

6. Louise's affected arm should be elevated on a pillow so that her:
   a. entire arm is in a horizontal plane.
   b. forearm is level with her heart.
   c. wrist is higher than her elbow, which should be higher than her shoulder.
   d. wrist is lower than her elbow so that circulation to her hand will not be decreased.

7. The nurse expects that Louise will be allowed out of bed in:

a. 1 to 2 days.

b. about 5 days.

c. about 1 week.

d. 1 to 2 weeks.

8. The nurse is aware that if a chemotherapy regime is prescribed, it most likely will include the following three drugs: _____, _____, and _____.

IDENTIFYING PATTERNS

Five figures of a woman performing breast self-examination follow. Start with the first figure and explain the activity associated with each step.

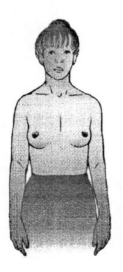

Step One

1. _____

2. _____

3. _____

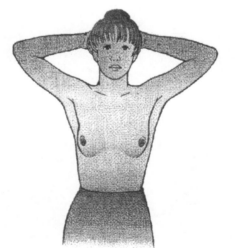

Step Two

1. _____

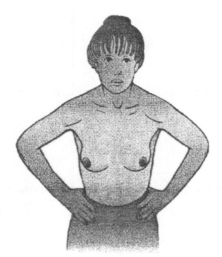

Step Three

1. _____

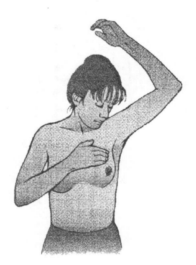

Step Four

1. _____

2. _____

3. _____

4. _____

5. _____

6. _____

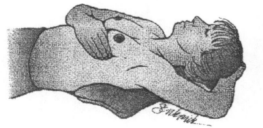

Step Five

1. _____

2. _____

3. _____

CHAPTER 49

Assessment and Management of Problems Related to Male Reproductive Processes

I. Interpretation, Completion, and Comparison

MULTIPLE CHOICE

Read each question carefully. Circle your answer.

1. Health education for a patient with prostatitis includes all of the following *except*:
   a. avoiding drinks that increase prostatic secretions.
   b. forcing fluids to prevent urine from backing up and distending the bladder.
   c. taking several hot sitz baths daily.
   d. using antibiotic therapy for 10 to 14 days.

2. Enlargement of the prostate gland, benign prostatic hyperplasia (BPH), is usually associated with:
   a. dysuria.
   b. dilation of the ureters.
   c. hydronephrosis.
   d. all of the above.

3. The incidence of BPH among men older than 60 years of age is:
   a. 35%.
   b. 50%.
   c. 65%.
   d. 80%.

4. As a cause of death in American men older than 55 years of age, cancer of the prostate ranks:
   a. first.
   b. second.
   c. third.
   d. fourth.

5. The racial group most likely to acquire and die from prostate cancer is:
   a. African Americans.
   b. Caucasians.
   c. Hispanics.
   d. Italians.

6. Prostatic cancer commonly metastasizes to the:
   a. bone and lymph nodes.
   b. liver and spleen.
   c. lungs and pancreas.
   d. brain and bladder.

7. The 10-year survival rate for prostate cancer is:
   a. 25%.
   b. 50%.
   c. 85%.
   d. 100%.

8. The concentration of prostate-specific antigen (PSA) is proportional to the total prostatic mass. As a diagnostic tool, PSA would indicate all of the following *except*:

   a. local progression of the disease.

   b. patient responsiveness to cancer therapy.

   c. recurrence of prostate cancer.

   d. the presence of malignancy.

9. The closed surgical procedure for a prostatectomy uses which approach?

   a. Perineal

   b. Suprapubic

   c. Retropubic

   d. Transurethral

10. Patients undergoing open surgical removal of the prostate, using the perineal approach, seem to experience a high incidence of:

    a. paralytic ileus.

    b. pneumonia.

    c. impotence.

    d. all of the above.

11. In most instances, patients can be advised that sex can resume, after a prostatectomy, in about:

    a. 4 weeks.

    b. 2 months.

    c. 10 weeks.

    d. 4 months.

12. An expected postoperative outcome of prostatectomy is light pink urine within:

    a. 24 hours.

    b. 48 hours.

    c. 3 days.

    d. 1 week.

13. During the 2 months it takes for the prostatic fossa to heal, the patient is advised not to:

    a. engage in strenuous exercise.

    b. perform the Valsalva maneuver.

    c. take long automobile rides.

    d. do all of the above.

14. In the 15- to 35-year-old age group, testicular cancer has a mortality rate of:

    a. 5%.

    b. 10%.

    c. 20%.

    d. 40%.

16. Retroperitoneal lymphadenectomy after orchiectomy would probably lead to:

    a. altered libido.

    b. inability to have orgasm.

    c. infertility.

    d. all of the above.

17. One cause of infertility in men is a:

    a. hydrocele.

    b. varicocele.

    c. paraphimosis.

    d. phimosis.

18. Neonatal circumcision is an important protective measure against carcinoma of the:

    a. penis.

    b. testes.

    c. scrotum.

    d. urethra.

19. All of the following are true of priapism *except* that it:

    a. is a urologic emergency.

    b. may result in gangrene.

    c. is painless.

    d. may result in impotence.

SHORT ANSWER

Read each statement carefully. Write your response in the space provided.

1. Two specific tests used to diagnose prostate cancer are: _____ and _____.

2. List 4 of a possible 17 medications associated with erectile dysfunction:

   _____, _____,

   _____, and _____.

3. The most common isolated organism that causes prostatitis is: _____.

4. List four of seven symptoms associated with prostatitis: _____,

   _____, _____, and _____.

5. List five symptoms found with BPH: _____, _____,

   _____, _____, and _____.

6. The most commonly used medication for estrogen therapy in the treatment of prostatic cancer is:

   _____; other hormonal therapies such as _____,

   _____, _____ , _____, and

   _____ suppress testicular androgen.

7. Five major, potential complications after prostatectomy are: _____,

   _____, _____, _____, and _____.

8. List the complication of prostatectomy that occurs in 80% to 95% of patients.

   _____.

9. Explain why low-dose heparin is usually given to patients undergoing prostatectomy.

   _____

10. Describe epididymitis and several of its common causes.

    _____

11. Two tumor markers that may be elevated in testicular cancer are:

    _____ and _____.

MATCHING

Match the term listed in column II with its description of disorder of the male reproductive system listed in column I.

Column I

1. _____ Collection of fluid in the testes
2. _____ An obstructive complex characterized by increased urinary frequency
3. _____ Constricted foreskin of the penis
4. _____ Failure of the testes to descend into the scrotum
5. _____ Inflammation of the testes
6. _____ Abnormal dilation of the veins in the scrotum
7. _____ Inflammation of the prostrate gland
8. _____ Infection of the epididymis

Column II

a. Cryptorchidism
b. Epididymitis
c. Hydrocele
d. Orchitis
e. Phimosis
f. Prostatism
g. Prostatitis
h. Variocele

II. Critical Thinking Questions and Exercises

DISCUSSION AND ANALYSIS

Discuss the following topics with your classmates.

1. Compare and contrast the etiology and clinical manifestations of orchitis and epididymitis.
2. Describe the psychogenic and organic causes of erectile dysfunction.
3. Compare and contrast the action, side effects, and contraindications of three medications used to treat erectile dysfunction: Viagra, Levita, and Cialis.
4. Describe the pathophysiology, clinical manifestations, and medical management for BPH.
5. Describe the benchmark surgical procedure for BPH.
6. Discuss five nursing diagnoses and related goals for a patient with prostate cancer.
7. Describe the physiologic changes in the male reproductive system that occurs with age.

CLINICAL SITUATIONS

Read the following case study. Fill in the blanks or circle the correct answer.

CASE STUDY: Prostatectomy

Tom is a 65-year-old college administrator who is schedule for a prostatectomy.

1. Preoperatively, two objectives to determine readiness for surgery are: _____ and _____.

2. Prostatectomy must be performed before: _____.

3. The most commonly performed surgical procedure that is carried out through endoscopy is:
   a. perineal approach.
   b. retropubic approach.
   c. suprapubic approach.
   d. transurethral approach.

4. List two possible postoperative complications of the transurethral resection of the prostate (TURP)
   approach: _____ and _____.

5. Explain why impotence may result from a prostatectomy.

   _____

6. List three possible preoperative nursing diagnoses: _____, _____, and

   _____.

7. Identify two nursing activities to help relieve postoperative bladder spasms: _____

   and _____.

8. Explain why the patient is advised not to sit for prolonged periods of time immediately after the operation.

   _____

9. Describe how you would teach a patient to do perineal exercises.

   _____

CHAPTER 50

Assessment of Immune Function

I. Interpretation, Completion, and Comparison

MULTIPLE CHOICE

Read each question carefully. Circle your answer.

1. A deficient immune system response that is congenital in origin would be classified as what kind of disorder?
   a. Autoimmune
   b. Gammopathy
   c. Natural deficiency
   d. Hypersensitivity

2. The immune system is essentially composed of:
   a. bone marrow.
   b. lymphoid tissue.
   c. white blood cells.
   d. all of the above components.

3. The primary production site of white blood cells involved in immunity is the:
   a. bone marrow.
   b. adenoids.
   c. thymus gland.
   d. spleen.

4. T lymphocytes, descendants of stem cells, mature in the:
   a. bone marrow.
   b. spleen.
   c. thymus.
   d. lymph nodes.

5. Granulocytes, which fight invasion by releasing histamine, do not include:
   a. basophils.
   b. eosinophils.
   c. lymphocytes.
   d. neutrophils.

6. The leukocytes that arrive first at a site where inflammation occurs are:
   a. B lymphocytes.
   b. cytotoxic T cells.
   c. helper T cells.
   d. neutrophils.

7. White blood cells that function as phagocytes are called:
   a. basophils.
   b. eosinophils.
   c. monocytes.
   d. lymphocytes.

8. An example of biologic response modifiers that interfere with viruses is:
   a. bradykinin.
   b. eosinophils.
   c. granulocytes.
   d. interferon.

9. The body's first line of defense is the:
   a. antibody response.
   b. cellular immune response.
   c. phagocytic immune response.
   d. white blood cell response.

10. The primary cells responsible for recognition of foreign antigens are:
    a. leukocytes.
    b. lymphocytes.
    c. monocytes.
    d. reticulocytes.

11. Lymphocytes interfere with disease by picking up specific antigens from organisms to alter their function during which stage of an immune response?
    a. Effector
    b. Proliferation
    c. Recognition
    d. Response

12. During the proliferation stage:
    a. antibody-producing plasma cells are produced.
    b. lymph nodes enlarge.
    c. lymphocytes rapidly increase.
    d. all of the above occur.

13. Antibodies are believed to be a type of:
    a. carbohydrate.
    b. fat.
    c. protein.
    d. sugar.

14. Cell-mediated immune responses are responsible for all of the following *except*:
    a. anaphylaxis.
    b. graft-versus-host reactions.
    c. transplant rejection.
    d. tumor destruction.

15. It is important to realize that cellular membrane damage results from all the following *except*:
    a. activation of complement.
    b. antibody–antigen binding.
    c. arrival of killer T cells.
    d. attraction of macrophages.

16. Effector T cells destroy foreign organisms by:
    a. altering the antigen's cell membrane.
    b. causing cellular lysis.
    c. producing lymphokines, which destroy invading organisms.
    d. all of the above mechanisms.

17. Helper T cells accomplish all of the following *except*:
    a. alter the cell membrane by causing cell lysis.
    b. produce lymphokines that activate T cells.
    c. produce cytokines.
    d. activate B cells and macrophages.

18. Complement acts by:
    a. attracting phagocytes to an antigen.
    b. destroying cells through destruction of the antigen's membrane.
    c. rendering the antigen vulnerable to phagocytosis.
    d. a combination of all of the above mechanisms.

19. Interferon is a lymphokine that exerts its effect by:
    a. increasing vascular permeability.
    b. inhibiting the growth of certain antigenic cells.
    c. stopping the spread of viral infections.
    d. suppressing the movement of macrophages.

20. Trace elements, essential for optimum immune function, include all of the following *except*:
    a. cholesterol.
    b. copper.
    c. manganese.
    d. selenium.

MATCHING

Match the immunoglobulin listed in column II with its associated immunoglobulin (Ig) activity listed in column I. An answer may be used more than once.

Column I

1. _____ Enhances phagocytosis
2. _____ Appears in intravascular serum
3. _____ Helps defend against parasites
4. _____ Activates complement system
5. _____ Protects against respiratory infections
6. _____ Influences B-lymphocyte differentiation
7. _____ Prevents absorption of antigens from food

Column II

a. IgA
b. IgD
c. IgE
d. IgG
e. IgM

Match the immune system effect listed in column II with its corresponding medication listed in column I. An answer may be used more than once.

Column I

1. _____ Cyclosporine
2. _____ Dactinomycin
3. _____ Indomethacin
4. _____ Methotrexate
5. _____ Mustargen
6. _____ Propylthiouracil
7. _____ Vancomycin

Column II

a. Agranulocytosis, leukopenia
b. Agranulocytosis, neutropenia
c. Leukopenia, aplastic bone marrow
d. Leukopenia, T-cell inhibition
e. Transient leukopenia

SCRAMBLEGRAM

Unscramble the letters to answer each statement.

1. A protein substance that responds to a specific antigen: _____

Y N I D T O A B

2. Enzymatic proteins that destroy bacteria: _____

T L P M N C E O E M

3. A substance that stimulates the production of antibodies: _____

G I N T E A N

4. Lymphocytes that directly attack antigens: _____

R P T E L H L E C L E S

5. Cells that engulf and destroy foreign bodies: _____

O G T A E Y P C S H

6. Proteins formed when cells are exposed to foreign agents: _____

F E O T N E S R I R N

II. Critical Thinking Questions and Exercises

DISCUSSION AND ANALYSIS

Discuss the following topics with your classmates.

1. Describe four ways that disorders of the immune system occur.
2. Distinguish between natural and acquired (active and passive) immunity.
3. Explain what "complement" is, how it is formed, and how it functions.
4. Explain how biologic response modifiers affect the immune response.
5. Explain what research has shown about the role of stem cells.
6. Discuss the age-related changes in immunologic function.
7. Compare and contrast the effects of adrenal corticosteroids, antimetabolites, and antibiotics on the immune system.
8. Describe the signs and symptoms that a nurse would assess for the cardiovascular, respiratory, and gastrointestinal system in the presence of immune system dysfunction.

CHAPTER 51

Management of Patients With Immunodeficiency

I. Interpretation, Completion, and Comparison

MULTIPLE CHOICE

Read each question carefully. Circle your answer.

1. Immunodeficiency disorders are caused by defects or deficiencies in:
   a. the complement system.
   b. B and T lymphocytes.
   c. phagocytic cells.
   d. all of the above.

2. The cardinal symptoms of immunodeficiency are:
   a. chronic diarrhea.
   b. chronic or recurrent severe infections.
   c. poor response to treatment of infections.
   d. inclusive of all the above.

3. The nitroblue tetrazolium reductase (NTR) test is used to diagnose immunodeficiency disorders related to:
   a. complement.
   b. B lymphocytes.
   c. T lymphocytes.
   d. phagocytic cells.

4. More than 50% of individuals with which disease develop pernicious anemia?
   a. Bruton disease
   b. Common variable immunodeficiency (CVID)
   c. DiGeorge syndrome
   d. Nezelaf syndrome

5. The most frequent presenting sign in patients with DiGeorge syndrome is:
   a. chronic diarrhea.
   b. hypocalcemia.
   c. neutropenia.
   d. pernicious anemia.

6. The primary cause of death for individuals with ataxia–telangiectasia is:
   a. acute renal failure.
   b. chronic lung disease.
   c. neurologic dysfunction.
   d. overwhelming infection.

7. The most common secondary immunodeficiency disorder is:
   a. AIDS.
   b. DAF.
   c. CVID.
   d. SCID.

8. The recommended dose of intravenous gamma globulin for a 60-kg man, given monthly, is:
   a. 15 g.
   b. 30 g.
   c. 45 g.
   d. 60 g.

9. When gamma globulin is infused intravenously, the rate should not exceed:
   a. 1.5 mL/min.
   b. 3 mL/min.
   c. 6 mL/min.
   d. 10 mL/min.

10. The nurse knows to stop an infusion of gamma globulin if the patient experiences:
    a. flank pain.
    b. shaking chills.
    c. tightness in the chest.
    d. any or all of the above.

SHORT ANSWER

Read each statement carefully. Write your response in the space provided.

1. Primary immunodeficiencies predispose people to three conditions: _____,
   _____, and _____.

2. List five disorders of common, primary immunodeficiencies: _____,
   _____, _____, _____, and _____.

3. The two types of inherited B-cell deficiencies result from lack of differentiation of B-cells into:
   _____ and _____.

4. More than 50% of patients with CVID develop which disorder? _____.

5. DiGeorge syndrome is an example of which immunodeficiency? _____.

6. The most prevalent cause of immunodeficiency worldwide is: _____.

II. Critical Thinking Questions and Exercises

INTERPRETING PATTERNS

For each group of clustered clues, write the corresponding immunodeficiency disorder.

Increased incidence of bacterial infections.

Readily develops fungal infections from candida organism.

Easily infected from herpes simplex.

Afflicted with chronic eczematoid dermatitis.

1. Disorder is: _____

   There is disappearance of germinal centers from lymphatic tissue.

   There is complete lack of antibody production.

   It is associated with the most common immunodeficiency seen in childhood.

   Disease onset occurs most often in the second decade of life.

2. Disorder is: _____

Lymphopenia is usually present.

Thymus gland fails to develop.

Chronic mucocutaneous candidiasis is an associated disorder.

3. Disorder is: _____

IgA deficiency is present in 40% of individuals.

T-cell deficiencies become more severe with age.

Neurologic symptoms usually occur before 5 years of age.

4. Disorder is: _____

It usually occurs as a result of underlying disease processes.

It frequently is caused by certain autoimmune disorders.

It may be caused by certain viruses.

5. Disorder is: _____

EXAMINING ASSOCIATIONS

Read each analogy. Fill in the space provided with the best response. Explain the correlation.

1. Job's syndrome : phagocytic dysfunction :: Bruton's disease : _____

2. Colony-stimulating factor : HIE syndrome :: Intravenous gamma globulin : _____

3. CVID : bacterial infections :: Ataxia–telangiectasia : _____

4. Angioneurotic edema : frequent episodes of edema :: Paroxysmal nocturnal hemoglobinuria :

_____

CHAPTER 52

Management of Patients With HIV Infection and AIDS

I. Interpretation, Completion, and Comparison

MULTIPLE CHOICE

Read each question carefully. Circle your answer.

1. The Centers for Disease Control and Prevention (CDC) approved the first antiretroviral drug for AIDS 6 years after the first cases were reported in:
   a. 1978.
   b. 1982.
   c. 1987.
   d. 1991.

2. After infection with HIV, the immune system responds by making antibodies against the virus, usually within how many weeks after infection?
   a. 1 to 2 weeks
   b. 3 to 6 weeks
   c. 3 to 12 weeks
   d. 6 to 18 weeks

3. Postexposure prophylaxis (PEP) medications should be started within _____ after exposure, but no longer than _____, to offer any benefit, and must be taken for _____.
   a. 1 hour; 72 hours; 4 weeks
   b. 4 days; 7 days; 2 weeks
   c. 1 week; 3 weeks; 3 months
   d. 1 month; 2 months; 6 months

4. Up to 85% of individuals infected with HIV will develop symptoms of AIDS within how many years after infection?
   a. 3 to 5 years
   b. 6 to 7 years
   c. 8 to 10 years
   d. 12 to 15 years

5. Abnormal laboratory findings seen with AIDS include:
   a. decreased CD4 and T-cell count.
   b. p24 antigen.
   c. positive EIA test.
   d. all of the above.

6. A widely used laboratory test that measures HIV-RNA levels and tracks the body's response to HIV infection is the:
   a. CD4/CD8 ratio.
   b. EIA test.
   c. viral load test.
   d. Western blot.

7. An example of an antiretroviral agent, classified as a fusion inhibitor, that must be injected subcutaneously twice a day is:
   a. Agenerase.
   b. Combivir.
   c. Fuzeon (T20).
   d. Retrovir.

8. A nurse knows that all of the following antiretroviral agents can be taken without regard to food intake *except* for:
   a. Hivid.
   b. Epivir.
   c. Sustiva.
   d. Videx.

9. One of the most frequent systemic side effects of anti-HIV drugs is:
   a. osteoporosis.
   b. hyperglycemia.
   c. lipodystrophy syndrome.
   d. pancreatitis.

10. A nurse would know that all of the following conditions are classified as HIV category B *except* for:
    a. candidiasis.
    b. herpes zoster.
    c. Kaposi's sarcoma.
    d. listeriosis.

11. The most common infection in persons with AIDS (80% occurrence) is:
    a. Cytomegalovirus.
    b. Legionnaire's disease.
    c. *Mycobacterium tuberculosis.*
    d. *Pneumocystis* pneumonia.

12. The most debilitating gastrointestinal condition found in up to 90% of all AIDS patients is:
    a. anorexia.
    b. chronic diarrhea.
    c. nausea.
    d. vomiting.

13. A diagnosis of "wasting syndrome" can be initially made when involuntary weight loss exceeds what percentage of baseline body weight?
    a. 10%
    b. 15%
    c. 20%
    d. 25%

14. The minimum number of daily calories recommended for a 70-kg individual with AIDS-related "wasting syndrome" is:
    a. 1,500 calories.
    b. 2,000 calories.
    c. 2,800 calories.
    d. 4,000 calories.

15. The minimum number of daily protein calories for a 70-kg individual with AIDS-related "wasting syndrome" is:
    a. 20 calories.
    b. 35 calories.
    c. 45 calories.
    d. 60 calories.

16. The most common malignancy seen with HIV infection is:
    a. carcinoma of the skin.
    b. Kaposi's sarcoma.
    c. pancreatic cancer.
    d. stomach cancer.

17. Long-term adherence to HIV treatment regimens remains at about:
    a. 10% compliance.
    b. 15% to 25% compliance.
    c. 30% to 50% compliance.
    d. greater than 75% compliance.

SHORT ANSWER

Read each statement carefully. Write your response in the space provided.

1. As of 2008, approximately _____ million people are living with HIV/AIDS. The percentage of women afflicted is what percent? _____. The most heavily afflicted country is _____, with _____% of all residents living with the disease.

2. The two major means of HIV transmission are: _____ and _____.

3. List five types of body fluids that can transmit HIV-1: _____, _____, _____, _____, and _____.

4. HIV belongs to a group of viruses known as: _____.

5. The standard new HIV testing method now used when information about HIV status is needed immediately (emergency room, labor, and delivery) is: _____.

6. Drug resistance can be defined as: _____.

7. A fungal infection present in nearly all patients with AIDS is: _____.

8. A recommended chemotherapeutic agent for Kaposi's sarcoma is: _____.

9. The second most common malignancy in people with AIDS is: _____.

MATCHING

Match the AIDS-indicated category listed in column II with its associated clinical condition listed in column I. An answer may be used more than once.

Column I

1. _____ Histoplasmosis
2. _____ Hairy leukoplakia
3. _____ Kaposi's sarcoma
4. _____ Acute primary HIV infection
5. _____ Pneumocystis carinii
6. _____ Bacillary angiomatosis
7. _____ Persistent generalized lymphadenopathy (PGL)
8. _____ Extrapulmonary cryptococcosis

Column II

a. Clinical category A
b. Clinical category B
c. Clinical category C

II. Critical Thinking Questions and Exercises

DISCUSSION AND ANALYSIS

Discuss the following topics with your classmates.

1. Discuss the safe sexual behaviors that a nurse should incorporate into an education plan to prevent HIV/AIDS.
2. Give specific examples of how health care providers can maintain "Standard Precautions" to prevent HIV transmission.
3. Explain the procedures that would be used for postexposure prophylaxis for health care providers.
4. Describe the stage of HIV disease known as *primary* infection.
5. Describe the clinical symptoms of a patient infected with acute HIV syndrome.
6. Describe some of the adverse effects associated with HIV treatment.
7. Describe the clinical manifestations of the immune reconstitution inflammatory syndrome (IRIS).
8. Describe the appearance of the cutaneous lesions seen with Kaposi's sarcoma.
9. Discuss nursing interventions for a patient with HIV encephalopathy.
10. Distinguish between the etiology and clinical manifestations of cryptococcal meningitis and cytomegalovirus retinitis.
11. Discuss at least eight nursing diagnoses and four collaborative problems for patients with AIDS and HIV infections.

CLINICAL SITUATIONS

Read the following case study. Fill in the blanks or circle the correct answer.

CASE STUDY: Acquired Immunodeficiency Syndrome

Brenden is a 39-year-old homosexual who has been recently diagnosed with AIDS.

1. On initial assessment, the nurse identifies two major potential risk factors associated with AIDS:

   _____ and _____.

2. As part of her assessment, the nurse checks Brenden for candidiasis. To do this, she would inspect Brenden's:
   a. heart.
   b. lungs.
   c. oral cavity.
   d. skin.

3. Assessment data indicated dehydration as evidenced by:
   a. bradycardia.
   b. hypertension.
   c. urine's specific gravity greater than 1.025.
   d. urine output greater than 70 mL/h.

4. List 3 of 11 potential nursing diagnoses: _____, _____, and

   _____.

5. List 2 of 5 possible collaborative problems that are indicated in the assessment data:

   _____ and _____.

6. List two common nutritional complications of HIV/AIDS: _____ and

   _____.

7. The nurse advises Brenden to avoid certain foods that are bowel irritants to prevent diarrhea. She advises him not to eat:

   a. bland foods.

   b. cooked cereal.

   c. jelly and pudding.

   d. popcorn.

8. To improve Brenden's nutritional status, the nurse would:

   a. encourage him to rest before eating.

   b. limit fluids 1 hour before meals.

   c. serve five to six small meals per day.

   d. do all of the above.

9. Identify the side effects a nurse should be aware of for a patient taking Epivir or Retrovir:

_____

CHAPTER 53

Assessment and Management of Patients With Allergic Disorders

I. Interpretation, Completion, and Comparison

MULTIPLE CHOICE

Read each question carefully. Circle your answer.

1. The body's first line of defense against potential invaders is the:
   a. gastrointestinal tract.
   b. respiratory tract.
   c. skin.
   d. combination of all the above.

2. An example of an incomplete protein antigen that triggers an allergic response is:
   a. animal dander.
   b. horse serum.
   c. medications.
   d. pollen.

3. The classification of immunoglobulin (Ig) that occupies certain receptors on mast cells and produces an inflammatory response is:
   a. IgA.
   b. IgD.
   c. IgE.
   d. IgG.

4. Histamine acts on major organs by:
   a. contracting bronchial smooth muscle.
   b. dilating small venules.
   c. increasing gastric secretions.
   d. stimulating all of the above mechanisms.

5. A popular medication that has an affinity for H_1 receptors is:
   a. Benadryl.
   b. Prilosec.
   c. Tagamet.
   d. Zantac.

6. A chemical mediator of hypersensitivity that is released during platelet aggregation and causes bronchial smooth muscle contraction is:
   a. bradykinin.
   b. histamine.
   c. prostaglandin.
   d. serotonin.

7. Hypersensitivity reactions follow reexposure and are classified by type of reaction. An anaphylactic reaction is usually identified as type:
   a. I.
   b. II.
   c. III.
   d. IV.

8. A type II hypersensitivity reaction occurs when a normal constituent is viewed as foreign by the body. An example of a type II reaction is:

   a. bacterial endocarditis.

   b. Rh-hemolytic disease (newborn).

   c. lupus erythematosus.

   d. rheumatoid arthritis.

9. Delayed hypersensitivity (type IV) is said to have occurred when the inflammatory response to an allergen peaks within:

   a. 4 to 8 hours.

   b. 24 to 72 hours.

   c. 4 to 6 days.

   d. 1 to 2 weeks.

10. The nurse monitors the patient's eosinophil level. She suspects a definite allergic disorder with an eosinophil value of what percentage of the total leukocyte count?

    a. 1% to 3%

    b. 3% to 4%

    c. 5% to 10%

    d. 15% to 40%

11. Atopic disorders that result from an allergic response to an allergen include:

    a. allergic rhinitis.

    b. atopic dermatitis.

    c. bronchial asthma.

    d. all of the above.

12. Pruritus and nasal congestion may be indicators of an impending anaphylactic reaction. These symptoms usually occur within how many hours after exposure?

    a. 2 hours

    b. 6 hours

    c. 12 hours

    d. 24 hours

13. When a patient is experiencing an allergic response, the nurse should initially assess the patient for:

    a. dyspnea, bronchospasm, and/or laryngeal edema.

    b. hypotension and tachycardia.

    c. the presence and location of pruritus.

    d. the severity of cutaneous warmth and flushing.

14. Allergic rhinitis is induced by:

    a. airborne pollens or molds.

    b. ingested foods.

    c. parenteral medications.

    d. topical creams or ointments.

15. Patients who are sensitive to ragweed should be advised that weed pollen begins to appear in:

    a. early spring.

    b. early fall.

    c. summer.

    d. midwinter.

16. A major side effect of antihistamines that requires accurate patient education is:

    a. dryness of the mouth.

    b. anorexia.

    c. palpitations.

    d. sedation.

17. An area of nursing concern when administering a sympathomimetic drug is the drug's ability to:

    a. cause bronchodilation.

    b. constrict integumentary smooth muscle.

    c. dilate the muscular vasculature.

    d. do all of the above.

18. Injected allergens are used for "hyposensitization" and may produce systemic reactions that can be harmful. The medication that should be on hand in case of an adverse reaction is:

    a. Dramamine.

    b. epinephrine.

    c. Phenergan hydrochloride.

    d. Pyribenzamine.

19. A type of contact dermatitis that requires the combination of sun exposure and a chemical is:
    a. allergic dermatitis.
    b. irritant dermatitis.
    c. photoallergic dermatitis.
    d. phototoxic dermatitis.

20. The most serious manifestation of hereditary angioedema is:
    a. abdominal pain.
    b. conjunctivitis.
    c. laryngeal edema.
    d. urticaria.

21. One of the most severe food allergies is caused by:
    a. chocolate.
    b. milk.
    c. peanuts.
    d. shrimp.

SHORT ANSWER

Read each statement carefully. Write your response in the space provided.

1. Antibodies, the most effective defense mechanisms in the body, react with antigens in three ways to prepare them for removal from the blood by phagocytes: _____, _____, and _____.

2. An allergic reaction occurs when:

   _____

   _____

   _____

3. Antibodies formed by lymphocytes and plasma cells, in response to an immunogenic stimulus, are called:

   _____.

4. Prostaglandins are primary chemical mediators that respond to a stimulus by contracting smooth muscle and increasing capillary permeability. This response causes: _____.

5. Type III hypersensitivity reactions involve the binding of antibodies to antigens. List two possible disorders: _____ and _____.

6. Two examples of a type IV hypersensitivity reaction (occurs 24 to 72 hours after exposure) are: _____ and _____.

7. Explain why the radioallergosorbent (RAST) test is so beneficial in diagnosis.

   _____

8. The most common cause of anaphylaxis that accounts for 75% of fatal reactions in the United States is:

   _____.

9. The initial medication of choice for a severe allergic reaction is: _____.

10. People need to be advised that a "rebound" anaphylactic reaction can occur _____ (hours) after an initial attack, even when epinephrine has been given.

II. Critical Thinking Questions and Exercises

DISCUSSION AND ANALYSIS

Discuss the following topics with your classmates.

1. Briefly describe the physiologic response that causes an allergic reaction.
2. Explain the production and function of immunoglobulins.
3. Describe the role and function of histamine in response to an allergic threat.
4. Distinguish among the four types of hypersensitivity reactions (types I to IV).
5. Distinguish among three types of allergy tests: skin tests, provocative testing, and a radioallergosorbent test.
6. Distinguish between an *atopic* and *nonatopic* IgE-mediated allergic reaction.
7. Describe the clinical manifestations that occur with a severe anaphylactic reaction.
8. Describe the pathophysiology and medical interventions for anaphylaxis.
9. Compare the actions and nursing implications for the *seven* antihistamines listed in Table 53-2 in the text.
10. Compare the etiology and clinical manifestations of four types of contact dermatitis.
11. Describe the clinical manifestations and medical/nursing management for a patient with a latex allergy reaction.

CLINICAL SITUATIONS

Read the following case study. Fill in the blanks or circle the correct answer.

CASE STUDY: Allergic Rhinitis

Chris is a 26-year-old contractor who specializes in finished basements. Because of his job, he is frequently working in environments where there are substances that stimulate an allergic reaction.

1. Based on assessment data, three likely nursing diagnoses would be: _____, _____, and _____.

2. Four probable patient goals would be: _____, _____, _____, and _____.

3. The nurse advises Chris that his attacks may be preceded by the symptoms of:
   a. breathing difficulty.
   b. pruritus.
   c. tingling sensations.
   d. all of the above.

4. The nurse also advises him that other symptoms may be more alarming, such as:
   a. hoarseness.
   b. a rash or hives.
   c. wheezing.
   d. all of the above.

5. A teaching plan for Chris would include information about:
   a. reducing exposure to allergens.
   b. desensitization procedures.
   c. correct use of medications.
   d. all of the above.

6. The nurse tells Chris that if the physician recommends a series of inoculations for desensitization, he should expect to receive injections every:
   a. day for 30 days.
   b. week for 1 year.
   c. 2 to 4 weeks.
   d. month for 4 years.

CHAPTER 54

Assessment and Management of Patients With Rheumatic Disorders

I. Interpretation, Completion, and Comparison

MULTIPLE CHOICE

Read each question carefully. Circle your answer.

1. The most common symptom of rheumatic disease that causes a patient to seek medical attention is:
   - a. joint swelling.
   - b. limited movement.
   - c. fatigue.
   - d. pain.

2. In the inflammatory process in rheumatic diseases, a triggering event (trauma, stress) starts the process by activating:
   - a. collagenase.
   - b. leukotrienes.
   - c. prostaglandins.
   - d. T lymphocytes.

3. All of the following blood studies are consistent with a positive diagnosis of rheumatoid arthritis (RA) *except* a(an):
   - a. positive C-reactive protein (CRP).
   - b. positive antinuclear antibody (ANA).
   - c. red blood cell count of <4.0 million/μL.
   - d. serum complement level (C3) of >130 mg/dL.

4. A serum study that is positive for the rheumatoid factor is:
   - a. diagnostic for Sjögren's syndrome.
   - b. diagnostic for systemic lupus erythematosus (SLE).
   - c. specific for RA.
   - d. suggestive of RA.

5. The nurse knows that a patient who is present with the symptom of "blanching of his fingers on exposure to cold" would be assessed for the rheumatic disease known as:
   - a. ankylosing spondylitis.
   - b. Raynaud's phenomenon.
   - c. Reiter's syndrome.
   - d. Sjögren's syndrome.

6. Synovial fluid from an inflamed joint is characteristically:
   - a. clear and pale.
   - b. milky, cloudy, and dark yellow.
   - c. scanty in volume.
   - d. straw-colored.

7. A patient is suspected of having *myositis*. The nurse prepares the patient for what procedure that will confirm the diagnosis?
   - a. bone scan.
   - b. computed tomography (CT).
   - c. magnetic resonance imaging (MRI).
   - d. muscle biopsy.

8. The RA reaction produces enzymes that break down:
   a. collagen.
   b. elastin.
   c. hematopoietic tissue.
   d. strong supporting tissue.

9. In RA, the autoimmune reaction primarily occurs in the:
   a. joint tendons.
   b. cartilage.
   c. synovial tissue.
   d. interstitial space.

10. In RA, the cartilage is replaced with fibrous connective tissue during the stage of synovial joint destruction known as:
    a. cartilage erosion.
    b. increased phagocytic production.
    c. lymphocyte infiltration.
    d. pannus formation.

11. A popular and effective COX-2 inhibitor that increases the patient's risk of stroke is:
    a. Bextra.
    b. Celebrex.
    c. Feldene.
    d. Tolectin.

12. A disease-modifying antirheumatic drug (DMARD) that is successful in the treatment of RA yet has retinal eye changes as a side effect is:
    a. Imuran.
    b. Aralen.
    c. Plaquenil.
    d. Solganal.

13. Nonsteroidal anti-inflammatory drugs (NSAIDs) used in rheumatic diseases include all of the following *except*:
    a. Clinoril.
    b. Cytoxan.
    c. Motrin.
    d. Celebrex.

14. Gold-containing compounds act by inhibiting:
    a. DNA synthesis.
    b. lysosomal enzymes.
    c. platelet aggregation.
    d. T- and B-cell activity.

15. When a person with arthritis is temporarily confined to bed, the position recommended to prevent flexion deformities is:
    a. prone.
    b. semi-Fowler's.
    c. side-lying with pillows supporting the shoulders and legs.
    d. supine with pillows under the knees.

16. To immobilize an inflamed wrist, the nurse should splint the joint in a position of:
    a. slight dorsiflexion.
    b. extension.
    c. hyperextension.
    d. internal rotation.

17. A characteristic cutaneous lesion, called the "butterfly rash," appears across the bridge of the nose in 50% of patients with:
    a. gout.
    b. rheumatoid arthritis.
    c. systemic sclerosis.
    d. systemic lupus erythematosus.

18. The single, most important medication for the treatment of systemic SLE is:
    a. immunosuppressants.
    b. corticosteroids.
    c. NSAIDs.
    d. salicylates.

19. Clinical manifestations of scleroderma include:
    a. decreased ventilation owing to lung scarring.
    b. dysphagia owing to hardening of the esophagus.
    c. dyspnea owing to fibrotic cardiac tissue.
    d. all of the above.

20. The most common type of disabling connective tissue disease in the United States is:
    a. carpal tunnel syndrome.
    b. degenerative joint disease.
    c. fibrositis.
    d. polymyositis.

21. Pathophysiologic changes seen with osteoarthritis include:
    a. joint cartilage degeneration.
    b. the formation of bony spurs at the edges of the joint surfaces.
    c. narrowing of the joint space.
    d. all of the above changes.

22. The nurse knows that a patient diagnosed with a spondyloarthropathy would not have:
    a. ankylosing spondylitis.
    b. Raynaud's phenomenon.
    c. reactive arthritis.
    d. psoriatic arthritis.

23. With a diagnosis of gout, a nurse should expect to find:
    a. glucosuria.
    b. hyperuricemia.
    c. hypoproteinuria.
    d. ketonuria.

24. A purine-restricted diet is prescribed for a patient. The nurse should recommend:
    a. dairy products.
    b. organ meats.
    c. raw vegetables.
    d. shellfish.

MATCHING

Match the clinical interpretation/laboratory significance listed in column II with its associated test listed in column I.

Column I

1. _____ Uric acid
2. _____ Complement
3. _____ Rheumatoid factor
4. _____ Hematocrit
5. _____ HLA-B27 antigen
6. _____ Antinuclear antibody (ANA)
7. _____ Creatinine
8. _____ C-Reactive protein (CRP)

Column II

a. A decrease can be seen in chronic inflammation
b. A positive test is associated with SLE, RA, and Raynaud's disease
c. An increase in this substance is seen with gout
d. This protein substance is decreased in RA and SLE
e. This is present in 80% of those who have RA
f. This is present in 85% of those with ankylosing spondylitis
g. Frequently positive for RA and SLE
h. An increase may indicate renal damage, as in scleroderma

II. Critical Thinking Questions and Exercises

DISCUSSION AND ANALYSIS

Discuss the following topics with your classmates.

1. Explain the theory of "degradation" as it relates to the pathophysiology of rheumatic diseases.
2. Explain the difference between *exacerbation* and *remission*.
3. Distinguish between the pathophysiology of inflammatory rheumatic disease and that of degenerative rheumatic disease.
4. Discuss the physiologic rationale supporting the management goals and strategies for the treatment of rheumatic diseases.
5. Describe the type of exercises and precautions used to promote mobility for a patient with a rheumatic disease.
6. Distinguish between the process and nursing implications for surgical procedures for RA: synovectomy, tenorrhaphy, arthrodesis, and arthroplasty.
7. Describe the pathophysiology and clinical manifestations of polymyalgia rheumatica.
8. Describe the pathophysiology and clinical manifestations of degenerative joint disease (osteoarthritis).
9. Explain the pathophysiology and clinical manifestations of gout.
10. Explain the etiology and nursing management for fibromyalgia.

CLINICAL SITUATIONS

Read the following case studies. Fill in the blanks or circle the correct answer.

CASE STUDY: Diffuse Connective Tissue Disease

Jane, a 33-year-old mother of two, has joint pain and stiffness, decreased mobility, and increased frequency of fatigue. She is depressed.

1. The physician immediately suspects a diagnosis of _____, a diffuse connective tissue disease that the nurse knows manifests itself primarily in women.

    a. polymyositis

    b. rheumatoid arthritis

    c. scleroderma

    d. systemic lupus erythematosus

2. On initial examination, the physician notes that Jane's knees are hot, swollen, and painful. The physician orders specific laboratory studies. The test result, which is not significant for a diagnosis of RA, is:

    a. a decreased red blood cell count.

    b. an elevated C4 complement component.

    c. an elevated erythrocyte sedimentation rate.

    d. a positive CRP.

3. The nurse also assesses the four systemic features usually found with RA: _____,

    _____, _____, and _____.

4. Jane is scheduled for an arthrocentesis. The nurse advises her that her knee joint will be anesthetized locally and a fluid specimen will be obtained. There is no special preparation or precautions after the procedure. Jane is told that a positive finding would be joint fluid that:

a. contains few inflammatory cells.

b. does not contain leukocytes.

c. is viscous and tan in color.

d. will not form a mucin clot.

5. A positive diagnosis of RA results in a multidisciplinary approach to treatment. Jane's pharmacotherapy regimen includes several drug classifications. A popular NSAID that may be prescribed is:

a. Aralen.

b. Imuran.

c. Motrin.

d. Ridaura.

6. If Jane experiences gastric irritation and/or ulceration, the physician may order a new class of NSAIDs called _____.

7. A low-dose corticosteroid regimen is begun for a short period. The nurse advises Jane to be aware of certain drug-induced side effects, such as:

a. elevated blood pressure.

b. gastric upset.

c. weight gain.

d. all of the above.

CASE STUDY: Systemic Lupus Erythematosus

Brooke is a 41-year-old mother of two teenagers who has had symptoms of joint tenderness for about 10 years. Lately, she has noticed significant morning stiffness and a slight rash over the bridge of her nose and cheeks. Her physician suspects a diagnosis of SLE.

1. Before beginning the assessment, the nurse knows that the etiology of SLE is an altered immune regulation that can be caused by disturbances in: _____, _____, _____, and _____.

2. The altered immune response can be described as: _____.

3. The nurse is aware that the physician will do a complete cardiovascular assessment, checking the patient for _____, _____, and _____.

4. Blood testing will be ordered to determine the presence of: _____, _____, _____, and _____.

5. The nurse knows that the physician may order _____ medications for treating Brooke's symptoms, if they are considered mild.

6. As part of health teaching, the nurse reminds Brooke that possible cardiovascular complications require periodic screening for _____ and _____.

INTERPRETING PATTERNS

Review Figure 54-1 in the text, which shows the pathophysiology of RA. Outline in detail the series of related steps that lead to the inflammation, beginning with the antigen stimulus that activates monocytes and T lymphocytes using the following flow chart.

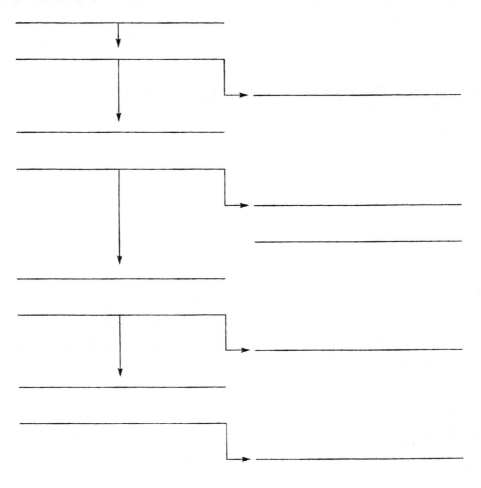

CHAPTER 55

Assessment of Integumentary Function

I. Interpretation, Completion, and Comparison

MULTIPLE CHOICE

Read each question carefully. Circle your answer.

1. For the average adult with a normal body temperature, a nurse needs to know that insensible water loss is approximately:
   a. 250 mL/day.
   b. 600 mL/day.
   c. 800 mL/day.
   d. 1,000 mL/day.

2. When a nurse applies a cold towel to a patient's neck to reduce body heat, heat is reduced by:
   a. conduction.
   b. convection.
   c. evaporation.
   d. radiation.

3. Sweating, a process by which the body regulates heat loss, does not occur until the core body temperature exceeds the base level of:
   a. 24°C.
   b. 37°C.
   c. 43°C.
   d. 51°C.

4. In a dark-skinned person, color change that occurs in the presence of shock can be evidenced when the skin appears:
   a. ashen gray and dull.
   b. dusky blue.
   c. reddish pink.
   d. whitish pink.

5. Dark-skinned patients who have cherry-red nail beds, lips, and oral mucosa may be exhibiting signs of:
   a. anemia.
   b. carbon monoxide poisoning.
   c. polycythemia.
   d. shock.

6. A clinical example of a primary skin lesion known as a macule is:
   a. hives.
   b. impetigo.
   c. port-wine stains.
   d. psoriasis.

7. A patient is examined and noted to have a herpes simplex/zoster skin lesion. The nurse knows to describe the lesion as a:
   a. macule.
   b. papule.
   c. vesicle.
   d. wheal.

SHORT ANSWER

Read each statement. Write your response in the space provided.

1. The epidermis, the outermost layer of epithelial cells, is composed of three types of cells: _____, _____, and _____.

2. The epidermis is almost completely replaced every _____.

3. The subcutaneous tissue, which is primarily composed of _____ tissue, has a major role in _____ regulation.

4. The term used to describe hair loss is: _____.

5. There are two types of skin glands: _____ and _____.

6. Skin needs to be exposed to sunlight to manufacture vitamin _____.

7. List 5 of 10 benign skin changes seen in the elderly: _____, _____, _____, _____, and _____.

8. Jaundice can first be observed by examining the _____ and _____.

9. The nurse should know that clubbing of the nails is usually a diagnostic sign of: _____.

II. Critical Thinking Questions and Exercises

ANALYZING COMPARISONS

Read each analogy. Fill in the space provided with the best response.

1. Keratin : skin hardening :: Melanin : _____

2. Bluish skin color : insufficient oxygenation :: Yellow-green skin : _____

3. Merkel cells : nervous system :: Langerhans cells : _____

4. Hirsutism : excessive hair growth :: _____ : hair loss

5. Vitamin D deficiency : rickets :: Vitamin C deficiency : _____

6. Palpation : skin turgor :: _____ : vesicle

7. Acne : a pustule :: Psoriasis : _____

IDENTIFYING PATTERNS

Consider the cutaneous manifestations of systemic disease listed in each grouping. Cluster the data to identify the skin manifestation.

Seen in systemic lupus erythematosus

Characterized by red, spidery lines

Appears in plaques on the nose and ears

Seen on scales on the cheek area

1. _____

Appears as an ulcerated lesion

Is a painless chancre

2. _____

Seen in platelet disorders

Associated with vessel fragility

Characterized by purpura

3. _____

Occurs in infections

Seen with allergic reactions

Characteristic of drug reactions

4. _____

Present as macules, papules, plaques, or nodules

Lesions are visually multiple

Lesions are characteristically blue-red or dark brown

Seen in AIDS

5. _____

IDENTIFYING PATTERNS

For each of the following eight primary or secondary lesions, document two defining characteristics.

1. Cherry angioma

    a. _____

    b. _____

2. Crust

    a. _____

    b. _____

3. Cyst

    a. _____

    b. _____

4. Fissure

    a. _____

    b. _____

5. Keloid

    a. _____

    b. _____

6. Telangiectasis

    a. _____

    b. _____

7. Petechia

    a. _____

    b. _____

8. Spider angioma

    a. _____

    b. _____

APPLYING CONCEPTS

For each pathophysiologic change in the skin that occurs with aging, list associated alterations in function.

1. Thinning of the dermis and epidermis at their junction (example)

    a. _____

    b. _____

    c. _____

    d. _____

2. Loss of subcutaneous tissue of elastin, fat, and collagen

    a. _____

    b. _____

    c. _____

3. Decreased cellular replacement

    a. _____

    b. _____

4. Decrease in the number and function of sweat and sebaceous glands

    a. _____

5. Reduced hormonal levels of androgens

    a. _____

CHAPTER 56

Management of Patients With Dermatologic Problems

I. Interpretation, Completion, and Comparison

MULTIPLE CHOICE

Read each question carefully. Circle your answer.

1. In the absence of infection or heavy discharge, chronic wounds should remain covered for:
   a. 6 to 12 hours.
   b. 12 to 24 hours.
   c. 24 to 36 hours.
   d. 48 to 72 hours.

2. Moisture-retentive dressings, more effective than wet compresses at removing exudate, should remain in place a minimum of:
   a. 6 hours.
   b. 12 hours.
   c. 18 hours.
   d. 24 hours.

3. A moisture-retentive dressing that promotes debridement and helps form granulation tissue is a:
   a. calcium alginate dressing.
   b. foam dressing.
   c. hydrocolloid dressing.
   d. hydrogel dressing.

4. Occlusive dressings applied to a dermatosis are used to:
   a. enhance the absorption of topical medications.
   b. improve hydration.
   c. increase the local skin temperature.
   d. do all of the above.

5. The patient is advised to apply a suspension-type lotion to a dermatosis site. The nurse advises the patient that the lotion must be applied how often to be effective?
   a. Every hour
   b. Every 3 hours
   c. Every 12 hours
   d. Day at the same time

6. The nurse knows to assess for which local side effect when corticosteroids are used for dermatologic conditions?
   a. Skin atrophy
   b. Striae
   c. Telangiectasia
   d. All of the above

7. An example of a very potent corticosteroid used for treating a dermatologic condition is:
   a. Aclovate.
   b. Aristocort.
   c. Temovate.
   d. Westcort.

8. The most common symptom of pruritus is:
   a. a rash.
   b. itching.
   c. flaking.
   d. pain.

9. A nurse should assess all possible causes of pruritus, including the presence of endocrine disease, such as:
   a. biliary cirrhosis.
   b. hypothyroidism.
   c. lymphoma.
   d. diabetes mellitus.

10. Nurses should advise patients with pruritus to avoid all of the following *except*:
    a. drying soaps.
    b. emollient lubricants.
    c. vigorous towel drying.
    d. warm to hot water.

11. A systemic pharmacologic agent prescribed for nodular cystic acne is:
    a. Accutane.
    b. benzoyl peroxide.
    c. Retin-A.
    d. salicylic acid.

12. Management of follicular disorders includes all of the following *except*:
    a. cleansing of the skin with an antibacterial soap to prevent spillage of bacteria to adjacent tissues.
    b. rupture of the boil or pimple to release the pus.
    c. systemic antibiotic therapy to treat the infection.
    d. warm, moist compresses to increase resolution of the furuncle or carbuncle.

13. Herpes Zoster (shingles) is:
    a. a varicella-zoster viral infection related to chickenpox.
    b. an inflammatory condition that produces vesicular eruptions along nerve pathways.
    c. manifested by pain, itching, and tenderness.
    d. characterized by all of the above.

14. Tinea capitis (ringworm of the scalp) can be identified by the presence of:
    a. papules at the edges of inflamed patches.
    b. circular areas of redness.
    c. scaling and spots of baldness.
    d. all of the above.

15. Patient education for the management of pediculosis capitis should include advising the patient to:
    a. comb his or her hair with a fine-toothed comb dipped in vinegar to remove nits.
    b. disinfect all combs and brushes.
    c. wash his or her hair with a shampoo containing lindane (Kwell).
    d. do all of the above.

16. A patient is complaining of severe itching that intensifies at night. The nurse decides to assess the skin using a magnifying glass and penlight to look for the "itch mite." The nurse suspects the skin condition known as:
    a. contact dermatitis.
    b. pediculosis.
    c. scabies.
    d. tinea corporis.

17. Psoriasis is an inflammatory dermatosis that results from:
    a. a superficial infection with *Staphylococcus aureus*.
    b. dermal abrasion.
    c. overproduction of keratin.
    d. excess deposition of subcutaneous fat.

18. The characteristic lesion of psoriasis is a:
    a. red, raised patch covered with silver scales.
    b. cluster of pustules.
    c. group of raised vesicles.
    d. pattern of bullae that rupture and form a scaly crust.

19. A new, nonsteroidal, topical treatment for psoriasis would be:
    a. Kenalog.
    b. Dovonex.
    c. Tegison.
    d. Valisone.

20. Exfoliate dermatitis is characterized by erythema and scaling and is associated with:
    a. a loss of stratum corneum.
    b. capillary leakage.
    c. hypoproteinemia.
    d. all of the above.

21. Nursing care for a patient with toxic epidermal necrolysis (TEN) should include:
    a. inspection of the oral cavity.
    b. assessment of urinary output.
    c. application of topical skin agents.
    d. all of the above actions.

22. The incidence of skin cancer in fair-skinned Americans is approximately:
    a. 8%.
    b. 12%.
    c. 20%.
    d. 35%.

23. Because sun damage is cumulative, the harmful effects of skin cancer may be severe by age:
    a. 20 years.
    b. 30 years.
    c. 40 years.
    d. 50 years.

24. Basal cell carcinoma tumors appear most frequently on the:
    a. face.
    b. chest.
    c. arms.
    d. hands.

25. Squamous cell metastases have a mortality rate of about:
    a. 25%.
    b. 40%.
    c. 60%.
    d. 75%.

26. The most lethal of all skin cancers is:
    a. basal cell.
    b. squamous cell.
    c. malignant melanoma.
    d. Kaposi's sarcoma.

27. Danger signals of melanoma include changes in a mole's:
    a. color.
    b. shape or outline.
    c. size or surface.
    d. all of the above.

28. The etiology of Kaposi's sarcoma is believed to be:
    a. environmental.
    b. genetic.
    c. viral.
    d. a combination of one or all of the above.

29. A living tissue transplant from the same person is known as a(an):
    a. allograft.
    b. alloplastic implant.
    c. autograft.
    d. xenograft.

30. For a graft to "take":
    a. the area must be free of infection.
    b. the recipient bed must have an adequate blood supply.
    c. immobilization must be ensured.
    d. all of the above conditions must be present.

SHORT ANSWER

Read each statement carefully. Write your response in the space provided.

1. List four major objectives of therapy for patients with dermatologic problems: _____, _____, _____, and _____.

2. Moisture-retentive dressings are very efficient at removing exudate because they:

   _____

   _____.

3. Cytokines, which have potent mitogenic activity, work by:

   _____

   _____.

4. A common nursing diagnosis for a patient with dermatosis would be:

   _____.

5. The most common skin condition in adolescents and young adults between the ages of 12 and 35 years is:

   _____.

6. Two common bacterial skin infections are: _____, and _____.

7. Bullous impetigo, a deep-seated infection characterized by large, fluid-filled blisters, is caused by the bacteria _____.

8. Two major complications of TEN and Stevens-Johnson syndrome (SJS) are: _____ and _____; the major cause of death is _____. The major sites of infection are the _____, _____, and _____.

9. The most common cancer in the United States is: _____. The most common types of this cancer are: _____ and _____ and diagnosis is made by _____.

10. A major risk factor for malignant melanoma for young women under 30 years of age is use of a tanning bed _____ times/year.

SCRAMBLEGRAM

Complete the following by circling the word or words that answer each statement below. Terms may be written in any direction.

S	C	U	F	A	M	V	I	R	S	O
A	L	A	U	O	X	C	Q	U	C	C
M	I	S	R	L	A	E	P	O	A	H
R	N	I	U	B	R	S	R	T	B	E
E	I	S	N	P	U	A	I	E	I	I
D	M	O	C	S	E	N	A	N	E	L
O	E	R	L	G	E	T	C	S	S	I
Y	N	E	E	A	E	Y	L	L	A	T
P	T	X	E	D	I	L	Y	A	E	I
S	S	C	O	M	E	D	O	N	E	S

DEFINITION OF TERMS

1. Primary lesion of acne
2. Dry, crackling skin at corners of mouth
3. Localized skin infection involving hair follicles
4. Localized skin infection involving only one hair follicle
5. The most common fungal infection of the skin or scalp
6. Bacterial skin infections
7. Lotions with added oil to soften skin
8. Overly dry skin
9. An enzymatic debriding agent
10. A semisolid emulsion that becomes liquid when applied to the skin or scalp
11. A topical corticosteroid with medium to high potency
12. An antiviral agent used to treat Herpes Zoster
13. An infestation of the skin caused by the itch mite
14. A prescription scabicide
15. A potentially fatal (35% mortality) skin disorder

II. Critical Thinking Questions and Exercises

DISCUSSION AND ANALYSIS

Discuss the following topics with your classmates.

1. Discuss the five rules of wound care that every nurse should know.
2. Explain why a foul odor would be expected when autolytic debridement is used.
3. Describe the advantages of moisture-retentive dressings over wet dressings.
4. Distinguish between a furuncle and a carbuncle. Discuss nursing and medical management.
5. Distinguish between Herpes Zoster and Herpes Simplex.
6. Discuss the clinical manifestations and medical and nursing management for a patient with genital herpes.

7. Discuss the use of biological agents as a new line of treatment for psoriasis.
8. Explain the process of photochemotherapy.
9. Discuss the nursing and medical management of patients with TEN and SJS skin disorders.
10. Explain the five risk factors for developing malignant melanoma.

CLINICAL SITUATIONS

Read the following case studies. Fill in the blank spaces or circle the correct answer.

CASE STUDY: Acne Vulgaris

Brian is a 15-year-old who has been experiencing facial eruptions of acne for about a year. The numerous lesions are inflamed and present on the face and neck. He has tried many over-the-counter medications and nothing seems to help. His father had a history of severe acne when he was a teenager.

1. On the basis of the knowledge of acne vulgaris, the nurse knows that the skin disorder is characterized by

   five types of lesions: _____, _____, _____,

   _____, and _____.

2. The etiology of acne stems from:
   a. genetic factors.
   b. bacterial factors.
   c. hormonal factors.
   d. an interplay of all of the above.

3. Acne, most prevalent at puberty, is the direct result of oversecretion of the _____ glands.
   a. exocrine
   b. lacrimal
   c. sebaceous
   d. mucous

4. Explain the rationale for using benzoyl peroxide.

   _____

5. Explain the rationale for using synthetic vitamin A compounds (retinoids).

   _____

6. A common antibiotic that is frequently prescribed for treatment of acne is:
   a. terbutaline.
   b. tamoxifen.
   c. tetracycline.
   d. terfenadine.

7. A common oral retinoid that is used for acne is:
   a. Accutane.
   b. Acne-Aid.
   c. Actinex.
   d. Adalat.

8. Based on assessment data, identify two collaborative problems:

   _____ and _____.

CASE STUDY: Malignant Melanoma

Steve is a 26-year-old professional baseball player for a Florida farm team. He spent many hours in the sun practicing between 9:00 AM and 4:00 PM. His V-neck uniform left little protection to his chest. Steve had a mole on his chest for 5 years. One day last October he noticed that the margins of the mole were elevated and palpable and the color had become darker. Since his father had malignant melanoma when he was 32 years old, Steve decided to see a physician.

1. Steve knows that malignant melanoma is currently responsible for 3% of all cancer deaths. Based on statistical predictions, the number of deaths in 10 years will be approximately:

   a. 2%.   c. 6%.

   b. 4%.   d. 10%.

2. Three criteria to support total body digital photography for assessment are: _____,

   _____, and _____.

3. The most common form of melanoma is _____, which is most commonly found on the

   _____ and _____.

4. On examination, the physician notes a circular lesion with irregular outer edges and a pinkish hue in the center. The physician suspected the lesion to be:

   a. an acral-lentiginous melanoma.   c. a nodular melanoma.

   b. a lentigo-maligna melanoma.   d. a superficial spreading melanoma.

5. The physician confirms the diagnosis by:

   a. complete blood cell count analysis.   c. excisional biopsy.

   b. computed tomography.   d. skin examination.

6. The lesion is greater than 14 mm in thickness and growing vertically. The physician knows that:

   a. dermal invasion is likely.   c. metastasis is probable.

   b. the prognosis is favorable.   d. peripheral growth will occur next.

7. The physician considers chemotherapy using:

   a. cisplatin.   c. nitrosoureas.

   b. dacarbazine.   d. all of the above.

8. The physician advises Steve that with lymph node involvement he only has a _____% chance of surviving 5 years.

Study Guide for Brunner and Suddarth's Textbook of Medical-Surgical Nursing, 12th edition.

CHAPTER 57

Management of Patients With Burn Injury

I. Interpretation, Completion, and Comparison

MULTIPLE CHOICE

Read each question carefully. Circle your answer.

1. A full-thickness burn is:
   a. classified by the appearance of blisters.
   b. identified by the destruction of the dermis and epidermis.
   c. not associated with edema formation.
   d. usually very painful because of exposed nerve endings.

2. With partial-thickness (second-degree) burns, skin regeneration begins to take place:
   a. within 7 days.
   b. in 2 to 4 weeks.
   c. after 2 months.
   d. between the third and sixth month.

3. Plasma seeps out into surrounding tissues after a burn. The greatest amount of fluid leaks out in:
   a. the first 2 hours.
   b. 4 to 8 hours.
   c. 12 hours.
   d. 24 to 36 hours.

4. As fluid is reabsorbed after injury, renal function maintains a diuresis for up to:
   a. 3 days.
   b. 1 week.
   c. 2 weeks.
   d. 1 month.

5. Fluid shifts during the first week of the acute phase of a burn injury that cause massive cell destruction result in:
   a. hypernatremia.
   b. hypokalemia.
   c. hyperkalemia.
   d. hypercalcemia.

6. An unexpected laboratory value during the fluid remobilization phase of a major burn is a:
   a. hematocrit level of 45%.
   b. a pH of 7.20; PaO_2 of 38 mm Hg; and bicarbonate level of 15 mEq/L.
   c. serum potassium level of 3.2 mEq/L.
   d. serum sodium level of 140 mEq/L.

7. Plasma leakage produces edema, which increases:
   a. circulating blood volume.
   b. the hematocrit level.
   c. systolic blood pressure.
   d. all of the above.

8. The leading cause of death in fire victims is believed to be:
   a. cardiac arrest.
   b. carbon monoxide intoxication.
   c. hypovolemic shock.
   d. septicemia.

9. A serious gastrointestinal disturbance that frequently occurs with a major burn is:
   a. diverticulitis.
   b. hematemesis.
   c. paralytic ileus.
   d. ulcerative colitis.

10. A child tips a pot of boiling water onto his bare legs. The mother should:
   a. avoid touching the burned skin, and take the child to the nearest emergency department.
   b. cover the child's legs with ice cubes secured with a towel.
   c. immerse the child's legs in cool water.
   d. liberally apply butter or shortening to the burned area.

11. A man suffers leg burns from spilled charcoal lighter fluid. His son extinguishes the flames. While waiting for an ambulance, the burn victim should:
   a. have someone assist him into a bath of cool water, where he can wait for emergency personnel.
   b. lie down, have someone cover him with a blanket, and cover his legs with petroleum jelly.
   c. remove his burned pants so that the air can help cool the wound.
   d. sit in a chair, elevate his legs, and have someone cut his pants off around the burned area.

12. As the first priority of care, a patient with a burn injury will initially need:
   a. a patent airway established.
   b. an indwelling catheter inserted.
   c. fluids replaced.
   d. pain medication administered.

13. Eyes that have been irritated or burned with a chemical should be flushed with cool, clean water:
   a. immediately.
   b. in 5 to 10 minutes.
   c. after an eye examination.
   d. after 24 hours.

14. Decreased urinary output during the first 48 hours of a major burn is secondary to all of the following *except*:
   a. decreased adrenocortical activity.
   b. hemolysis of red blood cells.
   c. hypovolemia.
   d. sodium retention.

15. Electrolyte changes in the first 48 hours of a major burn include:
   a. base bicarbonate deficit.
   b. hypernatremia.
   c. hypokalemia.
   d. all of the above.

16. The resuscitation formula for replacing fluid lost during the first 24 to 48 hours recommends the administration of:
   a. colloids.
   b. electrolytes.
   c. crystalloids.
   d. all of the above.

17. A sample consensus formula for fluid replacement recommends that a balanced salt solution be administered in the first 24 hours of a burn in the range of 2 to 4 mL/kg/% of burn with 50% of the total given in the first 8 hours postburn. A 176-lb (80-kg) man with a 30% burn should receive a minimum of how much fluid replacement in the first 8 hours?
   a. 1,200 mL
   b. 2,400 mL
   c. 3,600 mL
   d. 4,800 mL

18. Fluid and electrolyte changes in the emergent phase of burn injury include all of the following *except*:
   a. base-bicarbonate deficit.
   b. elevated hematocrit level.
   c. potassium deficit.
   d. sodium deficit.

19. During the acute phase of burn injury, the nurse knows to assess for signs of potassium shifting:
    a. within 24 hours.
    b. between 24 and 48 hours.
    c. at the beginning of the third day.
    d. beginning on day 4 or day 5.

20. One parameter of adequate fluid replacement is an hourly urinary output in the range of:
    a. 10 to 30 mL.
    b. 30 to 50 mL.
    c. 80 to 120 mL.
    d. 100 to 200 mL.

21. During the fluid remobilization phase, the nurse knows to expect all of the following *except*:
    a. hemodilution.
    b. increased urinary output.
    c. metabolic alkalosis.
    d. sodium deficit.

22. Fluid remobilization usually begins:
    a. within the first 24 hours, when massive amounts of fluid are being administered intravenously.
    b. after 48 hours, when fluid is moving from the interstitial to the intravascular compartment.
    c. after 1 week, when capillary permeability has returned to normal.
    d. after 1 month, when scar tissue covers the wound and prevents evaporative fluid loss.

23. Wound cleansing and surgical debridement may begin as early as:
    a. 72 hours.
    b. 1 week.
    c. 1.5 to 2 weeks.
    d. 1 month.

24. Leukopenia within 48 hours is a side effect associated with the topical antibacterial agent:
    a. cerium nitrate solution.
    b. gentamicin sulfate.
    c. sulfadiazine, silver (Silvadene).
    d. mafenide (Sulfamylon).

25. The nurse knows that the topical antibacterial agent that does not penetrate eschar is:
    a. Acticoat.
    b. mafenide acetate.
    c. silver nitrate 0.5%.
    d. silver sulfadiazine 1%.

26. The nurse knows to monitor sodium and potassium levels (drug is hypotonic) when a burn patient is being treated with:
    a. Silvadene.
    b. silver nitrate 0.5%.
    c. Sulfamylon.
    d. all of the above.

27. After an occlusive dressing is applied to a burned foot, the foot should be placed in the position of:
    a. adduction.
    b. dorsiflexion.
    c. external rotation.
    d. plantar flexion.

28. Biologic dressings that use skin from living or recently deceased humans are known as:
    a. autografts.
    b. heterografts.
    c. homografts.
    d. xenografts.

29. The nurse knows that the physician will most likely prescribe the analgesic of choice for treatment of acute burn pain which is:
    a. Demerol.
    b. Fentanyl.
    c. morphine sulfate.
    d. OxyContin.

30. The recommended route for administration of low-dose narcotics is:
    a. intramuscular.
    b. intravenous.
    c. oral.
    d. subcutaneous.

31. To meet his early nutritional demands for protein, a 198-lb (90-kg) burned patient will need to ingest a minimum of how much of protein every 24 hours?
    a. 90 g/day.
    b. 110 g/day.
    c. 180 g/day.
    d. 270 g/day.

32. Early indicators of late-stage septic shock include all of the following *except*:
    a. decreased pulse pressure.
    b. a full, bounding pulse.
    c. pale, cool skin.
    d. renal failure.

SHORT ANSWER

Read each statement carefully. Write your response in the space provided.

1. The two age groups that have increased morbidity and mortality from burn injuries are:
   _____ and _____.

2. The overall mortality rate (all ages and total body surface area for burn injuries) is:
   _____.

3. The severity of burn injury and likelihood of survival is dependent on seven factors. Name four:
   _____, _____, _____, and _____.

4. Burn injuries are classified according to: _____ and _____.

5. List two pulmonary complications that occur secondary to inhalation injuries:
   _____ and _____.

6. The leading cause of death in thermally injured patients is: _____.

7. The resuscitation goal of fluid replacement therapy, postburn injury, is a urinary output of:
   _____.

8. The three major bacteria responsible for infection in burn centers are: _____, _____, and _____.

9. Three commonly used topical antibacterials for skin care are: _____, _____, and _____.

10. List four signs of sepsis, postburn: _____, _____, _____, and _____.

II. Critical Thinking Questions and Exercises

DISCUSSION AND ANALYSIS

Discuss the following topics with your classmates.

1. Explain why the survival rate for burn victims has increased significantly over the last 10 years.
2. Compare and contrast the three methods used to estimate total body surface area (TBSA) affected by burns: Rule of Nines, Lund and Browder Method, and the Palmer Method.
3. Explain the pathophysiology of a burn injury specific to the following system alterations: cardiovascular, fluid and electrolyte, pulmonary, renal, and gastrointestinal.
4. Explain the pathophysiology of carbon monoxide poisoning.
5. Describe general emergency procedures that a nurse should employ at the burn scene.
6. Describe the nurses' role during the immediate burn injury phase using the ABCs of trauma care.
7. Discuss general nursing actions for six nursing diagnoses for care of a patient during the emergent phase of burn injury.
8. Distinguish between the purposes and nursing implications for biologic dressings (homografts and heterografts) and biosynthetic and synthetic dressings.
9. Describe the appearance of hypertrophic and keloid scars and measures to prevent their formation.
10. Discuss why congestive heart failure is a potential complication of an acute burn.

IDENTIFYING PATTERNS

Complete the following flow chart illustrating the pathophysiologic sequence of reactions that result from a systemic response to a burn injury. Refer to Figure 57-3 in the text.

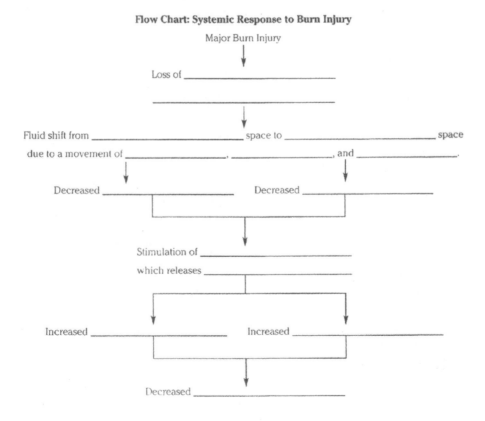

Flow Chart: Systemic Response to Burn Injury

Major Burn Injury

Loss of _____

_____

Fluid shift from _____ space to _____ space
due to a movement of _____, _____, and _____.

Decreased _____   Decreased _____

Stimulation of _____

which releases _____

Increased _____   Increased _____

Decreased _____

CLINICAL SITUATIONS

Develop a nursing care plan for each of the two situations below. For each nursing diagnosis, list goals, nursing actions, rationale, and expected outcomes. Refer to Chart 57-5 in the text.

1. Aimee, a 9-month-old child, climbed onto a stove where an electric range was on high. Her pajamas caught fire, and she was burned over 60% of her body (excluding her face and neck) with second- and third-degree burns. Her mother managed to extinguish the flames and immerse her in a sink of cool water before emergency help arrived. Aimee was transported to a burn treatment center. There are two other preschool children in her family.

2. Brad, a 12-year-old child, sustained full-thickness burns on his upper chest, face, and neck when he was trying to start a charcoal fire to prepare dinner for his father. His father sprayed him with water from a hose and took him to a hospital emergency department 3 miles away. On arrival, Brad was semiconscious and in extreme respiratory distress. He and his divorced father live together.

CHAPTER 58

Assessment and Management of Patients With Eye and Vision Disorders

I. Interpretation, Completion, and Comparison

MULTIPLE CHOICE

Read each question carefully. Circle your answer.

1. The muscles of the eyeball are innervated by all of the following cranial nerves *except* cranial nerve:
   a. III.
   b. IV.
   c. V.
   d. VI.

2. Vision becomes less efficient with age, because aging is associated with:
   a. a decrease in pupil size.
   b. a slowing of accommodation.
   c. an increase in lens opaqueness.
   d. all of the above.

3. During a routine eye examination, a patient complains that she is unable to read road signs at a distance when driving her car. The physician knows to check for:
   a. astigmatism.
   b. anisometropia.
   c. myopia.
   d. presbyopia.

4. Legal blindness refers to a best-corrected visual acuity (BCVA) that does not exceed what reading in the better eye?
   a. 20/50
   b. 20/100
   c. 20/150
   d. 20/200

5. Increased ocular pressure, resulting from optic nerve damage, is indicated by a reading of:
   a. 0 to 5 mm Hg.
   b. 6 to 10 mm Hg.
   c. 11 to 20 mm Hg.
   d. 21 mm Hg or higher.

6. A diagnostic clinical manifestation of glaucoma is:
   a. a significant loss of central vision.
   b. diminished acuity.
   c. pain associated with a purulent discharge.
   d. the presence of halos around lights.

7. When assessing the visual fields in acute glaucoma, the nurse would expect to find a:
   a. clear cornea.
   b. constricted pupil.
   c. marked blurring of vision.
   d. watery ocular discharge.

8. Pharmacotherapy for primary glaucoma that decreases the outflow of aqueous humor would include all of the following *except*:
   a. alpha-adrenergic agonists.
   b. carbonic anhydrase inhibitors.
   c. beta-blockers.
   d. miotics.

9. After cataract surgery, a patient is encouraged to:
   a. maintain bed rest for 1 week.
   b. lie on his or her stomach while sleeping.
   c. avoid bending his or her head below the waist.
   d. lift weights to increase muscle strength.

10. Clinical symptoms of a detached retina include:
    a. a sensation of floating particles.
    b. a definite area of blank vision.
    c. momentary flashes of light.
    d. all of the above.

11. The most common type of retinal detachment is:
    a. exudative.
    b. rhegmatogenous.
    c. traction.
    d. a combination of rhegmatogenous and traction.

12. The most common cause of visual loss in people older than 60 years of age is:
    a. macular degeneration.
    b. ocular trauma.
    c. retinal vascular disease.
    d. uveitis.

13. Chemical burns of the eye are immediately treated with:
    a. local anesthetics and antibacterial drops for 24 to 36 hours.
    b. hot compresses applied at 15-minute intervals.
    c. flushing of the lids, conjunctiva, and cornea with tap water or normal saline
    d. cleansing of the conjunctiva with a small cotton-tipped applicator.

14. Acute bacterial conjunctivitis is characterized by:
    a. blurred vision.
    b. elevated intraocular pressure.
    c. a mucopurulent ocular discharge.
    d. severe pain.

15. The most common neoplasm of the eyelids is:
    a. basal cell carcinoma.
    b. a chalazion.
    c. xanthelasmas.
    d. squamous cell carcinoma.

16. What type of medication is used in combination with mydriatics to dilate the patient's pupil?
    a. Anti-infectives
    b. Corticosteroids
    c. Cycloplegics
    d. NSAIDs

17. The most common antifungal agent used to treat eye infections is:
    a. acyclovir.
    b. amphotericin.
    c. ganciclovir.
    d. penicillin.

SHORT ANSWER

Read the statement carefully. Write your response in the space provided.

1. Normal intraocular pressure is: _____.

2. A visual acuity exam result of 20/100 is interpreted to mean:

   _____.

3. List four common causes of visual impairment or blindness in those over the age 40:

   _____, _____, _____, and

   _____.

4. The second leading cause of irreversible blindness in the world is:

   _____.

5. Two significant changes in the optic nerve in glaucoma are: _____ and _____.

6. The most common laser surgeries for glaucoma are: _____ and _____.

7. According to the World Health Organization, the leading cause of blindness in the world is:

   _____.

8. An initial treatment for a splash injury to the eye would be: _____.

9. Three microorganisms that most commonly cause bacterial conjunctivitis are: _____,

   _____, and _____.

10. A characteristic sign of viral conjunctivitis is _____.

11. One of the most serious ocular consequences of diabetes mellitus is: _____.

12. The most common cause of retinal inflammation in patients with AIDS is:

    _____.

MATCHING

Match the characteristic or function of the eye listed in column II with its associated structure listed in column I.

Column I

1. _____ Choroid
2. _____ Lens
3. _____ Pupil
4. _____ Retina
5. _____ Vitreous humor
6. _____ Cornea
7. _____ Sclera
8. _____ Iris
9. _____ Uvea
10. _____ Limbus

Column II

a. Maintains the form of the eyeball
b. Area where most of the blood vessels for the eye are located
c. Degree of convexity modified by contraction and relaxation of the ciliary muscles
d. Contractile membrane between the cornea and lens
e. Transparent part of the fibrous coat of the eyeball
f. Accommodates to the intensity of light by dilating or contracting
g. White part of the eye
h. The pigmented, vascular coating of the eye
i. The edge of the cornea where it joins the sclera
j. Contains nerve endings that transmit visual impulses to the brain

Match the term listed in column II with its associated definition listed in column I.

Column I   Column II

1. _____ Excessive production of tears   a. Iritis

2. _____ Another term for an external hordeolum   b. Keratitis

3. _____ The term oculus dexter refers to the _____ eye   c. Photophobia

4. _____ A term used to describe an inflammatory condition of the uveal tract   d. Aphakia

5. _____ Another term for nearsightedness   e. Right

6. _____ An inflammatory condition affecting the iris   f. Ptosis

7. _____ People who are photosensitive function better outdoors during this   g. Epiphora
           time of day   h. Strabismus

8. _____ Inflammation of the cornea   i. AM

9. _____ A loss of cornea substance or tissue as a result of inflammation   j. Laceration

10. _____ Abnormal sensitivity to light   k. Ulcer

11. _____ The term oculus sinister refers to the _____ eye   l. Left

12. _____ Absence of the lens   m. Uveitis

13. _____ Uneven curvature of the cornea   n. Astigmatism

14. _____ Drooping of the upper eyelid   o. Sty

15. _____ A tear in the eye tissue   p. Myopia

16. _____ A condition in which one eye deviates from the object at which the
            person is looking

II. Critical Thinking Questions and Exercises

EXTRACTING INFERENCES

Examine Figure 58-1 in the text. List the specific functions for each external structure of the eye listed below.

1. Lacrimal sac, gland, and duct: _____.

2. Pupil: _____.

3. Iris: _____.

4. Limbus: _____.

5. Sclera: _____.

6. Conjunctiva: _____.

7. Outer and inner canthus: _____.

8. Upper eyelid: _____.

9. Caruncle: _____.

DISCUSSION AND ANALYSIS

Discuss the following topics with your classmates.

1. Explain the pathophysiology associated with glaucoma.
2. Explain the clinical manifestations of altered vision seen in those with cataracts.
3. Distinguish between two types of refractive surgery: PRK and LASIK.
4. Describe the clinical manifestations and surgical management for retinal detachment.
5. Distinguish between dry and wet macular degeneration.
6. Describe dry eye syndrome.
7. Distinguish between the following surgical procedures: enucleation, evisceration, and exenteration.

IDENTIFYING PATTERNS

For each group of clustered clues, identify the specific disorder of the eye.

A chronic inflammation of the eyelid margins

Formation of scales and granulations on the eyelashes

White eyelashes may result from this condition

Staphylococcus aureus may be a primary infecting organism

1. _____

A superficial infection of the glands of the eyelids

Pain and swelling of the eyelids are characteristic signs

Warm, moist compresses on the eyelids facilitate healing

Topical sulfonamides may be prescribed

2. _____

Symptoms include hyperemia and edema of conjunctiva

Etiology may be bacterial, fungal, viral, or allergic

Lay person's term for condition is "pink-eye"

3. _____

Corneal edema is a common sign in this disorder

Ulceration and infection are associated with this disorder

Cycloplegics and mydriatics may be prescribed

Etiology is usually associated with trauma or compromise

Systemic or local defense mechanisms

4. _____

Characterized by an opacification of the lens

Usually associated with the aging process

Vision is clouded because light to the retina is blocked

Associated with compromised night vision

5. _____

CLINICAL SITUATIONS

Nursing Care Plan

Develop a nursing care plan based on the following clinical situation.

Elise is a 65-year-old woman who needs to have cataract surgery on her right eye. Elise lives with her daughter in a three-story house and has rheumatoid arthritis. She needs a cane to walk. Her daughter has a Down's syndrome child at home who requires constant care. Share your nursing care plan with your instructor for comments.

Nursing Diagnoses

Goals   Nursing Actions   Rationale   Expected Outcomes

CASE STUDY: Cataract Surgery

Marcella is a 75-year-old single woman who has had progressive diminished vision and increased difficulty with night driving. Her physician suspects that Marcella has a cataract. He does a complete eye examination and history.

1. As part of an oral history, the physician tries to determine whether Marcella has any of the common

   factors that contribute to cataract development, such as: _____, _____,

   _____, and _____.

2. Marcella, during her history, told the physician that she was experiencing the three common symptoms

   found with cataracts: _____, _____, and _____.

3. On ophthalmic examination, the physician noted the major objective finding seen with cataracts:

   _____.

4. When assessing the need for surgery, the physician determined that Marcella's best corrected vision was
   worse than the minimal standard of:
   a. 20/15.   c. 20/35.
   b. 20/25.   d. 20/50.

5. The physician decided to perform _____, the most preferred technique for cataract surgery.

6. Postoperatively, Marcella knows that she will need to avoid lying on the side of the affected eye for a

   period of _____.

CHAPTER 59

Assessment and Management of Patients With Hearing and Balance Disorders

I. Interpretation, Completion, and Comparison

MULTIPLE CHOICE

Read each question carefully. Circle your answer.

1. The organ of hearing is known as the:
   a. cochlea.
   b. eardrum.
   c. semicircular canal.
   d. stapes.

2. Mechanical vibrations are transformed into neural activity so that sounds can be differentiated by the:
   a. cochlea.
   b. organ of Corti.
   c. ossicles.
   d. semicircular canals.

3. To straighten the ear canal for examination, the nurse would grasp the auricle and pull it:
   a. backward.
   b. upward.
   c. slightly outward.
   d. in all of these directions.

4. A sensorineural (perceptive) hearing loss results from impairment of the:
   a. eighth cranial nerve.
   b. middle ear.
   c. outer ear.
   d. seventh cranial nerve.

5. The critical level of loudness that most people (without a hearing loss) are comfortable with is a decibel (dB) reading of:
   a. 15 dB.
   b. 30 dB.
   c. 45 dB.
   d. 60 dB.

6. Severe hearing loss is associated with a decibel loss in the range of:
   a. 25 to 40 dB.
   b. 40 to 55 dB.
   c. 70 to 90 dB.
   d. more than 90 dB.

7. The physician ordered an examination of the middle ear to assess muscle reflex to sound. The nurse knows to prepare the patient for a(an):
   a. electronystagmography.
   b. platform posturography.
   c. sinusoidal harmonic acceleration.
   d. tympanogram.

8. A hearing loss that is a manifestation of an emotional disturbance is known as what kind of hearing loss?
   a. Conductive
   b. Functional
   c. Mixed
   d. Sensorineural

9. The minimum noise level known to cause noise-induced hearing loss, regardless of duration, is:
   a. 55 to 60 dB.
   b. 65 to 70 dB.
   c. 75 to 80 dB.
   d. 85 to 90 dB.

10. What is the occurrence of hearing impairment, at birth, which is related to genetic factors 50% of the time?
   a. 1:100
   b. 3:100
   c. 5:100
   d. 10:1,000

11. It is projected that by 2050 what percentage of people over 55 years of age will have some form of hearing loss?
   a. 15%
   b. 30%
   c. 50%
   d. 75%

12. Changes in the ear that occur with aging may include:
   a. atrophy of the tympanic membrane.
   b. increased hardness of the cerumen.
   c. degeneration of cells at the base of the cochlea.
   d. all of the above.

13. The most common fungus associated with ear infections is:
   a. *Staphylococcus albus.*
   b. *Staphylococcus aureus.*
   c. *Aspergillus.*
   d. *Pseudomonas.*

14. Nursing instructions for a patient suffering from external otitis should include the:
   a. application of heat to the auricle.
   b. avoidance of swimming.
   c. ingestion of over-the-counter analgesics, such as aspirin.
   d. all of the above.

15. A tympanoplasty, the most common procedure for chronic otitis media, is surgically performed to:
   a. close a perforation.
   b. prevent recurrent infection.
   c. reestablish middle ear function.
   d. accomplish all of the above.

16. A symptom that is not usually found with acute otitis media is:
   a. aural tenderness.
   b. rhinitis.
   c. otalgia.
   d. otorrhea.

17. An incident of otitis media is usually associated with:
   a. ear canal swelling.
   b. discharge.
   c. intense ear pain.
   d. prominent localized tenderness.

18. A myringotomy is performed primarily to:
   a. drain purulent fluid.
   b. identify the infecting organism.
   c. relieve tympanic membrane pressure.
   d. accomplish all of the above.

19. Postoperative nursing assessment for a patient who has had a mastoidectomy should include observing for facial paralysis, which might indicate damage to which cranial nerve?
   a. First
   b. Fourth
   c. Seventh
   d. Tenth

20. A facial nerve neuroma is a tumor on which cranial nerve?
   a. Third
   b. Fifth
   c. Seventh
   d. Eighth

21. A dietary modification for a patient with Ménière's disease would be:
    a. a decrease in sodium intake to 1,500 mg daily.
    b. fluid restriction to 2.0 L/day.
    c. an increase in calcium to 1.0 g/day.
    d. an increase in vitamin C to 1.5 g/day.

22. An acoustic neuroma is a benign tumor of which cranial nerve?
    a. Fifth
    b. Sixth
    c. Seventh
    d. Eighth

II. Critical Thinking Questions and Exercises

DISCUSSION AND ANALYSIS

Discuss the following topics with your classmates.

1. Describe how sound is conducted and transmitted.
2. Distinguish between three tests used to evaluate gross auditory acuity: the Rhine test, the Weber Test, and the Whisper Test.
3. Discuss the age-related advancement of deafness in those over 65 years of age.
4. Distinguish between three inner ear conditions: vertigo, nystagmus, and motion sickness.
5. Distinguish between three types of hearing aids: behind the ear, in the ear, and in the canal.

EXAMINING ASSOCIATIONS

View the figure below. For each anatomic area labeled, write the associated physiologic function.

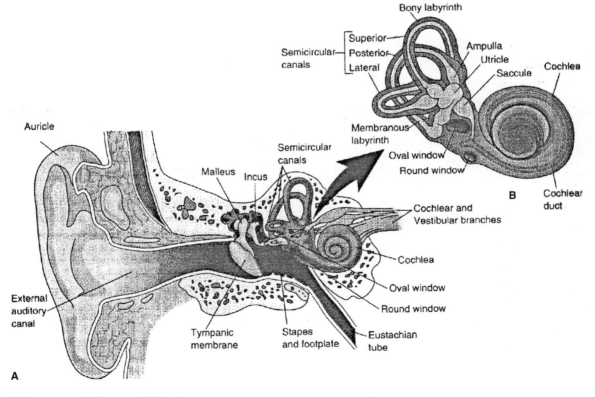

(A) Anatomy of the ear. **(B)** The inner ear.

1. Auricle: _____

2. Malleus: _____

3. Incus: _____

4. Semicircular canals: _____

5. Cochlea: _____

6. Oval window: _____

7. Round window: _____

8. Eustachian tube: _____

9. Stapes: _____

10. Tympanic membrane: _____

11. External auditory canal: _____

CLINICAL SITUATIONS

Read the following case studies. Fill in the blanks or circle the correct answer.

CASE STUDY: Mastoid Surgery

Amber is a 73-year-old grandmother who is scheduled for mastoid surgery to remove a cholesteatoma, a cystlike sac filled with keratin debris, which was large enough to occlude the ear canal.

1. Preoperatively, the physician reviews the results of the audiogram and assesses for the presence of associated ear problems, such as: _____, _____, _____, _____, _____, _____, _____, and _____.

2. Identify four major preoperative nursing goals for the patient: _____, _____, _____, and _____.

3. Postoperatively, it is common for the patient to experience: _____.

4. The patient is advised that the postauricular incision should be kept dry for:
   a. 7 days.
   b. 2 weeks.
   c. 6 weeks.
   d. 1 month.

5. Two important signs of infection are: _____ and _____.

6. Manipulation of the semicircular canals during surgery may result in the symptom of:
   a. sharp, shooting pain.
   b. inner ear fullness.
   c. purulent drainage.
   d. vertigo.

7. The patient is advised that it is normal to hear popping and crackling sounds in the affected ear for about:
   a. 3 days.
   b. 1 week.
   c. 3 to 5 weeks.
   d. 2 to 4 months.

8. The patient is taught to prevent activities that increase intracranial pressure for 2 to 3 weeks after surgery, such as: _____, _____, _____, and _____.

CASE STUDY: Ménière's Disease

David is a 42-year-old lawyer who travels internationally. He has recently been diagnosed with Ménière's disease.

1. The classic triad of symptoms that are diagnostic for Ménière's disease are: _____, _____, and _____.

2. The basic pathophysiology causing the triad of symptoms listed in the previous question is:

   _____.

3. The most common and disrupting clinical symptom of this disease is: _____.

4. A diet for Ménière's disease would include avoiding:
   a. bread.
   b. cheese.
   c. eggs.
   d. milk.

5. A popular medication prescribed to suppress the vestibular system is:
   a. Antivert.
   b. Lasix.
   c. Phenergan.
   d. Valium.

6. The most popular surgical procedure used to treat this disease is:
   a. endolymphatic sac decompression.
   b. labyrinthectomy.
   c. middle ear perfusion.
   d. vestibular nerve section.

CHAPTER 60

Assessment of Neurologic Function

I. Interpretation, Completion, and Comparison

MULTIPLE CHOICE

Read each question carefully. Circle your answer.

1. A neurotransmitter that helps control mood and sleep is:
   a. acetylcholine.
   b. dopamine.
   c. enkephalin.
   d. serotonin.

2. Parkinson's disease is caused by an imbalance in the neurotransmitter known as:
   a. acetylcholine.
   b. dopamine.
   c. GABA.
   d. endorphin.

3. A person's personality and judgment are controlled by that area of the brain known as the:
   a. frontal lobe.
   b. occipital lobe.
   c. parietal lobe.
   d. temporal lobe.

4. The lobe of the cerebral cortex that is responsible for the understanding of language and music is the:
   a. frontal lobe.
   b. occipital lobe.
   c. parietal lobe.
   d. temporal lobe.

5. Voluntary muscle control is governed by a vertical band of "motor cortex" located in the:
   a. frontal lobe.
   b. occipital lobe.
   c. parietal lobe.
   d. temporal lobe.

6. The sleep–wake cycle regulator and the site of the hunger center is known as the:
   a. hypothalamus.
   b. medulla oblongata.
   c. pituitary gland.
   d. thalamus.

7. The overall regulation of the autonomic nervous system is the function of the:
   a. cerebellum.
   b. hypothalamus.
   c. pons.
   d. temporal lobe of the cerebral cortex.

8. The "master gland" is also known as the:
   a. adrenal gland.
   b. thyroid gland.
   c. pineal gland.
   d. pituitary gland.

9. The major receiving and communication center for afferent sensory nerves is the:
   a. medulla oblongata.
   b. pineal body.
   c. pituitary gland.
   d. thalamus.

10. The normal adult produces about 150 mL of cerebrospinal fluid daily from the:
    a. ventricles.
    b. dura mater.
    c. circle of Willis.
    d. corpus callosum.

11. The spinal cord tapers off to a fibrous band of tissue at the level of the:
    a. coccygeal nerve.
    b. first lumbar vertebra.
    c. lateral ventricle.
    d. medulla oblongata.

12. The preganglionic fibers of the sympathetic neurons are located in those segments of the spinal cord identified as:
    a. C1 to T1.
    b. C3 to L1.
    c. C8 to L3.
    d. T1 to S5.

13. The parasympathetic division of the autonomic nervous system yields impulses that are mediated by the secretion of:
    a. acetylcholine.
    b. epinephrine.
    c. norepinephrine.
    d. all of the above.

14. Motor axons form pyramidal tracts that cross to the opposite side. This crossed pyramidal tract occurs in the brain in the area of the:
    a. frontal cerebrum.
    b. lateral portion of the cerebellum.
    c. medulla oblongata.
    d. pons.

15. The brain center responsible for balancing and coordination is the:
    a. cerebellum.
    b. second lumbar vertebra.
    c. first sacral nerve.
    d. sacrum.

16. The Romberg test is used to assess:
    a. balance and coordination.
    b. muscle strength.
    c. biceps reflex.
    d. muscle tone.

17. The Babinski reflex is used to assess:
    a. muscle strength.
    b. coordination.
    c. central nervous system disease.
    d. optical nerve damage.

18. To reduce leakage of cerebrospinal fluid after myelography with an oil-based medium, the patient lies down for 12 to 24 hours in what position?
    a. In high-Fowler's position
    b. In bed with head elevated 30 to 45 degrees
    c. Prone
    d. Recumbent

19. Patient preparation for electroencephalography includes omitting, for 24 hours before the test, all of the following *except*:
    a. coffee and tea.
    b. solid foods.
    c. stimulants.
    d. tranquilizers.

20. For a lumbar puncture, the nurse should assist the patient to flex his or her head and thighs while lying on the side so that the needle can be inserted between the:
    a. fourth and fifth cervical vertebrae.
    b. fifth and sixth thoracic vertebrae.
    c. third and fourth lumbar vertebrae.
    d. first and second sacral vertebrae.

21. After a lumbar puncture, the nurse knows to assess for the most common (30% occurrence) complication of a(an):
    a. epidural abscess.
    b. epidural hematoma.
    c. throbbing headache.
    d. meningitis.

MATCHING

Match the nervous system response listed in column II with the neurotransmitter listed in column I.

Column I

1. _____ Gamma-aminobutyric acid
2. _____ Enkephalin
3. _____ Norepinephrine
4. _____ Dopamine
5. _____ Acetylcholine
6. _____ Serotonin

Column II

a. Primarily excitatory; can produce vagal stimulation of heart
b. Inhibits pain pathways and can control sleep
c. Affects behavior, attention, and fine movement
d. Excitatory response, mostly affecting moods
e. Muscle and nerve inhibitory transmissions
f. Excitatory; inhibits pain transmission

II. Critical Thinking Questions and Exercises

DISCUSSION AND ANALYSIS

Discuss the following topics with your classmates.

1. Describe the blood–brain barrier.
2. Describe the role and functions of the hypothalamus.
3. Explain the role of the thalamus in integrating sensory impulses.
4. Conduct a health assessment of the nervous system on one of your classmates.
5. Demonstrate, on a classmate, how to examine the following reflexes: deep tendon, biceps, triceps, brachioradialis, patellar, and Achilles.
6. Distinguish between the purposes and techniques for magnetic resonance imaging (MRI) and positron emission tomography (PET) in neurological assessment.

EXAMINING ASSOCIATIONS

Write the effects produced by the parasympathetic and sympathetic nervous systems on each organ or tissue listed in column I. Use the terms provided, and document in the space below. The answers for the first organ or tissue are provided as an example.

Autonomic Nervous System

Terms to be used

Acceleration

Constriction

Dilation

Inhibition

Increased motility

Secretion

Organ or Tissue	Parasympathetic Effect	Sympathetic Effect
a. Bronchi	Constriction	Dilation
b. Cerebral vessels	_____	_____
c. Coronary vessels	_____	_____
d. Heart	_____	_____
e. Iris of the eye	_____	_____
f. Salivary glands	_____	_____
g. Smooth muscle of		
(1) Bladder wall	_____	_____
(2) Large intestine	_____	_____
(3) Small intestine	_____	_____

Cranial Nerves

Next to each cranial nerve listed by number, write the appropriate corresponding terminology in column I and a major associated function in column II. The answers for the first cranial nerve are provided as an example.

Nerve No.	Column I	Column II
I	Olfactory	Smell
II	_____	_____
III	_____	_____
IV	_____	_____
V	_____	_____
VI	_____	_____
VII	_____	_____
VIII	_____	_____
IX	_____	_____
	_____	
	_____	
	_____	

APPLYING CONCEPTS

Diagram of the Brain

View the diagram of the brain below and list the major functions of each identified area.

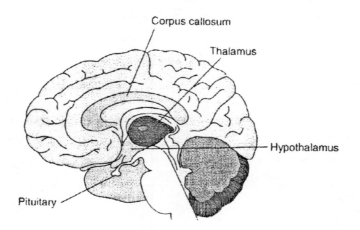

Medial view of the brain.

Thalamus

1. _____

2. _____

Hypothalamus

1. _____

2. _____

3. _____

4. _____

5. _____

6. _____

7. _____

8. _____

Pituitary

1. _____

2. _____

CHAPTER 61

Management of Patients With Neurologic Dysfunction

I. Interpretation, Completion, and Comparison

MULTIPLE CHOICE

Read each question carefully. Circle your answer.

1. Unconsciousness may have what type of origin?
   a. Neurologic
   b. Metabolic
   c. Toxicologic
   d. Multisystem involvement

2. The first priority of treatment for a patient with altered level of consciousness is:
   a. assessment of pupillary light reflexes.
   b. determination of the cause.
   c. positioning to prevent complications.
   d. maintenance of a patent airway.

3. A nurse assesses the patient's level of consciousness using the Glasgow Coma Scale. What score indicates severe impairment of neurologic function?
   a. 3
   b. 6
   c. 9
   d. 12

4. The most severe neurologic impairments are evidenced by abnormal body posturing defined as:
   a. decerebrate.
   b. decorticate.
   c. flaccid.
   d. rigid.

5. The normal range of intracranial pressure (ICP) is:
   a. 5 to 8 mm Hg.
   b. 0 to 10 mm Hg.
   c. 20 to 30 mm Hg.
   d. 25 to 40 mm Hg.

6. ICP can be increased by a:
   a. decrease in venous outflow.
   b. dilation of the cerebral blood vessels.
   c. rise in $PaCO_2$.
   d. change in all of the above.

7. Initial compensatory vital sign changes with increased ICP include all of the following *except*:
   a. a slow, bounding pulse.
   b. an increased systemic blood pressure.
   c. a decreased temperature.
   d. respiratory rate irregularities.

8. A patient is admitted to the hospital with an ICP reading of 20 mm Hg and a mean arterial pressure of 90 mm Hg. The nurse knows that the cerebral perfusion pressure (CPP) would be calculated at:
   a. 50 mm Hg.
   b. 60 mm Hg.
   c. 70 mm Hg.
   d. 80 mm Hg.

9. Irreversible neurologic dysfunction occurs when the CPP is:
   a. less than 50 mm Hg.
   b. 60 to 80 mm Hg.
   c. 75 to 95 mm Hg.
   d. greater than 100 mm Hg.

10. A nurse knows that a patient experiencing Cushing's triad would not exhibit:
    a. bradycardia.
    b. bradypnea.
    c. hypertension.
    d. tachycardia.

11. The earliest sign of serious impairment of brain circulation related to increasing ICP is:
    a. a bounding pulse.
    b. bradycardia.
    c. hypertension.
    d. lethargy and stupor.

12. As ICP rises, the nurse knows that she may be asked to give a commonly used osmotic diuretic:
    a. glycerin.
    b. isosorbide.
    c. mannitol.
    d. urea.

13. An indicator of compromised respiratory status significant enough to require mechanical ventilation for an average-weight adult patient with a neurologic dysfunction would be:
    a. an expiratory reserve volume of 1,300 mL.
    b. an inspiratory capacity of 3,000 mL.
    c. a residual volume of 1,400 mL.
    d. a vital capacity of 1,000 mL.

14. Nursing care activities for a patient with increased ICP would *not* include:
    a. assisting the patient with isometric exercises.
    b. avoiding activities that interfere with venous drainage of blood from the head.
    c. use of a cervical collar.
    d. teaching the patient to exhale when being turned (to avoid the Valsalva maneuver).

15. A nurse assessing urinary output as an indicator of diabetes insipidus knows that an hourly output of what volume over 2 hours may be a positive indicator?
    a. 50 to 100 mL/h
    b. 100 to 150 mL/h
    c. 150 to 200 mL/h
    d. More than 200 mL/h

16. Neurologic and neurosurgical approaches to pain relief would include:
    a. stimulation procedures.
    b. administration of intraspinal opiates.
    c. interruption of nerve tracts that conduct pain.
    d. all of the above mechanisms.

17. Postcraniotomy cerebral edema is at a maximum how long after brain surgery?
    a. 6 hours
    b. 12 to 20 hours
    c. 24 to 72 hours
    d. 3 to 5 days

18. The majority of cases of epilepsy occur in those:
    a. younger than 20 years of age.
    b. 25 to 35 years of age.
    c. approximately 45 years of age.
    d. older than 60 years of age.

19. Long-term use of antiseizure medication in women leads to an increased incidence of:
    a. anemia.
    b. osteoarthritis.
    c. osteoporosis.
    d. obesity.

20. Nursing care for a patient who is experiencing a convulsive seizure includes all of the following *except*:
    a. loosening constrictive clothing.
    b. opening the patient's jaw and inserting a mouth gag.
    c. positioning the patient on his or her side with head flexed forward.
    d. providing for privacy.

21. A seizure characterized by loss of consciousness and tonic spasms of the trunk and extremities, rapidly followed by repetitive generalized clonic jerking, is classified as a:
    a. focal seizure.
    b. generalized seizure.
    c. Jacksonian seizure.
    d. partial seizure.

22. A nutritional approach for seizure management includes a diet that is:
    a. low in fat.
    b. restricts protein to 10% of daily caloric intake.
    c. high in protein and low in carbohydrate.
    d. at least 50% carbohydrate.

23. Headaches classified as primary would include all of the following *except*:
    a. aneurysm.
    b. cluster.
    c. migraine.
    d. tension.

24. A beta-blocking agent commonly used for the treatment of a migraine headache is:
    a. Amerge.
    b. Inderal.
    c. Maxalt.
    d. Zomig.

SHORT ANSWER

Read each statement carefully. Write your response in the space provided.

1. Potential collaborative problems for a patient with an altered level of consciousness would include:

   _____, _____, _____, _____, and

   _____.

2. List three major potential complications in a patient with a depressed level of consciousness:

   _____, _____, and _____.

3. The earliest sign of increased ICP is: _____.

4. List three primary complications of increased ICP:

   _____, _____, and _____.

5. List six treatment goals for the prompt management of increased ICP:

   _____, _____, _____,

   _____, _____, and _____.

6. The primary, lethal complication of ICP is: _____.

7. Nursing postoperative management includes: detecting and reducing _____, relieving

   _____, preventing _____, and monitoring _____ and

   _____.

8. The leading cause of seizures in the elderly is: _____.

9. A major potential complication of epilepsy is: _____.

10. List six "triggers" known to cause migraine headaches:

_____, _____, _____,

_____, _____, and _____.

MATCHING

Match the neurologic dysfunction in column II with its associated nursing intervention found in column I. An answer may be used more than once.

Column I

1. _____ Assist with daily active or passive range of motion.

2. _____ Elevate the head of the bed 30 degrees.

3. _____ Institute a bowel-training program.

4. _____ Maintain dorsiflexion to affected area.

5. _____ Place the patient in a lateral position.

Column II

a. Footdrop
b. Incontinence
c. Impaired cough reflex
d. Keratitis
e. Paralyzed diaphragm
f. Paralyzed extremity

II. Critical Thinking Questions and Exercises

DISCUSSION AND ANALYSIS

Discuss the following topics with your classmates.

1. Describe several nursing interventions for maintaining the airway for a patient with an altered level of consciousness.
2. Discuss 6 of 12 major goals for a patient with an altered level of consciousness.
3. Describe Cushing's reflex, a phenomenon seen when cerebral blood flow decreases significantly.
4. Explain two trends in neurological monitoring: microdialysis and cerebral oxygenation monitoring.
5. Distinguish between the early and late signs of ICP that a nurse would be responsible for assessing.
6. Explain the rationale for regulating body temperature in patients with cerebral disorders.
7. Describe the nursing management of a patient during a seizure.
8. Describe the role of the nurse after a seizure has occurred.
9. Describe the pathophysiology, clinical manifestations, and medical/nursing interventions for epilepsy.
10. Describe the clinical manifestations of a migraine headache from prodrome phase to the recovery phase.

INTERPRETING PATTERNS

Complete the following analogies by inserting the word that reflects the association.

1. Craniotomy : surgery involving entry into the cranial vault :: Craniectomy : _____

2. Cushing's response : increased arterial pressure in response to increased ICP :: Cushing's triad:

_____

3. Decerebration : extreme extension of the upper and lower extremities :: _____ : abnormal flexion of the upper extremities

4. A primary headache : controllable localized pain :: Migraine headache : _____

5. Ataxic breathing : random sequences of deep and shallow breaths :: Cheyne–Stokes breathing :

_____

CLINICAL SITUATIONS

Read the following case study. Develop a nursing care plan using the format shown below.

Miss Potter, a 32-year-old , single, circus performer, has been unconscious since she was admitted to the hospital 1 week ago after falling from a high wire. Her family must leave the area to travel with the circus and is expected to return in 2 months.

Nursing Diagnoses

Goals   Nursing Actions   Rationale   Expected Outcomes

APPLYING CONCEPTS

Look at Table 61-1 , Nursing Assessment for the Unconscious Patient, in the text. For each of the two figures, list the clinical assessment technique in column I and the clinical significance in column II.

Eyes

Column I   Column II

1. Fixed, dilated pupils (example)   1. Injury at midbrain (example)

2. _____   2. _____

3. _____   3. _____

4. _____   4. _____

Foot

Column I   Column II

1. _____   1. _____

   _____

                                         2. _____

                                            _____

                                         3. _____

                                            _____

CHAPTER 62

Management of Patients With Cerebrovascular Disorders

I. Interpretation, Completion, and Comparison

MULTIPLE CHOICE

Read each question carefully. Circle your answer.

1. As a cause of death in the United States, stroke currently ranks:
   a. second.
   b. third.
   c. fourth.
   d. fifth.

2. The most common cause of cerebrovascular disease is:
   a. arteriosclerosis.
   b. embolism.
   c. hypertensive changes.
   d. vasospasm.

3. The etiology of an ischemic stroke would include a(an):
   a. cardiogenic emboli.
   b. cerebral aneurysm.
   c. arteriovenous malformation.
   d. intracerebral hemorrhage.

4. The majority of ischemic strokes have what type of origin?
   a. Cardiogenic embolic
   b. Cryptogenic
   c. Large artery thrombotic
   d. Small artery thrombotic

5. The nurse knows that symptoms associated with a transient ischemic attack (TIA), usually a precursor of a future stroke, usually subside in:
   a. 1 hour.
   b. 3 to 6 hours.
   c. 12 hours.
   d. 24 to 36 hours.

6. The degree of neurologic damage that occurs with an ischemic stroke depends on the:
   a. location of the lesion.
   b. size of the area of inadequate perfusion.
   c. amount of collateral blood flow.
   d. combination of the above factors.

7. A stroke victim is experiencing memory loss and impaired learning capacity. The nurse knows that brain damage has most likely occurred in which lobe?
   a. Frontal
   b. Occipital
   c. Parietal
   d. Temporal

8. The initial mortality rate for a stroke can be as high as:
   a. 10%.
   b. 20%.
   c. 30%.
   d. 50%.

9. The most common motor dysfunction of a stroke is:
   a. ataxia.
   b. diplopia.
   c. dysphagia.
   d. hemiplegia.

10. The initial diagnostic test for a stroke, usually performed in the emergency department, is a:
    a. 12-lead electrocardiogram.
    b. carotid ultrasound study.
    c. noncontrast computed tomogram.
    d. transcranial Doppler flow study.

11. An emergency department nurse understands that a 110-lb recent stroke victim will receive at least the minimum dose of recombinant tissue plasminogen activator (t-PA). The patient will receive a minimum dose of:
    a. 50 mg.
    b. 60 mg.
    c. 85 mg.
    d. 100 mg.

12. The most common side effect of t-PA is:
    a. an allergic reaction.
    b. bleeding.
    c. severe vomiting.
    d. a second stroke in 6 to 12 hours.

13. Eighty percent of hemorrhagic strokes are primarily caused by:
    a. an embolus.
    b. a cerebral thrombus.
    c. a brain tumor.
    d. uncontrolled hypertension.

14. A classic diagnostic system of hemorrhagic stroke is the patient's compliant of:
    a. numbness of an arm or leg.
    b. double vision.
    c. severe headache.
    d. dizziness and tinnitus.

15. Most patients with hemorrhagic strokes are placed in bed in which position?
    a. High-Fowler's
    b. Prone
    c. Supine
    d. Semi-Fowler's (head of bed at 15 to 30 degrees)

SHORT ANSWER

Read each statement carefully. Write your response in the space provided.

1. The primary cerebrovascular disorder in the United States is _____, which is also called a _____ to emphasize the urgency of its occurrence.

2 Since 1996, thrombolytic therapy with recombinant plasminogen activator (t-PA) for ischemic stroke has significantly decreased poststroke symptoms. However, the treatment challenge is that the therapy has to be given within what time period? _____

3. Four nonmodifiable risk factors for stroke are:
   _____, _____, _____, and
   _____.

4. The main surgical procedure for managing TIAs is: _____.

5. Four primary complications of carotid endarterectomy are: _____,

_____, _____, and _____.

6. Three possible collaborative problems for a patient recovering from an ischemic stroke are:

_____, _____, and _____.

7. Hemorrhagic strokes are caused by bleeding into: _____, _____, or _____.

8. Potential complications of a hemorrhagic stroke include: _____, _____,

_____, and _____.

9. The most common cause of intracerebral hemorrhage is: _____.

MATCHING

Match the clinical manifestations of specific neurologic deficits listed in column II with its associated cause listed in column I.

Column I

1. _____ Ataxia
2. _____ Receptive aphasia
3. _____ Dysphagia
4. _____ Homonymous hemianopsia
5. _____ Loss of peripheral vision
6. _____ Expressive aphasia
7. _____ Diplopia
8. _____ Paresthesia

Column II

a. Difficulty judging distances
b. Unaware of the borders of objects
c. Double vision
d. Staggering, unsteady gait
e. Difficulty in swallowing
f. Difficulty with proprioception
g. Unable to form words that are understandable
h. Unable to comprehend the spoken word

II. Critical Thinking Questions and Exercises

DISCUSSION AND ANALYSIS

Discuss the following topics with your classmates.

1. Compare the etiology and symptoms of two types of stroke: ischemic stroke and hemorrhagic stroke.
2. Explain the pathophysiology of a brain attack.
3. Describe clinical manifestations of a stroke that a nurse should interpret. Organize those symptoms according to classifications of deficits: visual field, motor and sensory loss, verbal, perceptual, cognitive and psychological effects.
4. Describe the focus of nursing interventions when helping a patient recover from an ischemic stroke.
5. Distinguish between the causes of four types of hemorrhagic stroke: intracerebral, intracranial, arteriovenous malformations, and subarachnoid hemorrhage.

CLINICAL SITUATIONS

Construct a nursing care plan for Mrs. Coe. Refer to Charts 62-3 and 62-4 in the text.

Mrs. Coe recently sustained an ischemic stroke. She is 41 years old and lives with her husband and three sons. Emphasize the rehabilitative phase, which should have begun with her diagnosis, and stress the retraining of her flaccid right upper and lower extremities. She also needs to be taught how to sit, stand, and walk with balance and how to use a wheelchair.

Nursing Diagnoses

Goals	Nursing Actions	Rationale	Expected Outcomes

CHAPTER 63

Management of Patients With Neurologic Trauma

I. Interpretation, Completion, and Comparison

MULTIPLE CHOICE

Read each question carefully. Circle your answer.

1. All of the following statements about the occurrence of head injuries are correct *except*:
   a. The majority of all victims are younger than 25 years of age.
   b. An estimated 50,000 persons die annually from these injuries.
   c. Motor vehicle crashes are the primary cause.
   d. The majority of injuries occur in females.

2. A cerebral hemorrhage located within the brain is classified as:
   a. an epidural hematoma.
   b. an extradural hematoma.
   c. an intracerebral hematoma.
   d. a subdural hematoma.

3. The Glasgow Coma Scale is used to determine the level of consciousness. A score considered indicative of a coma is:
   a. 1.
   b. 3.
   c. 5.
   d. 7.

4. Assessing the level of consciousness is an important nursing measure postinjury. Signs of increasing intracranial pressure (ICP) include:
   a. bradycardia.
   b. increased systolic blood pressure.
   c. widening pulse pressure.
   d. all of the above.

5. Comatose patients are mechanically ventilated to control ICP. Hypocapnia is a goal that can be achieved with a $PaCO_2$ in the range of:
   a. 10 to 25 mm Hg.
   b. 25 to 30 mm Hg.
   c. 30 to 35 mm Hg.
   d. 35 to 40 mm Hg.

6. An indicator of elevated body temperature in a head-injured patient is:
   a. cerebral irritation from hemorrhage.
   b. damage to the hypothalamus.
   c. infection.
   d. all of the above.

7. To prevent decreased cerebral perfusion pressure after brain injury, the nurse knows that cerebral perfusion pressure must be at a minimum reading of:
   a. 15 mm Hg.
   b. 30 mm Hg.
   c. 50 mm Hg.
   d. 60 mm Hg.

8. A common cause of increased ICP is cerebral edema and swelling that peaks how long after the injury?
   a. 12 hours
   b. 12 to 24 hours
   c. 2 to 3 days
   d. 7 days

9. Posttraumatic seizures that are classified as *late* occur how long after the injury?
   a. 48 hours
   b. 72 hours
   c. 4 to 6 days
   d. 7 days

10. More than 50% of new victims of spinal cord injury are:
    a. 30 years of age or younger.
    b. 30 to 40 years of age.
    c. 40 to 50 years of age.
    d. 50 years of age or older.

11. In the United States, the number of new spinal cord injuries each year is estimated to be about:
    a. 5,000 cases.
    b. 11,000 cases.
    c. 20,000 cases.
    d. 25,000 cases.

12. The primary cause (35%) of spinal cord injuries is:
    a. gunshot wounds.
    b. industrial accidents.
    c. sports activities.
    d. motor vehicle crashes.

13. Spinal cord injury can be classified according to the area of spinal cord damage. Motor deficits in the upper rather than the lower extremities, usually caused by edema in the cervical area, are classified as:
    a. anterior cord syndrome.
    b. Brown-Séquard syndrome.
    c. central cord syndrome.
    d. peripheral syndrome.

14. Respiratory difficulty and paralysis of all four extremities occur with spinal cord injury:
    a. above C2.
    b. at C6.
    c. at C7.
    d. around C8.

15. High doses of which drug have been found to reduce swelling and disability if given within 8 hours of injury even though its use is controversial?
    a. Mannitol
    b. Methylprednisolone sodium
    c. Naloxone
    d. Neomycin

16. Loss of autonomic nervous system function below the level of the lesion causes what kind of shock?
    a. Cardiac
    b. Hypovolemic
    c. Septic
    d. Neurogenic

17. Recovery of vital organ functions resulting from spinal shock can take up to:
    a. 4 months.
    b. 12 months.
    c. 2 years.
    d. 4 years.

18. Orthostatic hypotension is a common problem for spinal cord injuries at the level of:
    a. C4.
    b. T7.
    c. L4.
    d. S1.

19. A common complication of immobility in a spinal cord injury is:
    a. pressure ulcers.
    b. thrombophlebitis.
    c. urinary tract infections.
    d. pneumonia.

SHORT ANSWER

Read each statement carefully. Write your response in the space provided.

1. A characteristic sign of a basilar skull fracture is:

   _____.

2. A brain injury can cause serious brain damage because:

   _____

3. Five symptoms of postconcussion syndrome are:

   _____, _____, _____,

   _____, and _____.

4. After concussion, a patient needs to know to seek medical attention if any of the following six symptoms

   occur: _____, _____, _____,

   _____, _____, and _____.

5. The most serious brain injury that can develop within the cranial vault is a: _____.

6. Identify four signs of a rapidly expanding, acute subdural hematoma that would require immediate
   surgical intervention:

   _____, _____, _____, and _____.

7. The three cardinal signs of brain death are: _____, _____,

   and _____.

8. List five collaborative problems that a nurse should assess for a patient with a brain injury:

   _____, _____, _____,

   _____, and _____.

9. Name the three criteria used to assess level of consciousness using the Glasgow Coma Scale:

   _____, _____, and _____.

10. Complications after traumatic head injuries can be classified according to: _____,

    _____, and _____.

11. The five vertebrae most commonly involved in spinal cord injuries are the: _____,

    _____, _____, _____, and _____.

12. List four common manifestations of pulmonary embolism:

    _____, _____, _____, and _____.

13. Three potential complications that may develop in spinal cord injury are:

    _____, _____, and _____.

14. Patients with tetraplegia and paraplegia are at increased risk for infection and sepsis from three common

    sources: _____, _____, and _____.

II. Critical Thinking Questions and Exercises

DISCUSSION AND ANALYSIS

Discuss the following topics with your classmates.

1. Discuss the frequency of head injuries in the United States.
2. Describe the clinical manifestations of traumatic brain injury.
3. Distinguish between a cerebral concussion and a cerebral contusion.
4. Distinguish between three types of intracranial hemorrhage: epidural hematoma, subdural hematoma, and intracerebral hemorrhage.
5. Explain why the most important consideration in any head injury is whether the brain is injured.
6. Explain what the Uniform Determination of Brain Death Act regulates.
7. Discuss the nursing measures that should be used to control ICP in severely brain-injured patients.
8. Describe the pathophysiology and nursing interventions for autonomic dysreflexia.

CLINICAL SITUATIONS

Read the following case studies. Develop a plan of care as indicated below.

CASE STUDY: Cervical Spine Injury

Develop a nursing care plan for Katie, an 11-year-old child, who suffered a cervical spine injury after diving into a swimming pool. Katie is in traction applied by Crutchfield tongs and is on a Stryker frame. She is the oldest of three children and has never been hospitalized before. Complete your nursing care plan, and share it with your instructor for comments.

Nursing Diagnoses

Goals	Nursing Actions	Rationale	Expected Outcomes

CASE STUDY: Paraplegia

Matthew, a 29-year-old Navy pilot, was recently injured in a training maneuver. Matthew is a paraplegic. He has been hospitalized for 1 week. He was recently married, and his wife is expecting their first child in 2 months. Emphasize the following areas in your nursing care plan: psychological support, weight-bearing activities, muscle exercises, mobilization, and sexual needs. Share your work with your clinical instructor.

Nursing Diagnoses

Goals	Nursing Actions	Rationale	Expected Outcomes

CHAPTER 64

Management of Patients With Neurologic Infections, Autoimmune Disorders, and Neuropathies

I. Interpretation, Completion, and Comparison

MULTIPLE CHOICE

Read each question carefully. Circle your answer.

1. Identify the bacteria *not associated* with the cause of septic meningitis:
   a. *Cryptococcus neoformans.*
   b. *Haemophilus influenza.*
   c. *Neisseria meningitides.*
   d. *Streptococcus pneumoniae.*

2. The most severe form of meningitis is considered to be:
   a. bacterial.
   b. aseptic.
   c. septic.
   d. viral.

3. Bacterial meningitis alters intracranial physiology, causing:
   a. cerebral edema.
   b. increased permeability of the blood–brain barrier.
   c. raised intracranial pressure.
   d. all of the above changes.

4. A brain abscess is a collection of infectious material within the substance of the brain that is caused by:
   a. direct invasion of the brain.
   b. spread of infection from nearby sites.
   c. spread of infection by other organs.
   d. all of the above mechanisms.

5. During assessment, the nurse knows that the most frequently reported disabling symptom found in multiple sclerosis is:
   a. depression.
   b. double vision.
   c. fatigue.
   d. pain.

6. A positive diagnosis of myasthenia gravis can be reached using the following test:
   a. anticholinesterase levels.
   b. magnetic resonance imaging.
   c. computed tomography (CT) scan.
   d. electromyography.

7. A surgical intervention that can cause substantial remission of myasthenia gravis is:
   a. esophagostomy.
   b. myomectomy.
   c. thymectomy.
   d. splenectomy.

8. The initial neurologic symptom of Guillain-Barré syndrome is:
   a. absent tendon reflexes.
   b. dysrhythmias.
   c. paresthesia of the legs.
   d. transient hypertension.

9. Tic douloureux is characterized by paroxysms of pain and burning sensations. It is a disorder of which cranial nerve?
   a. Third
   b. Fifth
   c. Seventh
   d. Eighth

10. Bell's palsy is characterized by weakness or paralysis of the facial muscles. It is a disorder of which cranial nerve?
    a. Third
    b. Fifth
    c. Seventh
    d. Eighth

11. Tinnitus and vertigo are clinical manifestations of damage to which cranial nerve.
    a. Fourth
    b. Sixth
    c. Eighth
    d. Tenth

SHORT ANSWER

Read each statement carefully. Write your response in the space provided.

1. Name the five infectious disorders of the nervous system: _____, _____, _____, _____, and _____.

2. List six signs of bacterial meningitis that a nurse should assess:

   _____, _____, _____, _____, _____, and _____.

3. The most common cause of acute encephalitis in the United States is: _____. The two medications of choice for this disorder are: _____ and _____.

4. The diagnosis of Creutzfeldt–Jakob disease can now be supported by the presence of: _____ in the cerebrospinal fluid.

5. The primary pathology of multiple sclerosis is damage to the: _____.

6. List the three forms of multiple sclerosis based on the frequency and progression of symptoms:
   _____, _____, and _____.

7. Myasthenia gravis is considered an autoimmune disease in which antibodies are directed against

   _____.

8. The majority of patients with myasthenia gravis exhibit these two clinical signs: _____ and

   _____.

9. The most common cause of peripheral neuropathy is: _____.

MATCHING

Match the cranial nerve listed in column II with its associated clinical disorder listed in column I. An answer may be used more than once.

Column I

1. _____ Optic neuritis
2. _____ Pituitary tumor
3. _____ Brain stem ischemia
4. _____ Trigeminal neuralgia
5. _____ Bell's palsy
6. _____ Herpes Zoster
7. _____ Ménière's syndrome
8. _____ Guillain-Barré syndrome
9. _____ Vagal body tumors
10. _____ Sinus tract tumor

Column II

a. I
b. II
c. IV
d. V
e. VI
f. VII
g. VIII
h. X

II. Critical Thinking Questions and Exercises

DISCUSSION AND ANALYSIS

Discuss the following topics with your classmates.

1. Demonstrate how to assess for the Kernig sign and the Brudzinski sign to determine a diagnosis of bacterial meningitis.
2. Distinguish between the clinical manifestations and medical/nursing interventions for arthropod-borne virus encephalitis and fungal encephalitis.
3. Explain what *demyelination* refers to in reference to multiple sclerosis.
4. Explain the etiology and clinical manifestations of myasthenic crises.
5. Discuss the clinical manifestations, pathophysiology, and medical/nursing interventions for Guillain-Barré syndrome.

CLINICAL SITUATIONS

Read the following case study. Circle the correct answer.

CASE STUDY: Multiple Sclerosis

Toni, a 32-year-old mother of two, has had multiple sclerosis for 5 years. She is currently enrolled in a school of nursing. Her husband is supportive and helps with the care of their preschool sons. Toni has been admitted to the clinical area for diagnostic studies related to symptoms of visual disturbances.

1. The nurse is aware that multiple sclerosis is a progressive disease of the central nervous system characterized by:

   a. axon degeneration.

   b. demyelination of the brain and the spinal cord.

   c. sclerosed patches of neural tissue.

   d. all of the above.

2. During the physical assessment, the nurse recalls that the areas most frequently affected by multiple sclerosis are the:

   a. lateral, third, and fourth ventricles.

   b. optic nerve and chiasm.

   c. pons, medulla, and cerebellar peduncles.

   d. above areas.

3. The nurse knows that the two most common clinical symptoms are: _____ and _____.

4. During the nursing interview, Toni minimizes her visual problems, talks about remaining in school to attempt advanced degrees, requests information about full-time jobs in nursing, and mentions her desire to have several more children. The nurse recognizes Toni's emotional responses as being:

   a. an example of inappropriate euphoria characteristic of the disease process.

   b. a reflection of coping mechanisms used to deal with the exacerbation of her illness.

   c. indicative of the remission phase of her chronic illness.

   d. realistic for her current level of physical functioning.

5. Toni's disease process involves a sacral plexus. Assessment should include:

   a. bladder problems or urinary tract infections.

   b. bowel management.

   c. sex.

   d. all of the above.

6. The nurse knows that disease-modifying pharmacologic therapy can reduce the frequency and duration of

   relapse. List five probable medications: _____, _____, _____,

   _____, and _____.

CHAPTER 65

Management of Patients With Oncologic or Degenerative Neurologic Disorders

I. Interpretation, Completion, and Comparison

MULTIPLE CHOICE

Read each question carefully. Circle your answer.

1. The highest incidence of brain tumors occurs during which decades of life?
   a. Earlier than the third
   b. In the third
   c. In the fourth
   d. Between the fifth and seventh

2. The most frequently seen intracerebral brain neoplasm is:
   a. an acoustic neuroma.
   b. an angioma.
   c. a glioma.
   d. a meningioma.

3. A patient is diagnosed with an intracerebral tumor. The nurse knows that the diagnosis may include all of the following *except* a(an):
   a. astrocytoma.
   b. ependymoma.
   c. medulloblastoma.
   d. meningioma.

4. The most common benign encapsulated brain tumor (representing 15% of primary brain tumors) is a(an):
   a. angioma.
   b. glioblastoma multiforme.
   c. meningioma.
   d. neuroma.

5. A nurse knows that a patient exhibiting seizurelike movements localized to one side of the body most likely has:
   a. a cerebellar tumor.
   b. a frontal lobe tumor.
   c. a motor cortex tumor.
   d. an occipital lobe tumor.

6. All of the following tumor types are commonly seen in the elderly *except*:
   a. anaplastic astrocytoma.
   b. cerebral metastasis from other sites.
   c. glioblastoma multiforme.
   d. medulloblastoma.

7. The majority of brain tumors are treated by:
   a. neurosurgery.
   b. chemotherapy.
   c. radioisotope implants.
   d. all of the above mechanisms.

8. Metastatic brain lesions occur in what percentage of patients with cancer?
   a. 10%
   b. 25%
   c. 40%
   d. 50% to 70%

9. The median survival time for patients with brain lesion metastasis, when no surgery is performed and radiation therapy is used, is:

   a. 3 to 6 months.

   b. 9 to 12 months.

   c. 18 months.

   d. 24 months.

10. Parkinsonian symptoms usually appear during which decade of life?

   a. Fourth

   b. Fifth

   c. Sixth

   d. Seventh

11. The clinical manifestations of Parkinson's disease (bradykinesia, rigidity, and tremors) are directly related to a decreased level of:

   a. acetylcholine.

   b. dopamine.

   c. serotonin.

   d. phenylalanine.

12. The most effective drug currently used to control the tremor of parkinsonism is:

   a. Requip.

   b. Levodopa.

   c. Symmetrel.

   d. Permax.

13. Clinical manifestations of Huntington's disease include:

   a. abnormal involuntary movements (chorea).

   b. emotional disturbances.

   c. intellectual decline.

   d. all of the above.

14. The average time from onset to death for patients diagnosed with amyotrophic lateral sclerosis (ALS) is:

   a. 3 to 5 years.

   b. 6 to 8 years.

   c. 10 years.

   d. 15 to 20 years.

15. The majority of lumbar disc herniations occur at the level of:

   a. L1 to L2.

   b. L3 to L4.

   c. L4 to L5.

   d. S1 to S2.

SHORT ANSWER

Read each statement carefully. Write your response in the space provided.

1. The majority of metastatic lesions to the brain occur from six areas: _____, _____, _____, _____, _____, and _____.

2. Name the three most common systemic signs of increased intracranial pressure: _____, _____, and _____.

3. List three common focal or localized symptoms of increased intracranial pressure: _____, _____, and _____.

4. A spinal cord tumor located within the spinal cord is classified as: _____.

5. List five degenerative disorders of the central and peripheral nervous system: _____, _____, _____, _____, and _____.

6. Identify the four cardinal signs of Parkinson's disease:

_____, _____, _____, and

_____.

7. List the five chief symptoms of amyotrophic lateral sclerosis:

_____, _____, _____,

_____, and _____.

8. Identify two common characteristics of muscular dystrophies: _____ and _____.

9. Cervical disk herniation usually occurs at the _____ interspaces.

10. Identify two major collaborative problems for patients with a cervical discectomy: _____ and _____.

MATCHING

Match the term of a neurologic disorder listed in column II with its associated disorder listed in column I.

Column I

1. _____ Impaired ability to execute voluntary movements
2. _____ Rapid, jerky, purposeless movements of extremities of facial muscles
3. _____ A sensation of "pins and needles"
4. _____ Restlessness and agitation
5. _____ Disease of the spinal nerve root
6. _____ Minute and illegible handwriting
7. _____ Very slow voluntary movements and speech
8. _____ Abnormal voice quality caused by incoordination of speech muscles

Column II

a. Akathisia
b. Bradykinesia
c. Chorea
d. Dyskinesia
e. Dysphonia
f. Micrographia
g. Paresthesia
h. Radiculopathy

II. Critical Thinking Questions and Exercises

DISCUSSION AND ANALYSIS

Discuss the following topics with your classmates.

1. Discuss a variety of physiologic changes that result from the infiltration of tissue subsequent to the growth of a brain tumor.
2. Describe the various classifications of brain tumors based on their pathophysiology.
3. Discuss the primary nursing diagnoses and interventions for a patient with cerebral metastases or an incurable brain tumor.
4. Describe the benefits and limitations of thalamotomy and pallidotomy in the treatment of Parkinson's disease.
5. Explain the basic pathophysiology and clinical manifestations of Huntington's disease.

CLINICAL SITUATIONS

CASE STUDY: Parkinson's Disease

Charles is a 76-year-old retired professional golfer. He has recently been diagnosed as having Parkinson's disease.

1. The nurse knows that Parkinson's disease, a progressive neurologic disorder, is characterized by:
   - a. bradykinesia.
   - b. muscle rigidity.
   - c. tremor.
   - d. all of the above.

2. The nurse assesses for the characteristic movement of Parkinson's disease, which is:
   - a. an exaggerated muscle flaccidity that leads to frequent falls.
   - b. a hyperextension of the back and neck that alters normal movements.
   - c. a pronation–supination of the hand and forearm that interferes with normal hand activities.
   - d. a combination of all of the above.

3. Charles is started on chemotherapy, which is aimed at restoring dopaminergic activities. An example of such a drug is:
   - a. Artane.
   - b. Benadryl.
   - c. Elavil.
   - d. Levodopa.

4. Nutritional considerations as part of the nursing care plan would include all of the following *except*:
   - a. the diet should be semisolid to facilitate the passage of food.
   - b. calcium should be avoided.
   - c. the patient should be sitting in an upright position during feeding.
   - d. thick fluids should be encouraged to provide additional calories.

CASE STUDY: Huntington's Disease

Develop a nursing care plan for the patient described below.

Mike is a 49-year-old television producer who has been diagnosed as having Huntington's disease. He lives alone in a penthouse apartment and is extremely busy and successful in his business. He has no living relatives. He is experiencing uncontrollable movements and difficulties feeding himself. He recently started chemotherapy with haloperidol (Haldol). Share your care plan with your instructor for comments.

Nursing Diagnosis: Potential for accidental injury related to abnormal involuntary movements.

Goals	Nursing Actions	Rationale	Expected Outcomes

EXTRACTING INFERENCES

View Figure 65-1 in the text. For each brain tumor site, describe the expected clinical symptoms, nursing assessments and medical/surgical interventions.

CHAPTER 66

Assessment of Musculoskeletal Function

I. Interpretation, Completion, and Comparison

MULTIPLE CHOICE

Read each question carefully. Circle your answer.

1. The vertebrae can be classified as a type of:
   a. flat bone.
   b. irregular bone.
   c. long bone.
   d. short bone.

2. The sternum, a bone that is a site for hematopoiesis, is classified as a:
   a. flat bone.
   b. irregular bone.
   c. long bone.
   d. short bone.

3. The basic cells responsible only for the formation of bone matrix are:
   a. osteoblasts.
   b. osteoclasts.
   c. osteocytes.
   d. all of the above.

4. About 3 weeks after fracture, an internal bridge of fibrous material, cartilage, and immature bone joins bone fragments so that ossification can occur. The building of a "fracture bridge" occurs during the stage of bone healing known as:
   a. inflammation.
   b. cellular proliferation.
   c. callus formation.
   d. ossification.

5. The hip and shoulder are examples of diarthroses joints that are classified as:
   a. ball-and-socket joints.
   b. hinge joints.
   c. pivot joints.
   d. saddle joints.

6. The primary energy source for muscle cells is:
   a. adenosine triphosphate (ATP).
   b. creatine phosphate.
   c. glucose.
   d. glycogen.

7. Isometric contraction of the vastus lateralis is part of the exercises known as:
   a. biceps-tightening exercises.
   b. triceps-resisting exercises.
   c. gluteal-setting exercises.
   d. quadriceps exercises.

8. Patient education for musculoskeletal conditions for the aging is based on the understanding that there is a gradual loss of bone after a peak of bone mass at age:
   a. 20 years.
   b. 35 years.
   c. 40 years.
   d. 50 years.

9. By age 75 years, the average woman is susceptible to bone fractures and has lost about what percentage of cancellous bone?

   a. 15%

   b. 40%

   c. 60%

   d. 75%

10. The removal of synovial fluid from a joint is called:

   a. arthrectomy.

   b. arthrocentesis.

   c. arthrography.

   d. arthroscopy.

MATCHING

Match the range-of-motion term listed in column II with its associated description listed in column I.

Column I

1. _____ Pulling down toward the midline of the body

2. _____ The act of turning the foot inward

3. _____ The opposite movement of flexion

4. _____ Turning around on an axis

5. _____ Turning the palms down

6. _____ Pulling the jaw forward

7. _____ Moving away from the midline

8. _____ Conelike circular movement

9. _____ Turning the palm up

10. _____ Turning the foot outward

Column II

a. Supination

b. Extension

c. Circumduction

d. Abduction

e. Protraction

f. Eversion

g. Pronation

h. Adduction

i. Inversion

j. Rotation

SHORT ANSWER

Read each statement carefully. Write the best response in the space provided.

1. The leading cause of disability in the United States is: _____.

2. The most common musculoskeletal condition that necessitates hospitalization in those over 65 years of age

   is: _____.

3. The approximate percentage of total body calcium present in the bones is: _____.

4. In the human body, there are _____ bones.

5. Approximately _____ mg of calcium daily is essential to maintain adult bone mass.

6. Red bone marrow is located in the shaft of four long and flat bones: _____, _____,

   _____, and _____.

7. The major hormonal regulators of calcium homeostasis are: _____ and

   _____.

8. Ossification for major adult long bone fractures can take up to: _____.

9. The term used to describe the grating, crackling sound heard over irregular joint surfaces like the knee is:

_____.

SCRAMBLEGRAM

Unscramble the letters to answer each statement.

1. The fibrous membrane that covers the bone: _____

E O P T R M E S U I

2. These connect muscles to muscles: _____

A N S I G M L T E

3. The contractile unit of skeletal muscle: _____

O E S E A R M R C

4. These attach muscles to bone: _____

N T S O E D N

5. Loss of bone mass common in postmenopausal women: _____

I S S T P O O R E O O S

6. A lateral curving deviation of the spine: _____

L S O S O S I I C

7. Excessive fluid within a joint capsule: _____

N E O F I F S U

8. Aspiration of a joint to obtain synovial fluid: _____

S A I R E T T H N R E O C

II. Critical Thinking Questions and Exercises

DISCUSSION AND ANALYSIS

Discuss the following topics with your classmates.

1. List several general functions of the musculoskeletal system.
2. Compare and contrast the function of osteoblasts, osteocytes, and osteoclasts. Include a description of the Haversian system.
3. Describe the process of osteogenesis.
4. Explain how vitamin D regulates the balance between bone formation and bone resorption.
5. Explain the role of the sex hormones testosterone and estrogen on bone remodeling.

6. Describe the process of fracture healing mentioning the six stages of progression.
7. Contrast the difference between isotonic and isometric contractions.
8. Describe the age-related changes of the musculoskeletal system specific to bones, muscles, joints, and ligaments.
9. Distinguish between three common deformities of the spine: kyphosis, lordosis, and scoliosis.
10. Compare and contrast the purpose of three diagnostic procedures commonly prescribed for musculoskeletal conditions: computed tomography, magnetic resonance imaging, and arthrography.

EXTRACTING INFERENCES

View Figure 66-2 in the text and describe the physiologic function of listed structures.

1. Synovial cavity: _____.

2. Bursa: _____.

3. Patella: _____.

4. Fat pad: _____.

5. Articular cartilage: _____.

6. Medial meniscus: _____.

7. Intrapatellar bursa: _____.

CHAPTER 67

Musculoskeletal Care Modalities

I. Interpretation, Completion, and Comparison

MULTIPLE CHOICE

Read each question carefully. Circle your answer.

1. Choose the *incorrect* statement about the traditional plaster cast. After a plaster cast has been set, it:
   a. will take 1 to 3 days to dry.
   b. should be resonant to percussion.
   c. should be covered with a blanket to promote quick drying.
   d. will not have maximum strength until it is dry.

2. A patient with an arm cast complains of pain. The nurse should do all of the following *except*:
   a. assess the fingers for color and temperature.
   b. administer a prescribed analgesic to promote comfort and allay anxiety.
   c. suspect that the patient may have a pressure sore.
   d. determine the exact site of the pain.

3. The nurse who assesses bone fracture pain expects the patient to describe the pain as:
   a. a dull, deep, boring ache.
   b. sharp and piercing.
   c. similar to "muscle cramps."
   d. sore and aching.

4. The nurse suspects "compartment syndrome" for a casted extremity. She would assess for characteristic symptoms such as:
   a. decreased sensory function.
   b. excruciating pain.
   c. loss of motion.
   d. all of the above.

5. The nurse knows to assess the patient in an arm cast for possible pressure ulcers in the following area:
   a. lateral malleolus.
   b. olecranon.
   c. radial styloid.
   d. ulna styloid.

6. After removal of a cast, the patient needs to be instructed to do all of the following *except*:
   a. apply an emollient lotion to soften the skin.
   b. control swelling with elastic bandages, as directed.
   c. gradually resume activities and exercise.
   d. use friction to remove dead surface skin by rubbing the area with a towel.

7. A common pressure problem area for a long leg cast is the:
   a. dorsalis pedis.
   b. peroneal nerve.
   c. popliteal artery.
   d. posterior tibialis.

8. The nurse assesses for peroneal nerve injury by checking the patient's casted leg for the primary symptom of:
   a. burning.
   b. numbness.
   c. tingling.
   d. all of the above indicators.

9. The nurse is very concerned about the potential debilitating complication of peroneal nerve injury, which is:
   a. permanent paresthesias.
   b. footdrop.
   c. deep vein thrombosis (DVT).
   d. infection.

10. Choose the *incorrect* statement about turning a patient in a hip spica cast.
    a. A minimum of three persons are needed so that the cast can be adequately supported by their palms.
    b. Points over body pressure areas need to be supported to prevent the cast from cracking.
    c. The abduction bar should be used to ensure that the lower extremity can be moved as a unit.
    d. The patient should be encouraged to use the trapeze or side rail during repositioning.

11. Skin traction is limited to a weight between:
    a. 1 to 3 lb.
    b. 4.5 to 8 lb.
    c. 10 to 12 lb.
    d. 13 to 15 lb.

12. A patient in pelvic traction needs his or her circulatory status assessed. The nurse should check for a positive (1) Homans' sign by asking the patient to:
    a. extend both hands while the nurse compares the volume of both radial pulses.
    b. extend each leg and dorsiflex each foot to determine if pain or tenderness is present in the lower leg.
    c. plantar flex both feet while the nurse performs the blanch test on all of the patient's toes.
    d. squeeze the nurse's hands with his or her hands to evaluate any difference in strength.

13. Nursing assessment of a patient in traction should include:
    a. lung sounds and bowel sounds.
    b. circulation, sensation, and motion of the extremities in traction.
    c. the patient's level of anxiety and apprehension.
    d. all of the above interventions.

14. The nurse expects that up to how much weight can be used for a patient in skeletal traction?
    a. 10 lb
    b. 25 lb
    c. 40 lb
    d. 60 lb

15. When a patient is in continuous skeletal leg traction, it is important for the nurse to remember to do all of the following *except*:
    a. encourage the patient to use the trapeze bar.
    b. maintain adequate countertraction.
    c. remove the weights when pulling the patient up in bed to prevent unnecessary pulling on the fracture site.
    d. use a fracture bedpan to prevent soiling and to maintain patient comfort.

16. Patients with a hip and knee replacement begin ambulation with a walker or crutches how long after surgery?
    a. 24 hours
    b. 72 hours
    c. 1 week
    d. 2 to 3 weeks

17. An artificial joint for total hip replacement involves an implant that consists of:
    a. an acetabular socket.
    b. a femoral shaft.
    c. a spherical ball.
    d. all of the above.

18. The recommended leg position to prevent prosthesis dislocation after a total hip replacement is:
    a. abduction.
    b. adduction.
    c. flexion.
    d. internal rotation.

19. Postoperatively a patient with a total hip replacement is allowed to turn:
    a. 45 degrees onto his or her unoperated side if the affected hip is kept abducted.
    b. from the prone to the supine position only, and the patient must keep the affected hip extended and abducted.
    c. to any comfortable position as long as the affected leg is extended.
    d. to the operative side if his or her affected hip remains extended.

20. The nurse caring for a postoperative hip-replacement patient knows that the patient should not cross his or her legs, at any time, for how long after surgery?
    a. 2 months
    b. 3 months
    c. 4 months
    d. 6 months

21. One of the most dangerous of all postoperative complications is:
    a. atelectasis.
    b. hypovolemia.
    c. pulmonary embolism.
    d. urinary tract infection.

22. After a total hip replacement, stair climbing is kept to a minimum for:
    a. 1 month.
    b. 2 months.
    c. 3 to 6 months.
    d. 6 to 8 months.

23. After a total hip replacement, the patient is usually able to resume daily activities after:
    a. 3 months.
    b. 6 months.
    c. 9 months.
    d. 1 year.

24. Preoperative nursing measures that are appropriate for an orthopedic patient should include:
    a. encouraging fluids to prevent a urinary tract infection.
    b. teaching isometric exercises and encouraging active range of motion.
    c. discouraging smoking to improve respiratory function.
    d. all of the above interventions.

25. Postoperative nursing concerns when caring for an orthopedic patient should include:
    a. determining that the patient's pain is controlled by administering prescribed analgesics.
    b. observing for signs of shock, such as hypotension and tachycardia.
    c. preventing infection by using aseptic technique when giving wound care.
    d. all of the above interventions.

SHORT ANSWER

Read each statement carefully. Write your response in the space provided.

1. List four purposes for using a cast:

   _____, _____, _____, and _____.

2. The advantages of a fiberglass cast compared to a plaster cast are:

   _____

3. Unrelieved pain for a patient in a cast must be *immediately reported* to avoid four possible and serious potential problems:

   _____, _____, _____, and _____.

4. The nurse completes a neurovascular assessment of either the fingers or toes of a casted extremity to determine circulatory status. Describe expected outcomes. Which capillary refill test should be performed?

   _____

5. List the five "Ps" that should be assessed as part of the neurovascular check: _____,

   _____, _____, _____, and

   _____.

6. List several danger signs of possible circulatory constriction for a casted extremity:

   _____

7. List three major complications of an extremity that is casted, braced, or splinted.

   _____, _____, and _____.

8. Name four purposes for traction application:

   _____, _____, _____, and _____.

9. The most effective cleansing solution for care of a pin site is: _____.

10. A nursing goal for a patient with skeletal traction is to avoid infection and the development of

    _____ at the site of pin insertion.

11. List seven potential immobility-related complications that may develop when a patient is in skeletal

    traction: _____, _____, _____,

    _____, _____, _____, and

    _____.

12. The nurse knows to assess a patient for DVT by assessing the lower extremities for:

    _____, _____, _____, and

    _____.

II. Critical Thinking Questions and Exercises

DISCUSSION AND ANALYSIS

Discuss the following topics with your classmates.

1. Discuss four potential collaborative problems for a patient with a cast.
2. Discuss the major nursing goals for a patient with a cast.
3. Describe the complication of compartment syndrome and its recommended treatment.
4. Demonstrate muscle-setting (quadriceps and gluteal) and isometric exercises used to prevent disuse syndrome.
5. Describe the serious complication, Volkmann's contracture.
6. Describe the psychological behavior and the physiologic symptoms seen in patients with cast syndrome.

7. Describe the purpose of an external fixator device and the nursing management necessary to prevent complications.
8. Discuss principles to be followed when caring for a patient in traction.
9. Discuss the major nursing goals for a patient in traction.
10. Demonstrate the seven methods for preventing hip prosthesis dislocation that a nurse would teach a patient.
11. Outline in detail the patient education guidelines for home care after hip replacement.
12. Describe the nursing interventions, including patient teaching about the use of a continuous passive motion (CPM) device, for a total knee replacement.
13. Discuss five nursing diagnoses for the patient undergoing orthopedic surgery.

CLINICAL SITUATIONS

Read the following case studies. Fill in the blanks or circle the correct answer.

CASE STUDY: Buck's Traction

Bernadette is a 32-year-old bank secretary who was admitted to the hospital for unilateral Buck's extension traction to the left leg after a hip injury. Bernadette is the single parent of three children younger than 12 years of age.

1. On the basis of her knowledge of running traction, the nurse knows to expect that:
   a. the patient's leg will be flat on the bed to allow for a straight pulling force.
   b. the patient's leg will be flexed at the knee to allow for mobility without disruption of the pulling force.
   c. the traction will be applied directly to the bony skeleton to maintain a constant pulling force.
   d. the traction will allow the patient's leg to be suspended off the bed so that no further damage can occur to the hip.

2. The nurse knows that countertraction must be considered whenever traction is applied. Countertraction for Buck's traction is provided by: _____ and _____.

3. In preparing the patient's skin for Buck's traction application, the nurse knows that it is necessary to: _____ and _____.

4. The nurse makes certain that the weights applied will not exceed:
   a. 2 lb.
   b. 4 lb.
   c. 6 lb.
   d. 8 lb.

5. The nurse consistently assesses neurovascular status when traction is in place. List seven indicators that the nurse would evaluate.

_____

6. To prevent pressure ulcers and nerve damage, excessive pressure is avoided over the _____ and _____.

7. On assessment, the nurse notes a positive Homans' sign. Explain what this means.

_____

CASE STUDY: Total Hip Replacement

Tom is a 62-year-old athletic coach at a high school. Sports activities, especially baseball, have been the focus of his energies since he was in high school and college. Because of prior hip joint injuries and degenerative joint disease, he is scheduled for a total hip replacement.

1. Preoperatively, the nurse assesses the status of the cardiovascular system based on the knowledge that mortality for patients over 60 years is directly related to the complications of: _____ and _____.

2. As part of preoperative teaching, the nurse makes the patient aware of five major potential complications of hip replacement: _____, _____, _____, _____, and _____.

3. On the basis of knowledge that limited hip flexion decreases hip prosthesis dislocation, the nurse knows to:
   a. keep the patient flat in bed with the leg extended.
   b. gatch the knees to decrease the effect of pulling force on the hip.
   c. raise the head of the bed between 30 and 45 degrees.
   d. maintain the patient in semi-Fowler's position.

4. The nurse teaches Tom how to minimize hip extension during transfers and while sitting. The nurse should encourage him to:
   a. rotate the hip inward slightly during sitting to prevent pressure on the external border of the hip.
   b. hyperextend the leg during transfers so the hip socket will not "pop out."
   c. maintain adduction and flexion when moving around to minimize strain at the surgical site.
   d. always pivot on the unoperated leg to protect the operated leg from unnecessary work.

5. A dislocated prosthesis is evidenced by any of the following six indicators:
   _____, _____, _____, _____, _____, and _____.

6. In assessing postoperative wound drainage, the nurse knows that Tom's drainage of how much in the first 24 hours is within normal range?
   a. 150 mL
   b. 350 mL
   c. 600 mL
   d. 1,000 mL

7. The nurse is careful to assess for evidence of DVT (3% mortality), which occurs in approximately what percentage of patients who have not had any type of preventive mechanical or pharmacologic prophylaxis?
   a. 30%
   b. 48%
   c. 60%
   d. 75%

8. The nurse advises the patient that an acute infection may occur within how many months of surgery with delayed infections occurring up to how many months?

   _____.

CHAPTER 68

Management of Patients With Musculoskeletal Disorders

I. Interpretation, Completion, and Comparison

MULTIPLE CHOICE

Read each question carefully. Circle your answer.

1. The intervertebral disks that are subject to the greatest mechanical stress and greatest degenerative changes are:
   a. C3, C4, and L2.
   b. L1, L2, and L4.
   c. L2, L3, and L5.
   d. L4, L5, and S1.

2. Back pain is classified as "chronic" when the pain lasts without improvement for longer than:
   a. 4 weeks.
   b. 3 months.
   c. 6 months.
   d. 1 year.

3. The best position to ease low back pain is:
   a. high-Fowler's to allow for maximum hip flexion.
   b. supine with the knees slightly flexed and the head of the bed elevated 30 degrees.
   c. prone with a pillow under the shoulders.
   d. supine with the bed flat and a firm mattress in place.

4. When lifting objects, patients with low back pain should be encouraged to maximize the use of the following muscles:
   a. gastrocnemius.
   b. latissimus dorsi.
   c. quadriceps.
   d. rectus abdominis.

5. The nurse should encourage a patient with low back pain to do all of the following *except*:
   a. lie prone with legs slightly elevated.
   b. strengthen abdominal muscles.
   c. avoid prolonged sitting or walking.
   d. maintain appropriate weight.

6. Carpal tunnel syndrome is a neuropathy characterized by:
   a. bursitis and tendonitis.
   b. flexion contracture of the fourth and fifth fingers.
   c. median nerve compression at the wrist.
   d. pannus formation in the shoulder.

7. The term for onychocryptosis, a common foot condition, is:
   a. callus.
   b. bunion.
   c. flatfoot.
   d. ingrown toenail.

8. An overgrowth of the horny layer of epidermis on the foot is called a:
   a. bunion.
   b. clawfoot.
   c. corn.
   d. hammer toe.

9. The average 75-year-old woman with osteoporosis has lost how much of her cortical bone?
   a. 5%
   b. 10%
   c. 25%
   d. 40%

10. The estimated intake of calcium to prevent bone loss for a postmenopausal woman is _____ mg/day. The actual intake is about _____ mg/day.
    a. 600/200
    b. 900/300
    c. 1,200/400
    d. 1,500/600

11. Bone formation is enhanced by:
    a. calcium intake.
    b. muscular activity.
    c. weight bearing.
    d. all of the above.

12. The most common symptoms of osteomalacia are:
    a. bone fractures and kyphosis.
    b. bone pain and tenderness.
    c. muscle weakness and spasms.
    d. softened and compressed vertebrae.

13. Most cases of osteomyelitis are caused by:
    a. *Proteus.*
    b. *Pseudomonas.*
    c. *Salmonella.*
    d. *Staphylococcus aureus.*

14. Signs and symptoms of osteomyelitis may include all of the following *except*:
    a. pain, erythema, and fever.
    b. leukopenia, swelling, and purulent drainage.
    c. elevated erythrocyte sedimentation rate and increased white blood cell count.
    d. positive wound cultures and localized discomfort.

15. The specific treatment for chronic osteomyelitis would probably be:
    a. antibiotic therapy.
    b. drainage of localized foci of infection.
    c. immobilization.
    d. surgical removal of the sequestrum.

16. The most common benign bone tumor is:
    a. an enchondroma.
    b. a giant cell tumor.
    c. an osteochondroma.
    d. an osteoid osteoma.

17. Appropriate nursing actions when caring for a patient with a primary malignant bone tumor would include all of the following *except*:
    a. allowing the patient to independently plan his or her daily routine.
    b. estimating the size and location of the mass daily by vigorously palpating the affected area.
    c. assuring the patient receiving chemotherapy that alopecia, if it occurs, is temporary.
    d. encouraging range-of-motion exercises to prevent atrophy of unaffected muscles.

SHORT ANSWER

Read each statement carefully. Write the best response in the space provided.

1. Identify at least five musculoskeletal problems that cause acute low back pain.

   _____, _____, _____,
   _____, and _____.

2. List four nursing diagnoses for a patient undergoing foot surgery: _____,
   _____, _____, and _____.

3. Three significant characteristics of osteoporosis are: _____, _____, and
   _____.

4. Primary osteoporosis in women usually begins between the ages of: _____.

5. Explain the effects of the following on the development of age-related osteoporosis:

   a. Calcitonin: _____

   b. Estrogen: _____

   c. Parathyroid hormone: _____

6. The primary deficit in osteomalacia is: _____.

7. Three medications used to treat Paget's disease are: _____, _____,
   and _____.

II. Critical Thinking Questions and Exercises

DISCUSSION AND ANALYSIS

Discuss the following topics with your classmates.

1. Discuss the major nursing goals for a patient with low back pain.
2. Distinguish between the two inflammatory conditions: bursitis and tendonitis.
3. Describe "impingement syndrome" and the measures necessary to promote shoulder healing.
4. Explain the pathophysiology of carpal tunnel syndrome and Dupuytren's disease.
5. Discuss the etiology and medical treatment for the nine common foot problems listed in the chapter; for example, plantar fascitis, corn, and hammer toe.
6. Demonstrate assessment for Tinel's sign.
7. Describe the risk factors (modifiable and nonmodifiable) that are associated with osteoporosis.
8. Describe the pathophysiology of Paget's disease.
9. Describe the clinical manifestations and medical and nursing interventions for septic arthritis.

APPLYING CONCEPTS

Review the pictures of common foot deformities found in Figure 68-6 in the text and complete the exercises.

1. Identify each foot ailment and list the associated clinical manifestations.
2. For each ailment, list associated nursing diagnoses.
3. From each diagnosis, draft a nursing plan of care.
4. Broadly explain the medical/surgical management for each ailment.

CLINICAL SITUATIONS

Read the following case study. Fill in the blanks or circle the correct answer.

CASE STUDY: Osteoporosis

Emily is a 49-year-old administrative assistant at a community college who has just been diagnosed with osteoporosis. The physician has asked you to answer some of Emily's questions and explain the physician's directions for her level of activity and her nutritional needs.

1. Emily asks the nurse to explain why she is losing her bone mass. The nurse's explanation is based on the

   physiologic rationale that bone mass loss occurs when _____.

2. What two reasons could the nurse use to explain why women develop osteoporosis more frequently than

   men: _____ and _____.

3. The nurse advises Emily that about _____ of Caucasian women older than 50 years of age have some
   degree of osteoporosis.
   a. 10%   c. 50%
   b. 25%   d. 80%

4. The nurse advises Emily that the development of osteoporosis is significantly dependent on:
   a. decreased estrogen, which inhibits bone   c. increased vitamin D use, which interferes with
      breakdown.   calcium use.
   b. increased calcitonin, which enhances bone   d. increased parathyroid hormone, which
      resorption.   decreases with aging.

5. Part of Emily's teaching plan includes nutritional information about dietary calcium and vitamin D. The

   nurse advises Emily that she needs _____ mg of calcium a day.
   a. 500   c. 1,200
   b. 1,000   d. 1,500

6. Emily is told that her x-ray results indicated bone radiolucency. The nurse knows that Emily has probably

   already exhibited _____ demineralization.
   a. 5%   c. 20%
   b. 10%   d. 30%

CHAPTER 69

Management of Patients With Musculoskeletal Trauma

I. Interpretation, Completion, and Comparison

MULTIPLE CHOICE

Read each question carefully. Circle your answer.

1. A muscle tear that is microscopic and due to overuse is called a:
   a. contusion.
   b. dislocation.
   c. sprain.
   d. strain.

2. The acute inflammatory stage of a strain or sprain usually lasts:
   a. less than 24 hours.
   b. between 24 and 48 hours.
   c. about 72 hours.
   d. at least 1 week.

3. After arthroscopic surgery for a rotator cuff tear, a patient can usually resume full activity in:
   a. 3 to 4 weeks.
   b. 8 weeks.
   c. 3 to 4 months.
   d. 6 to 12 months.

4. A patient who has a meniscectomy by arthroscopic surgery needs to know that normal athletic activities can usually be resumed after:
   a. 2 weeks.
   b. 3 weeks.
   c. 2 months.
   d. 6 months.

5. An open fracture with extensive soft tissue damage is classified as a what grade fracture?
   a. I
   b. II
   c. III
   d. IV

6. Emergency management of a fracture should include:
   a. covering the area with a clean dressing if the fracture is open.
   b. immobilizing the affected site.
   c. splinting the injured limb.
   d. all of the above nursing interventions.

7. The most serious complication of an open fracture is:
   a. infection.
   b. muscle atrophy caused by loss of supporting bone structure.
   c. necrosis of adjacent soft tissue caused by blood loss.
   d. nerve damage.

8. Shock, as an immediate complication of fractures, is usually classified as:
   a. cardiogenic.
   b. hypovolemic.
   c. neurogenic.
   d. septicemic.

9. As a complication of fractures, fat emboli:
   a. represent the major cause of death in fracture patients.
   b. result in symptoms of decreased mental alertness.
   c. may compromise the patient's respiratory status, necessitating ventilator support.
   d. are characterized by all of the above.

10. After a fracture, the onset of symptoms for fat embolism syndrome occurs:
    a. within 1 to 2 days.
    b. 1 to 2 weeks after the fracture is set.
    c. about 4 weeks after the bone fragments solidify.
    d. immediately after the fracture heals, when activity begins.

11. The femur fracture that commonly leads to avascular necrosis or nonunion because of an abundant supply of blood vessels in the area is a fracture of the:
    a. condylar area.
    b. neck.
    c. shaft.
    d. trochanteric region.

12. Patients who experience a fracture of the humeral neck are advised that healing will take an average of _____ weeks, with restricted vigorous activity for an additional _____ weeks.
    a. 6, 2
    b. 10, 4
    c. 10, 6
    d. 16, 2

13. After an arm fracture, pendulum exercises are begun:
    a. as soon as tolerated, after a reasonable period of immobilization.
    b. in 2 to 3 weeks, when callus ossification prevents easy movements of bony fragments.
    c. in about 4 to 5 weeks, after new bone is well established.
    d. in 2 to 3 months, after normal activities are resumed.

14. The most serious complication of a supracondylar fracture of the humerus is:
    a. hemarthrosis.
    b. paresthesia.
    c. malunion.
    d. Volkmann's ischemic contracture.

15. The two most serious complications of pelvic fractures are:
    a. paresthesia and ischemia.
    b. hemorrhage and shock.
    c. paralytic ileus and a lacerated urethra.
    d. thrombophlebitis and infection.

16. Nursing assessment for a pelvic fracture includes:
    a. checking the urine for hematuria.
    b. palpating peripheral pulses in both lower extremities.
    c. testing the stool for occult blood.
    d. all of the above.

17. An acetabular fracture of the femur involves the:
    a. neck of the femur.
    b. shaft of the femur.
    c. supracondylar area of the femur.
    d. trochanteric region of the femur.

18. The most common complication of a hip fracture in the elderly is:
    a. avascular necrosis.
    b. infection.
    c. nonunion.
    d. pneumonia.

19. An immediate nursing concern for a patient who has suffered a femoral shaft fracture is assessment for:
    a. hypovolemic shock.
    b. infection.
    c. knee and hip dislocation.
    d. pain resulting from muscle spasm.

20. The longest immobilization time necessary for fracture union occurs with a fracture of the:
    a. intratrochanteric area of the femur.
    b. midshaft of the humerus.
    c. pelvis.
    d. tibial shaft.

21. The major indicator of lower extremity amputation is:
    a. congenital deformity.
    b. malignant tumor.
    c. peripheral vascular disease.
    d. trauma.

22. A nurse can foster a positive self-image in a patient who has had an amputation by all of the following *except*:
    a. encouraging the patient to care for the residual limb.
    b. allowing the expression of grief.
    c. introducing the patient to local amputee support groups.
    d. encouraging family and friends to refrain from visiting temporarily because this may increase the patient's embarrassment.

MATCHING

Match the type of fracture in column II with its descriptive terminology listed in column I.

PART I

Column I

1. _____ A break occurs across the entire section of the bone
2. _____ A fragment of the bone is pulled off by a ligament or tendon
3. _____ Bone is splintered into several fragments
4. _____ One side of a bone is broken and the other side is bent

Column II

a. Avulsion
b. Comminuted
c. Complete
d. Epiphyseal
e. Greenstick

PART II

Column I

1. _____ A fracture occurs at an angle across the bone
2. _____ Fragments are driven inward
3. _____ The fractured bone is compressed by another bone
4. _____ The fracture extends through the skin

Column II

a. Compressed
b. Depressed
c. Oblique
d. Open
e. Pathologic

SHORT ANSWER

Read each statement carefully. Write your response in the space provided.

1. Joint dislocations can lead to avascular necrosis if it is not treated. Avascular necrosis is:

   _____.

2. Crepitus, a grating sensation felt when the hands are placed over an extremity, is caused by:

   _____.

3. Patients with open fractures risk three major complications:

   _____, _____, and _____.

4. List three early and delayed complications of fractures:

   Early: _____, _____, and _____.

   Delayed: _____, _____, and _____.

5. Treatment of early shock in fractures consists of five activities:

   _____, _____, _____, _____, and

   _____.

6. List three early and serious complications associated with bed rest and reduced skeletal muscle contractions for a patient with an open fracture:

   _____, _____, and _____.

7. The most common fracture of the distal radius is: _____.

8. The most common complication of hip fractures in the elderly is:

   _____.

9. Common pulmonary complications, after hip fracture, for the elderly include:

   _____ and _____.

10. Three range-of-motion activities are avoided for a patient with a lower extremity amputation:

    _____, _____, and _____.

11. The residual limb should never be placed on a pillow to avoid:

    _____.

II. Critical Thinking Questions and Exercises

EXAMINING ASSOCIATIONS

Read each analogy. Fill in the space provided with the best response. Explain the correlation.

1. A strain : a microscopic muscle tear :: A sprain : _____.

2. A dislocation : lack of contact between the articular surfaces of bones :: _____ : partial dislocation of associated joint structures.

3. Closed reduction : the alignment of bone fragments into opposition :: open reduction :

_____.

4. Delayed union : delayed healing due to infection or poor nutrition :: nonunion :

_____.

5. Autograft : donor-to-donor tissue :: _____ : tissue from donor or other.

6. Intracapsular fracture : neck of the femur :: extracapsular fracture : _____.

DISCUSSION AND ANALYSIS

Discuss the following topics with your classmates.

1. Compare the nursing assessment and medical management for first-, second-, and third-degree strains and sprains.
2. Describe immediate nursing and medical management for an open fracture.
3. Distinguish between open and closed reduction as a management technique for fractures.
4. Discuss in detail those factors that enhance and inhibit fracture healing.
5. Explain the clinical manifestations and underlying pathophysiology of fat embolism.
6. Explain the etiology, clinical manifestations, and medical management for compartment syndrome.
7. Describe avascular necrosis of the bone.
8. Distinguish between the clinical manifestations and medical and nursing management of intracapsular and extracapsular fractures.

EXTRACTING INFERENCES

Examine Figure 69-1 in the text and answer the following questions.

1. The foot is firmly planted and the knee is struck laterally, as in basketball or soccer. This hit can result in a torn _____. The patient will immediately experience _____, _____, _____, and the inability to walk without assistance. Bleeding into the joint, _____, may occur.

2. The foot is firmly planted and the knee is hyperextended as in football. A "pop" sound is heard. This indicates a possible tear to the _____. Surgical reconstruction can be scheduled after _____. Rehabilitation takes _____ to _____ months.

3. Patients who report that their knees "give way" or "lock" after twisting or repetitive squatting are most likely experiencing a _____. Diagnosis is confirmed by _____. The most common postoperative complication is _____. Normal activities can be resumed in _____ (weeks/months).

CLINICAL SITUATIONS

Read the following case study. Circle the correct answer.

CASE STUDY: Above-the-Knee Amputation

William, a 70-year-old Catholic priest, lives in a center city rectory. He is scheduled to have an above-the-knee amputation of his left leg because of peripheral vascular disease.

1. Preoperatively, the nurse knows that the circulatory status of the affected limb should be evaluated by assessing for:
   a. color and temperature.
   b. palpable pulses.
   c. positioning responses.
   d. all of the above.

2. The level of William's amputation was determined after assessing:
   a. the circulatory status of the affected limb.
   b. the type of prosthesis to be used.
   c. William's ability to understand and use the prosthetic device.
   d. all of the above.

3. Preoperatively, the nurse needs to assist William in exercising the muscles needed for crutch walking. The major muscle to be strengthened is the:
   a. pectoralis major.
   b. gastrocnemius.
   c. quadriceps femoris.
   d. triceps brachii.

4. Postoperatively, William experiences phantom limb sensations. The most appropriate nursing response is to:
   a. agree with his statements, recognizing that he is expressing a psychological need.
   b. consistently stress the absence of the lower leg.
   c. disagree with him and reorient him to reality.
   d. keep him as active as possible and encourage self-expression.

5. William's amputation is treated with a soft compression dressing. Nursing care would include all of the following *except*:
   a. keeping the residual limb slightly elevated on a pillow to decrease edema.
   b. monitoring vital signs to detect any indication of bleeding.
   c. placing the residual limb in an extended position, with brief periods of elevation.
   d. keeping a tourniquet nearby in case of hemorrhage.

6. Preprosthetic nursing care should attempt to avoid any problem that can delay prosthetic fitting, such as:
   a. abduction deformities of the hip.
   b. flexion deformities.
   c. nonshrinkage of the residual limb.
   d. all of the above.

7. The nurse who is preparing to apply a bandage to William's residual limb knows that she should:
   a. anchor the bandage on the posterior surface of the residual limb.
   b. begin the vertical turns on the anterior surface of the residual limb.
   c. maintain the residual limb in a position of flexion while bandaging.
   d. use circular turns that run in a horizontal plane from the proximal to the distal segment.

8. The nurse teaches William to massage his residual limb to:
   a. decrease local tenderness.
   b. improve vascularity.
   c. mobilize the scar.
   d. accomplish all of the above.

CHAPTER 70

Management of Patients With Infectious Diseases

I. Interpretation, Completion, and Comparison

MULTIPLE CHOICE

Read each question carefully. Circle your answer.

1. The single, most important means of preventing the spread of infection is:
   a. antibiotic therapy.
   b. gowning and gloving.
   c. hand washing.
   d. isolation measures.

2. The bacterium with significant health care-associated infection (HAI) potential that is gram-positive, spore-forming, and highly resistant to antimicrobial therapy is:
   a. *Clostridium difficile.*
   b. methicillin-resistant *Staphylococcus aureus* (MRSA).
   c. *Staphylococcus aureus.*
   d. vancomycin-resistant enterococcus (VRE).

3. MRSA is a common HAI. The most frequently occurring pathogen identified with this disorder is:
   a. *Escherichia coli.*
   b. *Proteus.*
   c. *Pseudomonas aeruginosa.*
   d. *Staphylococcus aureus.*

4. A gram-positive organism that is less virulent than a gram-negative organism is:
   a. *Escherichia coli.*
   b. *Pseudomonas aeruginosa.*
   c. *Proteus.*
   d. *Staphylococcus aureus.*

5. It is recommended that the measles, mumps, and rubella (MMR) vaccine should be initially given to children at age:
   a. 2 months.
   b. 6 months.
   c. 12 to 15 months.
   d. 18 to 24 months.

6. Chickenpox and Herpes Zoster (also known as Shingles) are both caused by the same viral agent:
   a. *Clostridium difficile.*
   b. *Shigella.*
   c. *Plasmodium vivax.*
   d. *Varicella zoster.*

7. The most frequent bacterial cause of diarrhea worldwide is:
   a. *Campylobacter.*
   b. *Escherichia coli.*
   c. *Shigella.*
   d. *Yersinia.*

8. A gram-negative bacillus, linked to contaminated eggs or chicken, that causes diarrhea is:
   a. *Calicivirus.*
   b. *Campylobacter.*
   c. *Salmonella.*
   d. *Shigella.*

9. A common bacterial cause of diarrhea that has been linked to the ingestion of undercooked beef is:
   a. *Escherichia coli.*
   b. *Campylobacter.*
   c. *Salmonella.*
   d. *Shigella.*

10. The most common viral cause of diarrhea in children is:
   a. *Campylobacter.*
   b. *Shigella.*
   c. rotavirus.
   d. *Salmonella.*

11. The rehydration goal for a 70-kg patient who has moderate dehydration would be how many milliliters of oral rehydration solution (ORS) over 4 hours?
   a. 3,000 mL
   b. 5,000 mL
   c. 7,000 mL
   d. 9,000 mL

12. The transmission route for human immunodeficiency virus (HIV) is through:
   a. contaminated blood.
   b. semen and vaginal secretions.
   c. maternal–fetal blood.
   d. all of the above.

13. A chancre initially appears 2 to 3 weeks after inoculation with the spirochete, *Treponema pallidum*, in the sexually transmitted disease known as:
   a. chlamydia.
   b. gonorrhea.
   c. HIV/AIDS.
   d. syphilis.

14. Latent syphilitic lesions may still be treated with penicillin G benzathine for up to:
   a. 2 to 3 months.
   b. 3 to 6 months.
   c. 6 to 9 months.
   d. 1 year.

15. Gonorrhea is a sexually transmitted infection that involves the mucosal surface of the:
   a. genitourinary tract.
   b. pharynx.
   c. rectum.
   d. all of the above.

16. The primary site for gonorrhea in women is the:
   a. urethra.
   b. kidney.
   c. vagina.
   d. uterine cervix.

17. Choose the *incorrect* statement about West Nile virus infection.
   a. It was first seen in the United States in 1999.
   b. It is caused by an infected mosquito.
   c. It is treated successfully by intravenous antibiotics if diagnosed within 72 hours after symptoms onset.
   d. Its symptoms are similar to those of meningitis.

18. A person diagnosed with Legionnaire's disease would have a primary infection in his or her:
   a. bloodstream.
   b. central nervous system.
   c. gastrointestinal tract.
   d. lungs.

19. The antibiotic of choice for Legionnaire's disease is:
   a. Biaxin.
   b. Ilotycin.
   c. Levaquin.
   d. Zithromax.

SHORT ANSWER

Read each statement carefully. Write your response in the space provided.

1. Define the term *colonization*: _____.

2. Define the term *infection*: _____.

3. List the three components of a microbiology report, the primary source of information about most bacterial infection: _____, _____, and

   _____.

4. The two primary agencies involved in setting guidelines about infection prevention are: the

   _____ and the _____.

5. Two bacteria that are part of normal skin flora are: _____ and _____, whereas _____ and _____, considered transient flora, have increased pathogenic potential.

6. List the three primary organisms responsible for HAI potential: _____,

   _____, and _____.

7. Immunosuppressed adults should be vaccinated for: _____ and _____.

8. List at least six infectious diseases that have been controlled by successful vaccine programs:

   _____, _____, _____,

   _____, _____, and _____.

9. The two types of antiviral therapy available to treat a pandemic are: _____ and _____.

10. Identify 5 of 10 conditions classified as sexually transmitted diseases: _____,

    _____, _____, _____, and _____.

11. The most common infectious diseases in the United States are: _____, infecting approximately _____ million Americans annually. Of these, the two most commonly reported are: _____ and _____.

12. According to the Centers for Disease Control and Prevention (CDC), there are five emerging infectious diseases that have increased in the past two decades and are expected to increase in the near future. They are: _____, _____, _____, _____, and _____.

13. Pertussis (whooping cough) has recently reemerged as a childhood disease. The most common complication of infection is _____, which is usually treated with one of three antibiotics: _____, _____, and _____.

14. The most well-known viral hemorrhagic fever viruses are: _____ and

    _____.

MATCHING

Match the disease or condition listed in column II with its associated causative organism listed in column I.

Column I

1. _____ Varicella zoster
2. _____ *Neisseria gonorrhoeae*
3. _____ Hepatitis B virus
4. _____ *Staphylococcus aureus*
5. _____ Epstein-Barr virus
6. _____ Salmonella species
7. _____ *Streptococcus pneumoniae*
8. _____ *Microsporum* species

Column II

a. Chickenpox
b. Bloodborne hepatitis
c. Diarrheal disease
d. Gonorrhea
e. Impetigo
f. Mononucleosis
g. Pneumococcal pneumonia
h. Ringworm

II. Critical Thinking Questions and Exercises

EXAMINING ASSOCIATIONS

Examine the figure below. For each of the six links in the infection cycle, describe specific nursing interventions that can be used to break transmission. The first entry is filled in as an example.

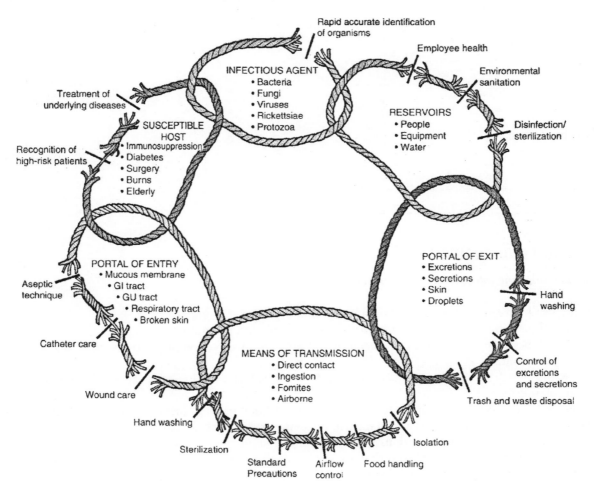

1. Infectious agent

    a. Educate patient about immunization (example)

    b. _____

    c. _____

2. Reservoirs

    a. _____

    b. _____

    c. _____

3. Portal of exit

    a. _____

    b. _____

    c. _____

4. Means of transmission

    a. _____

    b. _____

    c. _____

5. Portal of entry

    a. _____

    b. _____

    c. _____

6. Susceptible host

    a. _____

    b. _____

    c. _____

DISCUSSION AND ANALYSIS

Discuss the following topics with your classmates.

1. Distinguish between the terms *infection* and *infectious disease*.
2. Distinguish between *standard* and *transmission-based* isolation precautions.
3. Distinguish between the activities associated with four types of infection precautions: standard, airborne, droplet, and contact.
4. Review the CDC's standard recommended vaccination schedule and discuss the ages for initial and catch-up vaccinations.
5. Discuss general ways a nurse can help the community respond to an influenza pandemic. Describe local responses put into place in your community in response to the swine flu pandemic in 2009.
6. Describe specific nursing interventions for a patient with an infectious disease.
7. Discuss eight potential complications that a nurse needs to be aware of when treating and educating a patient with a sexually transmitted disease.

CHAPTER 71

Emergency Nursing

I. Interpretation, Completion, and Comparison

MULTIPLE CHOICE

Read each question carefully. Circle your answer.

1. In the United States, the elderly, who are major consumers of emergency health care, account for about how many million visits to the emergency department annually?
   a. 20 million
   b. 50 million
   c. 100 million
   d. 150 million

2. John, a 16-year-old boy, is brought to the emergency department after a vehicular accident. He is pronounced dead on arrival (DOA). When his parents arrive at the hospital, the nurse should:
   a. ask them to sit in the waiting room until she can spend time alone with them.
   b. speak to both parents together and encourage them to support each other and express their emotions freely.
   c. speak to one parent at a time in a private setting so that each can ventilate feelings of loss without upsetting the other.
   d. ask the emergency physician to medicate the parents so that they can handle their son's unexpected death quietly and without hysteria.

3. A triage nurse in the emergency department determines that a patient with dyspnea and dehydration is not in a life-threatening situation. The triage category that the nurse would choose is:
   a. delayed.
   b. emergent.
   c. immediate.
   d. urgent.

4. A nurse at the scene of an industrial explosion uses "field triage" to categorize victims for treatment. A patient in need of emergent care would be tagged using the color:
   a. blue.
   b. green.
   c. red.
   d. yellow.

5. The first priority in treating any patient in the emergency department is:
   a. controlling hemorrhage.
   b. establishing an airway.
   c. obtaining consent for treatment.
   d. restoring cardiac output.

6. An oropharyngeal airway should be inserted:
   a. at an angle of 90 degrees.
   b. upside down and then rotated 180 degrees.
   c. with the concave portion touching the posterior pharynx.
   d. with the convex portion facing upward.

7. Clinical indicators for emergency endotracheal intubation include:
   a. airway obstruction.
   b. respiratory arrest.
   c. respiratory insufficiency.
   d. all of the above.

8. The initial nursing measure for the control of hemorrhage caused by trauma is to:
   a. apply a tourniquet.
   b. apply firm pressure over the involved area or artery.
   c. elevate the injured part.
   d. immobilize the area to control blood loss.

9. The most common cause of shock in emergency situations is:
   a. cardiac failure.
   b. decreased arterial resistance.
   c. hypovolemia.
   d. septicemia.

10. Indicators of hypovolemic shock associated with internal bleeding include all of the following *except*:
    a. bradycardia.
    b. cool, moist skin.
    c. hypotension.
    d. thirst.

11. The leading cause of death in children and adults younger than 44 years of age is:
    a. cancer.
    b. drowning.
    c. pneumonia.
    d. trauma.

12. Nursing measures for a penetrating abdominal injury (gunshot and stab wound) would include:
    a. assessing for manifestations of hemorrhage.
    b. covering any protruding viscera with sterile dressings soaked in normal saline solution.
    c. looking for any associated chest injuries.
    d. all of the above actions.

13. A patient has experienced blunt abdominal trauma from a motor vehicle crash. The nurse assesses the patient with the knowledge that the most frequently injured solid abdominal organ is the:
    a. duodenum.
    b. large bowel.
    c. liver.
    d. pancreas.

14. Nursing management for a crushing lower extremity wound includes:
    a. applying a clean dressing to protect the wound.
    b. elevating the site to limit the accumulation of fluid in the interstitial spaces.
    c. splinting the wound in a position of rest to prevent motion.
    d. all of the above measures.

15. Identify the sequence of medical or nursing management for a patient who experiences multiple injuries.
    a. Assess for head injuries, control hemorrhage, establish an airway, prevent hypovolemic shock
    b. Control hemorrhage, prevent hypovolemic shock, establish an airway, assess for head injuries
    c. Establish an airway, control hemorrhage, prevent hypovolemic shock, assess for head injuries
    d. Prevent hypovolemic shock, assess for head injuries, establish an airway, control hemorrhage

16. Nursing measures for an extremity fracture would include:
    a. assessing for manifestations of shock.
    b. immobilizing the fracture site.
    c. palpating peripheral pulses.
    d. all of the above actions.

17. Progressive deterioration of body systems occurs when hypothermia lowers the body temperature to:
    a. 98°F.
    b. 97°F.
    c. 96°F.
    d. 95°F.

18. Approximately how many million women experience domestic violence every year?
    a. 2 million
    b. 3 million
    c. 4 million
    d. 5 million

19. Rose, a 19-year-old student, has been sexually assaulted. When assisting with the physical examination, the nurse should do all of the following *except*:
    a. have the patient shower or wash the perineal area before the examination.
    b. assess and document any bruises and lacerations.
    c. record a history of the event, using the patient's own words.
    d. label all torn or bloody clothes and place each item in a separate brown bag so that any evidence can be given to the police.

SHORT ANSWER

Read each question carefully. Write your response in the space provided.

1. Emergency department visits have increased by _____% since 1995, with injuries accounting for ___% of visits. For those over age 65, _____% of emergency department visits account for hospital admissions.

2. Emergency department personnel are at increased risk for exposure to communicable disease through blood or body fluids because of the number of people infected with _____, _____, and _____.

3. A patient with a foreign body airway obstruction typically demonstrates the inability to: _____, _____, or _____. With complete obstruction, permanent brain injury will occur in _____ minutes.

4. List six clinical signs/symptoms of probable internal hemorrhage: _____, _____, _____, _____, _____, and _____.

5. Heat stroke is a medical emergency evidenced by symptoms such as: _____, _____, _____, and _____. The body temperature may reach _____°F.

6. The second most common cause of unintentional death in children younger than 14 years of age is: _____.

7. The most common victims of snakebites are those between the ages of: _____ and _____ years of age.

8. Antivenin to treat snakebites must be administered within a time frame of: _____ to _____ hours.

9. An easy and immediate treatment for an ingested poison that is not caustic is _____, which immediately induces vomiting.

II. Critical Thinking Questions and Exercises

DISCUSSION AND ANALYSIS

Discuss the following topics with your classmates.

1. Using three examples provided by your classmates, describe some activities an emergency department nurse would employ to provide patient- and family-focused holistic care.
2. Describe the criteria distinguishing the five levels of a comprehensive triage system: resuscitation, emergent, urgent, nonurgent, and minor. Explain what "fast track" means.
3. Demonstrate the nursing management role in establishing an airway using the abdominal thrust, the head-tilt-chin-lift maneuver, the jaw-thrust maneuver, and oropharyngeal airway insertion.
4. Describe the immediate nursing intervention for a patient hemorrhaging externally from an extremity injury.
5. Explain why lactated Ringer's solution is initially useful as fluid replacement for a patient experiencing hypovolemic shock.
6. Describe the nursing assessment and management for a patient experiencing a crush injury.
7. Describe the immediate nursing and medical interventions for a patient with heat stroke.
8. Describe the nursing assessment activities for evaluating the signs and symptoms of anaphylaxis.
9. Explain the immediate nursing and medical management for someone who has swallowed a corrosive poison.
10. Explain the immediate intervention for a victim of carbon monoxide poisoning.
11. Describe the immediate nursing and medical management for a patient experiencing delirium tremors.
12. Describe the nurse's role in assessment, physical examination, and specimen collection for a victim of sexual assault.
13. Describe the clinical symptoms of posttraumatic stress disorder.

APPLYING CONCEPTS

For each of the following situations, identify a nursing action with supporting rationale for managing a foreign body obstruction.

Condition	Action	Rationale
Heimlich maneuver for standing or sitting conscious patient	1. _____	_____
	2. _____	_____
Heimlich maneuver with patient lying unconscious	1. _____	_____
	2. _____	_____
	3. _____	_____
	4. _____	_____
Finger sweep	1. _____	_____
	2. _____	_____
	3. _____	_____
Chest thrusts with conscious patient standing or sitting	1. _____	_____
	2. _____	_____
	3. _____	_____

CLINICAL SITUATIONS

For each of the following situations, supply nursing diagnoses, nursing interventions, and supporting rationales for intervention.

1. Consider a patient who has experienced blunt, abdominal trauma. Formulate nursing diagnoses and nursing interventions for the patient in the emergency department. Cite a rationale for each nursing action. List interventions in order of priority.
2. List the emergency nursing measures you would carry out if you were present when someone experienced an anaphylactic reaction to a bee sting. Formulate nursing diagnoses, list nursing interventions, and cite supporting rationales for your actions.
3. Ann is admitted to the emergency department because she ingested approximately 30 diet capsules 1 hour before admission. The nurse is to assist with gastric lavage. State nursing diagnoses with nursing interventions and supporting rationale for each action.

Read each question and write the answers in the spaces provided.

4. List specific nursing interventions that can be used for drug abuse with each of the following drugs. It is assumed that the patient is presenting to the emergency department for treatment.

Drug	Nursing Interventions
a. Cocaine	_____
b. Dexedrine	_____
c. Valium	_____
d. Aspirin	_____

5. Compare nursing actions for psychiatric emergencies in dealing with the following patients.

Psychiatric Patients	Nursing Actions
a. An overactive patient	_____
b. A violent patient	_____
c. A depressed patient	_____
d. A suicidal patient	_____

CHAPTER 72

Terrorism, Mass Casualty, and Disaster Nursing

I. Interpretation, Completion, and Comparison

MULTIPLE CHOICE

Read each question carefully. Circle the correct answer.

1. Disasters are assigned level designations based on the anticipated level of response needed. A disaster that requires statewide and federal assistance would be classified as:
   a. Level I.
   b. Level II.
   c. Level III.
   d. Level IV.

2. The National Medical Response Team for Weapons of Mass Destruction is a subbranch of the:
   a. Department of Health and Human Services.
   b. Department of Justice.
   c. Federal Emergency Management Agency.
   d. National Disaster Medical System.

3. The Department of Homeland Security issues a code "blue" relative to a situation. The nurse knows that this indicates a:
   a. perceived low risk.
   b. guarded risk.
   c. possible risk but ill-defined.
   d. high risk with no specific site.

4. The NATO triage system uses color-coded tagging to identify severity of injuries. A patient with survivable but life-threatening injuries (i.e., incomplete amputation) would be color-tagged with:
   a. black.
   b. green.
   c. red.
   d. yellow.

5. A triaged patient with psychological disturbances would be color-tagged with:
   a. black.
   b. green.
   c. red.
   d. yellow.

6. A triaged patient, with a significant injury that can wait several hours for treatment, would be assigned:
   a. priority 1.
   b. priority 2.
   c. priority 3.
   d. priority 4.

7. Those patients in a disaster who are unlikely to survive are triaged as:
   a. priority 1.
   b. priority 2.
   c. priority 3.
   d. priority 4.

8. The Environmental Protection Agency has identified four categories of personal protection equipment for health care workers in response to biological, chemical, or radiation exposure. The highest level of respiratory protection that includes a self-contained breathing apparatus and a chemical resistant suit is:
   a. level A.
   b. level B.
   c. level C.
   d. level D.

9. In natural disasters, what percentage of trapped victims survive up to 6 hours?
   a. 80%
   b. 60%
   c. Less than 50%
   d. Greater than 80%

10. The most severe form of anthrax exposure is through:
    a. skin contact.
    b. inhalation.
    c. ingestion.
    d. open wounds or sores.

11. An example of a chemical agent that acts by inhibiting acetylcholinesterase is a:
    a. nerve agent.
    b. blood agent.
    c. corrosive acid.
    d. vesicant.

12. The type of chemical agents that *do not* act within seconds (latency period) are:
    a. cyanide-based.
    b. sulfur mustards.
    c. nerve agents.
    d. vesicants.

13. An example of the most toxic chemical agent in existence is:
    a. chlorine.
    b. cyanide.
    c. mustard nitrogen.
    d. sarin.

14. A common chemical agent that causes harm by separating the alveoli from the capillary bed is:
    a. chlorine.
    b. cyanide.
    c. phosgene.
    d. sarin.

SHORT ANSWER

Complete each statement by filling in the blank space.

1. An example of a biological weapon of mass destruction is: _____; an example of a chemical weapon of mass destruction is: _____.

2. Four federal agencies that provide disaster assistance are: _____, _____, _____, and _____.

3. Only three states and the District of Columbia have locations for Disaster Medical Assistance Teams. These states are:

   _____, _____, and _____.

4. Describe the Incident Command System.

   _____

   _____

5. Identify five factors that influence an individual's response to disaster: _____,

   _____, _____, _____, and _____.

6. Distinguish between the terms *defusing* and *debriefing* as they relate to the Critical Incident Stress Management process.

   _____

   _____

7. Two biological agents most likely to be used during a terrorist attack are: _____ and

   _____.

8. Exposure to anthrax, without clinical signs and symptoms of the disease, requires a 60-day treatment

   with one of two antibiotics: _____ or _____. The mortality

   rate associated with respiratory distress is: _____%.

9. Smallpox has a case fatality rate of _____%.

10. Explain how pulmonary chemical agents (i.e., phosgene) act.

    _____

    _____

II. Critical Thinking Questions and Exercises

DISCUSSION AND ANALYSIS

Discuss the following topics with your classmates.

1. Compare and contrast the emergency responses for the three disaster levels.
2. Discuss the 13 components of an emergency operations plan and give examples relative to your local community.
3. Explain why patients who are most critically ill, with a high mortality rate, would be assigned a low triage priority in a disaster situation.
4. Discuss some of the cultural variables that health care providers need to consider in any disaster situation where a large number of diverse religious and ethnic groups of patients need to be treated.
5. Describe common behavioral responses seen in victims of mass disaster.
6. Describe the four effects that a blast wave has on a victim.
7. Outline the clinical manifestations and medical treatment for anthrax exposure.
8. Describe the clinical manifestations and medical treatment for smallpox.
9. Describe the clinical manifestations of nerve gas exposure.
10. Distinguish between the three types of radiation-induced injury.
11. Describe the phases of acute radiation syndrome.

Answer Key

Chapter 1

I. Interpretation, Completion, and Comparison

MULTIPLE CHOICE

1. d
2. a
3. d
4. b
5. c
6. d
7. c
8. d
9. d
10. c

SHORT ANSWER

1. Refer to chapter heading "Nursing Defined" under "The Health Care Industry and the Nursing Profession" in the text for phenomena.
2. Six significant changes are an increase in the aging population, increased cultural diversity, the changing patterns of diseases, increased technology, increased consumer expectations, and the higher costs for health care.
3. Four major health care concerns are emerging infectious diseases, trauma, obesity, and bioterrorism.
4. Human responses requiring nursing intervention should include self-image changes, impaired ventilation, and anxiety and fear. Answer may also include pain and discomfort, grief, and impaired functioning in areas such as rest and sleep.
5. Four major concepts are the capacity to perform to the best of one's ability, the flexibility of adjusting and adapting to various situations, a reported feeling of well-being and a feeling of "harmony," that everything is together.
6. In Maslow's hierarchy of needs, needs are ranked as follows. Refer to Figure 1-1 in the text.

Need	Example
Physiologic	Food and water
Safety and security	Financial security
Belongingness and affection	Companionship
Esteem and self-respect	Recognition by society
Self-actualization	Achieved potential in an area
Self-fulfillment	Creativity (painting)
Knowledge and understanding	Information and explanation
Aesthetics	Attractive environment

7. Answer should include six of these seven: stress, improper diet, lack of exercise, smoking, illicit drugs, high-risk behaviors (including risky sexual practices), and poor hygiene.
8. Tuberculosis, acquired immunodeficiency syndrome (AIDS), and sexually transmitted diseases
9. hypertension, heart disease, diabetes, and cancer
10. Evidence-based practice includes using current literature and research, outcomes assessment, and standardized plans of care (clinical guidelines and pathways, algorithms) to improve patient care.
11. Clinical pathways are tools for tracking a patient's progress toward positive outcomes within a specific period of time. Pathways include tests, treatments, activities, medications, consultations, and education within a set time period to achieve desired outcomes.
12. care mapping, multidisciplinary action plans (MAPs), clinical guidelines, and algorithms
13. Care mapping is more beneficial than a clinical pathway when a patient's complex condition defines prediction and a specific timeframe for achieving outcomes is excluded.
14. Managed care is characterized by prenegotiated payment rates, mandatory precertification, utilization review, limited choice of provider, and fixed-price reimbursement.
15. Case management is a system where one person or team coordinates the care for the patient and family. The goals include quality care, appropriate and timely care delivery, and cost reduction.
16. Four categories of advanced practice nurses are nurse practitioner, clinical nurse specialist, certified nurse-midwife, and certified registered anesthetist

II. Critical Thinking Questions and Exercises

DISCUSSION AND ANALYSIS

1. Refer to Appendix B in the text.
2. Community-based nursing and home health care is directed toward specific patient groups. Community-oriented or public health nursing focuses on groups of citizens or the community at large. Its emphasis is primary, secondary, and tertiary prevention.
3. The advanced practice nurse is able to perform functions that were previously restricted to the practice of medicine. Such functions include the performance of selected invasive procedures and the prescription of medications and treatments. Scope of practice is stipulated by individual state nurse practice acts.

SUPPORTING ARGUMENTS

1. Share your data and discuss your response with your instructor and classmates. There are no specific right or wrong answers. The validity of your response is determined by your ability to consciously support your argument. Refer to chapter heading "Health Care in Transition" in the text.

RECOGNIZING CONTRADICTIONS

1. The <u>majority</u> of health problems today are <u>chronic</u> in nature.
2. A person with chronic illness <u>can attain a high level of wellness</u> if he or she is successful in meeting his or her health potential within the limits of the chronic illness.
3. By 2030, it is predicted that the elderly in the United States will constitute <u>20%</u> of the total population; racial and ethnic minorities could constitute <u>50%</u> of the population.
4. Those with <u>chronic illnesses</u> are the largest group of health care consumers.
5. The second <u>largest</u> group of health care consumers in the United States is children.

6. Home health care nursing is a major component of <u>community-based nursing</u>.

EXAMINING ASSOCIATIONS

1. The answer should describe the severity of the patient's physical symptoms and his or her ability to address higher level needs. For example, the patient is unable, either physically, mentally, or emotionally, to address the need for safety and security.
2. The collaborative model of clinical decision making is usually found in a decentralized organizational structure in which shared participation, responsibility, and accountability are promoted. Physicians, nurses, and other health care workers participate collaboratively in decision making.
3. The primary nurse is in charge of a patient's complete nursing care. With patient-focused care, a nurse is assigned a caseload of patients during a work shift.

CLINICAL SITUATIONS

1. *FLOW CHART: RADIAL PULSE ASSESSMENT*

Refer to your knowledge of fundamental skills.

2. Radial Pulse Assessment

1.0	*2.0*	*3.0*	*4.0*	*5.0*
Patient ID	Explain Procedure	Identify Site	Palpate Pulse	Document Results
1.1 ID Patient 1.2 Ask patient's name 1.3 Check patient's name on bed	2.1 Give instruction at level of patient's learning.	3.1 Extend patient's forearm 3.2 Locate pulse on inner thumb-side of wrist	4.1 Place pads of index and middle fingers over radial artery. 4.2 Palpate for rate, rhythm, amplitude, and symmetry. 4.3 Count rate for 60 seconds if irregular, 30 seconds × 2, if regular. 4.4 Reassess for any abnormalities	5.1 Note rate and character of pulse 5.2 Record on graphic sheet on patient's chart 5.3 Report appropriate information

2. *FLOW CHART: CQI CAUSE AND EFFECT DIAGRAM: DELAYED MEDICATION*

CQI Cause and Effect Diagram: Delayed Medication
Possible Causes

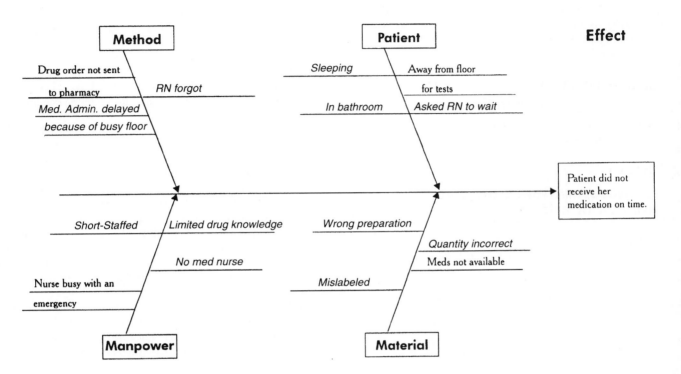

Chapter 2

I. Interpretation, Completion, and Comparison

MULTIPLE CHOICE

1. d   4. d
2. d   5. c
3. c   6. c

SHORT ANSWER

1. hypertension, diabetes, and obesity
2. federal legislation, tighter insurance regulations, decreasing hospital revenues, and alternate health care delivery systems
3. Nurses will need to be expert, independent decision makers who are self-directed, flexible, adaptable, and competent in critical thinking, physical assessment, health education, and basic nursing care.
4. Community-based nursing practice focuses on promoting and maintaining the health of individuals and families, preventing and minimizing the progression of disease, and improving the quality of life.
5. self-care, preventive care, continuity of care, and collaboration

6. Skilled nursing services may include intravenous therapy, injections, parenteral nutrition, venipuncture, catheter insertion, pressure ulcer and wound care, and ostomy care.
7. call the patient to obtain permission for a visit, schedule the visit, and verify the address
8. During the initial home visit, the patient is evaluated and a plan of care is established.
9. Nursing responsibilities include direct patient care, assessment and screening, treatment (acute, chronic, or emergency conditions), referral to other agencies, and health education.
10. trauma, tuberculosis, upper respiratory tract infections, poor nutrition and anemia, lice, scabies, peripheral vascular disease, hypothermia, arthritis, skin disorders, dental and foot problems, sexually transmitted diseases, and mental illness.

II. Critical Thinking Questions and Exercises

DISCUSSION AND ANALYSIS

1. *Primary* prevention focuses on health promotion and disease prevention (e.g., diabetic counseling). *Secondary* prevention focuses on health maintenance,

early detection, and prompt intervention (e.g., health care screening). *Tertiary* prevention focuses on minimizing deterioration and improving the quality of life (e.g., health care screening, rehabilitation).

2. Because hospitals are reimbursed a fixed rate per diagnosis-related group (DRG), patients are being discharged prior to full recovery. This issue is compounded by the growth in the aging population.

3. Refer to book, *Community and Public Health Nursing,* by M. Stanhope and J. Lancaster, 2008, St. Louis, Mosby.

CLINICAL SITUATIONS

CASE STUDY: ASSESSING THE NEED FOR A HOME VISIT

Refer to chapter heading "Home Health Visits" and Chart 2-2 in the text to complete the case study.

Chapter 3

I. Interpretation, Completion, and Comparison

MULTIPLE CHOICE

1. b	7. d	13. c
2. c	8. d	14. a
3. b	9. c	15. a
4. d	10. b	16. d
5. a	11. d	17. b
6. a	12. d	

SHORT ANSWER

1. A strong formal and informal foundation of knowledge, a willingness to pursue or ask questions, and an ability to develop solutions that are new, even if different from the current set of standards.

2. Answer may include active thinker, fair, independent and open-minded, persistent, empathic, honest, organized and systematic, proactive, flexible, realistic, humble, logical, curious, and insightful. Critical thinkers are good communicators and are committed to excellence.

3. Analysis, evaluation, explanation, inference, interpretation, and self-regulation.

4. Critical thinking is influenced by the culture, attitude, and experiences of the individual, who sees the situation through the lens of his or her experiences.

5. A *moral dilemma* is a conflict between two or more moral principles (choose between the lesser of two evils). A *moral problem* occurs when moral claims/principles are competing but one claim/principle is dominant. *Moral uncertainty* occurs when there is confusion about a principle and there is a strong feeling that something is not right. *Moral distress* results when constraints stand in the way of pursuing the correct action.

6. Nursing practice encompasses the protection, promotion, and optimization of health and abilities, prevention of illness and injury, alleviation of suffering through the diagnosis and treatment of human response, and advocacy in the care of individuals, families, communities, and populations.

7. confidentiality, use of restraints, trust, refusing care, and end-of-life concerns

8. Two types of "advanced directives" are a living will and a durable power of attorney.

9. A "durable power of attorney" exists when a person identifies another person to make health care decisions on his or her behalf.

10. Suggested statements include "Please tell me what brought you to the hospital," "Please tell me what you think your needs are," and "Please tell me about your past history."

11. A *nursing diagnosis* identifies actual or potential health problems that guide nurses in the development of a plan of care and is amenable to resolution by nursing actions. *Collaborative problems* are potential problems or complications that are medical in origin and require collaborative interventions with the physician and the health care team. The nursing diagnosis and collaborative problems are the patient's nursing problems. A medical diagnosis identifies diseases, conditions, or pathology that can be medically managed. Refer to Figure 3-2 in the text.

12. Expected outcomes of nursing intervention should be stated in behavioral terms and should be realistic as well as measurable. Expected behavioral outcomes serve as the basis for evaluating the effectiveness of nursing intervention.

NURSING OR COLLABORATIVE PROBLEMS

Refer to Figures 3-1 and 3-2 and Charts 3-6 and 3-7 in the text.

1. N	6. N
2. N	7. C
3. C	8. C
4. C	9. N
5. N	10. C

MATCHING (CRITICAL THINKING)

Refer to Chart 3-1 in the text.

1. e	5. a
2. g	6. c
3. f	7. b
4. d	

MATCHING (ETHICAL PRINCIPLES)

Refer to Chart 3-2 in the text.

1. d	4. f
2. e	5. a
3. b	6. c

II. Critical Thinking Questions and Exercises

DISCUSSION AND ANALYSIS
Refer to chapter heading "Planning" under "Using the Nursing Process" for questions 1 to 3 and Chart 3-9 in the text.

RECOGNIZING CONTRADICTIONS
1. Nursing ethics is a <u>distinct form of applied ethics</u> because <u>nursing is its own separate profession</u>.
2. <u>Moral distress exists</u> when a nurse is prevented from doing what he or she believes is correct.
3. A request for withdrawal of food and hydration necessitates an evaluation of harm and <u>may not be routinely supported</u> even for competent patients.
4. <u>Living wills are not always honored</u> because they refer to terminal illnesses and patients frequently change their perspective as they become sicker.

SUPPORTING ARGUMENTS
Answers are individualized; there are no right or wrong responses. Refer to chapter heading "Ethical Nursing Care" in the text for questions 1 to 3.

CLINICAL SITUATIONS
Outcomes per Nursing Diagnosis (Refer to NOC, Chart 3-6 in the text).
1. Patient will be able to walk from his room to the nursing station every morning with respiratory rate within normal limits.
2. Patient will move from bed to chair on second postoperative day with legs abducted.
3. Patient will achieve a balance between fluid intake and output with a weight gain no greater than 1 lb/week.
4. Patient will eat 1800 cal/day to maintain a desired weight of 135 lb.
5. Patient will sleep 6 to 8 hours, without interruption, every evening.

CASE STUDY: ETHICAL ANALYSIS
Assessment
Your answer should include the conflict between the nurse's professional obligation to provide treatment to all and the unpleasant outcome of choosing "the lesser of two evils."

Planning
You should be able to analyze the medical and political data that influence the treatment options. Because of the vast numbers of infected citizens relative to available treatment, not everyone can be cared for.

Implementation
You need to carefully analyze the outcomes of both theories for your decision making. There is no right or

wrong answer. You just need to support your decision with an ethical theory.

Evaluation
Your evaluation needs to show logical sequencing of problem solving based on an ethical theory. There is no right or wrong response.

Chapter 4

I. Interpretation, Completion, and Comparison

MULTIPLE CHOICE
1. d	5. a	9. b
2. d	6. a	10. a
3. d	7. a	11. a
4. b	8. a	12. c

SHORT ANSWER
1. Significant factors are the availability of health care outside the hospital setting, the employment of diverse health care providers to accomplish care management goals, and the increased use of alternative strategies other than the traditional approaches to care.
2. People with a chronic illness need as much health care information as possible to actively participate in and assume responsibility for the management of their own care. Health education can help the patient adapt to illness and cooperate with a treatment regimen. The goal of health education is to teach people to maximize their health potential.
3. Answer may include five of the following: medication compliance, maintaining a healthy diet, increasing daily exercise, self-monitoring for signs of illness, practicing good overall hygiene, seeking health screenings and evaluations and performing therapeutic, preventive measures.
4. Adherence implies that a patient makes one or more lifestyle changes to carry out specific activities to promote and maintain health.
5. Factors influencing adherence include demographic variables such as age, sex, and education; illness variables such as the severity of illness and the effects of therapy; psychosocial variables such as intelligence and attitudes toward illness; financial variables; and therapeutic regimen variables
6. choice, establishment of agreed upon goals, and the quality of the patient–provider relationship
7. Refer to the "Transtheoretical Model of Change" adapted from Miller (2009) and DiClemente (2007). Refer to Table 4-2 in the text.
8. The teaching–learning process requires the active involvement of teacher and learner, in an effort to reach the desired outcome—a change in behavior. The teacher serves as a facilitator of learning.
9. Answer may include six of the following: The elderly have difficulty adhering to a therapeutic regimen

because of increased sensitivity to medications, difficulty in adjusting to change and stress, financial constraints, forgetfulness, inadequate support systems, lifetime habits of self-medication, visual impairments, hearing deficits, and mobility limitations.

10. The elderly's ability to draw inferences, apply information, and understand major teaching points

11. The effects of a learning situation are influenced by a person's physical, emotional, and experiential readiness to learn. *Physical readiness* implies the physical ability of a person to attend to a learning situation. Basic physiologic needs are met so that higher-level needs can be addressed. *Emotional readiness* involves the patient's motivation to learn and can be encouraged by providing realistic goals that can be easily achieved so that self-esteem needs can be met. A person needs to be ready to accept the emotional changes (anxiety, stress) that accompany behavior modification resulting from the learning process. *Experiential readiness* refers to a person's past experiences that influence his or her approach to the learning process. Previous positive feedback and improved self-image reinforce experiential readiness.

12. lecture method, group teaching, demonstrations, use of teaching aids, reinforcement, and follow-up

13. increase the quality and years of healthy life for people and eliminate health disparities among various segments of the population

14. self-responsibility, nutritional awareness, stress reduction and management, and physical fitness

II. Critical Thinking Questions and Exercises

DISCUSSION AND ANALYSIS

1. Refer to Table 4-1 in the text.
2. Exercise can promote health by improving the function of the circulatory system and lungs, decrease cholesterol and low-density lipoproteins, decrease body weight, delay degenerative changes (osteoporosis), and improve muscle strength, endurance, and flexibility.

RECOGNIZING CONTRADICTIONS

1. Health education is an independent function of nursing practice that is a primary responsibility of the nursing profession.
2. Although diseases in children and those of an infectious nature are of utmost concern, the largest groups of people today who need health education are those with chronic illnesses and disabilities.
3. Patients are encouraged to adhere to their therapeutic regimen. Adherence connotes active, voluntary, collaborative patient *efforts*, whereas compliance is a more passive role.
4. Evaluation should be continuous throughout the teaching process so that the information gathered can be used to improve teaching activities.

5. The elderly usually experience significant gains from health promotion activities.
6. About 80% of those older than 65 years of age have one or more chronic illnesses.

EXAMINING ASSOCIATIONS

Refer to content as well as Chart 4-3 throughout the text to complete.

Chapter 5

I. Interpretation, Completion, and Comparison

MULTIPLE CHOICE

1. d
2. d
3. d
4. b
5. b
6. c
7. b
8. d (Chart 5-1 in the text.)
9. b
10. a
11. d
12. a
13. a
14. a
15. a

SHORT ANSWER

1. obtaining a patient health history, and performing a physical examination
2. the nurse needs to establish rapport, put the patient at ease, encourage honest communication, make eye contact, and listen carefully
3. When an atmosphere of mutual trust and confidence exists between an interviewer and a patient, the patient becomes more open and honest and is more likely to share personal concerns and problems.
4. The term *chief complaint* refers to that issue that brings the patient to the attention of the health care provider. When documenting a patient's chief complaint, exact words should be recorded in quotation marks.
5. Answer may include six of the following: cancer, hypertension, heart disease, diabetes, epilepsy, mental illness, tuberculosis, kidney disease, arthritis, allergies, asthma, alcoholism, and obesity.
6. Answer may include five of the following: patterns of sleep, exercise, nutrition, recreation, and personal habits such as smoking, the use of illicit drugs, alcohol, and caffeine.
7. heart disease, cancer, and stroke
8. Grains (6 oz), vegetables: (2.5 cups), fruits (2 cups), milk (3 cups), and meat and beans: (5.5 oz).
9. The score of 25 to 29 (overweight); 30 to 39 (obese); greater than, 40 (extremely obese). A score below 24 indicates risk for poor nutritional status. Refer to Figure 5-5 in the text.
10. men, greater than 40 in; women, greater than 35 in.
11. Negative nitrogen balance occurs when nitrogen output (urine, feces, perspiration) exceeds nitrogen intake

(food). When this happens, tissue is breaking down faster than it is being replaced.
12. iron, folate, and calcium
13. Correlation
    a. Inspection
    b. Inspection
    c. Palpation
    d. Palpation
    e. Percussion
    f. Auscultation
    g. Auscultation
    h. Palpation

MATCHING

Refer to Table 5-1 in the text.

1. h
2. c
3. d
4. e
5. g
6. b

II. Critical Thinking Questions and Exercises

DISCUSSION AND ANALYSIS

1. Refer to Chart 5-3 in the text.
2. Refer to Figures 5-3 and 5-4 in the text.

CLINICAL SITUATIONS

CASE STUDY: CALCULATE A HEALTHY DIET

Part I: Estimate Ideal Body Weight.

1. b, medium frame (height-to-wrist circumference is 10.4)
2. IBW is 130 lb; needs to lose, 50 lb (Refer to Chart 5-5 in the text.)
3. BMI is 29; overweight

Part II: Calculate a Balanced Diet Using the Food Guide Pyramid as a Reference (Chart 5-5 in the text).

1. 50 kg
2. 1418 calories
3. 1985 calories (1418 + 567)
4. 993 calories from carbohydrates, 595 calories from fat, 397 calories from protein
5. 248 g of carbohydrates, 66 g of fat, 99 g of protein

Part III: Using the USDA's Food Pyramid Guide (Figure 5-6 in the text), design a 2000-calorie diet for Mrs. Allred.

1. fruits, nuts and vegetable oils
2. whole grains
3. 2.5 cups
4. meat and beans
5. low or fat-free
6. 2 cups

Chapter 6

I. Interpretation, Completion, and Comparison

MULTIPLE CHOICE

1. d
2. d
3. b
4. a
5. d
6. d
7. d
8. b
9. a
10. b
11. c
12. a
13. b
14. b
15. d
16. d
17. a
18. d
19. b
20. d
21. d
22. c
23. d
24. d
25. d
26. b
27. b
28. a
29. c
30. a
31. d

SHORT ANSWER

1. constancy, homeostasis, stress, and adaptation
2. When the body suffers an injury, the response is maladaptive if the defense mechanisms have a negative effect on health.
3. Hyperpnea is the body's development of rapid breathing after intense exercise in response to an accumulation of lactic acid in muscle tissue and a deficit of oxygen.
4. Examples of acute, time-limited stressors may include taking an examination, giving a speech, or driving in a snowstorm. Examples of chronic, enduring stressors may include poverty, a handicap or disability, or living with an alcoholic.
5. Answer may include any of the following: traffic jam, sick child, missed appointment, car would not start, train is late (day-to-day stressors), earthquakes, wars, terrorism, events of history (major events that affect large groups of people); marriage, birth, death, retirement (infrequently occurring major stressors).
6. Adolph Meyer, in the 1930s, first showed a correlation between illness and critical life events. A Recent Life Changes Questionnaire (RLCQ) was developed by Holmes and Rahe (1967) that assigned numerical values to life events that require a change in an individual's life pattern. A correlation was seen between illness and the number of stressful events; the higher the numerical value, the greater the chance for becoming ill.
7. Cognitive appraisal refers to the evaluation of an event relative to what is at stake and what coping resources are available. External resources consist of money to purchase services and materials and social support systems that provide emotional and esteem support.

8. Hans Selye stated that "stress is essentially the rate of wear and tear on the body." He also defined stress as being a "nonspecific response" of the body regardless of the stimulus producing the response.
9. Answer should include six of the following: hypertension, diseases of the heart and blood vessels, kidney diseases, rheumatic and rheumatoid arthritis, inflammation of the skin and eyes, infections, allergic and hypersensitivity diseases, nervous and mental diseases, sexual dysfunction, digestive diseases, metabolic diseases, and cancer.
10. blood pressure, acid–base balance, blood glucose levels, body temperature, and fluids and electrolyte balance
11. redness, heat, swelling, pain, and loss of function
12. Answer can include anxiety, ineffective coping patterns, impaired thought processes, disrupted relationships, impaired adjustment, ineffective coping, social isolation, risk for spiritual distress, decisional conflict, etc.

MATCHING

1. b		5. b	
2. a		6. a	
3. a		7. b	
4. a		8. a	

II. Critical Thinking Questions and Exercises

DISCUSSION AND ANALYSIS

1. Refer to chapter heading "Stress and Adaptation" in the text.
2. Refer to chapter heading "Appraisal of the Stressful Event" in the text.
3. Refer to chapter heading "Stress: Threats to the Steady State" in the text.
4. People with positive energy and a healthy outlook on life typically perceive stressors as interesting, challenging, meaningful, and opportunities for change and growth.
5. Refer to chapter heading "Psychological Responses to Stress" in the text.
6. Refer to chapter heading "Selye's Theory of Adaptation" in the text.
7. Refer to Table 6-2 in the text.

CLINICAL SITUATIONS

FLOW CHART: THE SYMPATHETIC–ADRENAL–MEDULLARY RESPONSE TO STRESS

Refer to Table 6-1 in the text for flow chart of physiologic reactions.

General body arousal

↑Norepinephrine =

	Rationale
↑blood coagulability	↑cardiac output
↑heart rate	↑myocardial contractility
↑blood pressure	↑peripheral vasoconstriction
↑blood glucose levels	↑glycogen breakdown

Effects on:

Skeletal muscles	↑increased tension	↑increased excitation of muscles
Pupils	dilated	↑contraction of radial muscle of iris
Ventilation	rapid and shallow	↑oxygen preservation; bronchodilation

CASE STUDY: HYPERTENSIVE HEART DISEASE

Refer to Figure 6-2 in the text for nursing implications and rationales.

Selected Compensatory Mechanisms	*Nursing Implications*	*Rationale*
Renal blood flow is decreased as a result of hypertensive heart disease	**Assessment**	
	A. Blood pressure	A. Changes in the cardiovascular system are reflected in the blood pressure

	B. Urinary output
	  1. Amount
		B.
		  1. Output decreased with decreased blood flow

	2. Characteristics	2. Color changes occur with increased blood flow

	3. Urine chemistry values
	  a. Osmolality
		
		  a. Osmolality increases with heart failure

	b. Electrolytes	b. Potassium increases with renal failure
	C. Ability to cope with stress	C. Stress results in increased resistance to cardiac output
	Nursing Diagnoses/ Collaborative Problem	
	A. Fluid volume excess related to renin–angiotensin stimulation	A. Renin-angiotensin has a direct vasoconstriction effect on arterioles which leads to water retention
	Planning	
	A. Plan time for assessment around patient's need for rest.	A. Rest lowers metabolic rate and facilitates the healing process
	B. Plan an individual program of stress reduction	B. Compliance with a stress-management program will be higher if the program is individualized
	Implementation	
	A. Teach various relaxation techniques	A. Stress tends to increase epinephrine secretion, which causes vasoconstriction; this, in turn, increases the heart rate and resistance to cardiac output
	B. Develop specific ways to help the patient cope with and reduce stress	B. Stress reduction tends to reduce epinephrine secretion
	C. Modify diet to reduce sodium intake	C. Lowered sodium levels tend to decrease fluid retention, which decreases the work load of the heart
	Evaluation	
	A. Stress-reduction measures	A. Blood pressure reduction may be indicative of successful stress-reduction measures
	B. Dietary compliance relative to lowered sodium intake	B. Weight estimates, serum sodium levels, and the presence of edema are indicators of fluid retention and possible excess intake of sodium.

IDENTIFYING PATTERNS

FLOW CHART: SYMPATHETIC–ADRENAL AND HYPOTHALAMIC–PITUITARY RESPONSE

Refer to Figure 6-2 and chapter heading "Interpretation of Stressful Stimuli by the Brain" in the text.

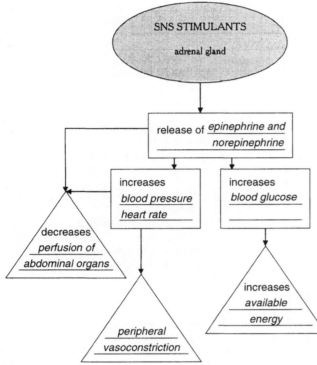

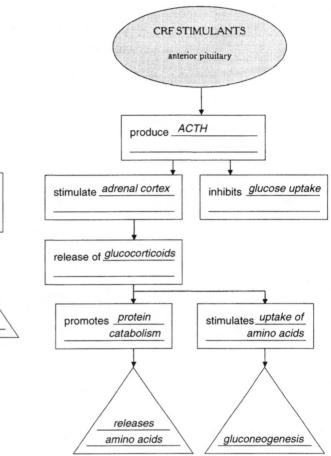

Chapter 7

I. Interpretation, Completion, and Comparison

MULTIPLE CHOICE

1. d
2. d
3. d
4. b
5. c
6. c

7. d (See Chart 7-9 in the text.)
8. b
9. a
10. b
11. c

SHORT ANSWER

1. 35% to 45%
2. The most common definition of a mental disorder is from the American Psychiatric Association (2000): "a group of behavioral or psychological symptoms or a pattern that manifests itself in significant distress, impaired functioning, or accentuated risk of enduring severe suffering or possible death."
3. Anxiety, anger, aggression, depression, suspicion, threats to a person's sense of self, and interference with ADL
4. Activity of the sympathetic nervous system; increased plasma catecholamine levels, and increased urinary epinephrine and norepinephrine levels.
5. Examples would include life events such as: rape; family violence; torture; earthquake; terrorism; fire; and military combat.
6. duration, greater than 2 weeks; and severity are the two criteria.
7. Answer should include four of these seven: headache, backache, abdominal pain, fatigue, malaise, anxiety, and sexual problems.
8. sadness, worthlessness, fatigue, guilt, and difficulty concentrating or making decisions
9. Intoxication and withdrawal are two common substance abuse problems.
10. Five significant family functions are (a) management, the use of power, decision making about resources, the establishment of rules, and provision of finances and future planning; (b) boundary setting, where the roles of adults and children are clear; (c) communication; (d) education, family support,

and appropriate modeling skills for living; and (e) socialization, acceptable behaviors for life and the transmission of culture.
11. acceptance of loss, acknowledgement of the intensity of the pain, adaptation to life after the loss, and cultivation of new relationships and activities

II. Critical Thinking Questions and Exercises

DISCUSSION AND ANALYSIS

1. Refer to chapter heading "Mental Health and Emotional Distress" and Chart 7-2 in the text.
2. Refer to Chart 7-3 in the text.
3. Refer to Chart 7-4 in the text.
4. Refer to Chart 7-10 in the text.
5. Refer to Chart 7-11 in the text.

RECOGNIZING CONTRADICTIONS

1. Since the 1980s there has been an increase in the use of holistic health care. Presently, >50% of people supplement traditional health care with alternative therapies.
2. The holistic approach to health care reconnects the mind and body traditionally separated by medicine.
3. Sadness, anxiety, and fatigue are common responses to health problems and are not age specific. Clinical depression is distinguished from everyday feelings of sadness by duration and severity.
4. A diagnosis of clinical depression requires the presence of five out of nine diagnostic criteria with depression and loss of pleasure present most of the time. (See Chart 7-6 in the text.)

CLINICAL SITUATIONS

CASE STUDY: HODGKIN'S DISEASE

1. a
2. b
3. d

CASE STUDY: RADICAL MASTECTOMY

1. a
2. b
3. b
4. d

Chapter 8

I. Interpretation, Completion, and Comparison

MULTIPLE CHOICE

1. d	3. d	5. a
2. d	4. d	6. d

7. b	10. a	13. b
8. c	11. a	14. c
9. a.	12. c	15. b

SHORT ANSWER

1. The founder of transcultural nursing is Madeleine Leininger.
2. The four basic characteristics of culture are: it is learned from birth through language and socialization, it is shared by all members of the same cultural group, it is influenced by specific environmental and technical factors, and it is dynamic and ever-changing.
3. Frequently differences in skin color, religion, and geographic areaaare the only elements used to identify diversity.
4. *Culturally competent nursing care* is effective, individualized care that shows respect for the dignity, personal rights, preferences, beliefs, and practices of people receiving care while acknowledging the biases of the caregiver and preventing that bias from interfering with care.
5. Four sample American subcultures are Black/African American, Hispanic/Latino Americans, Asian/Pacific Islanders, and Native Americans (American Indians and Alaska Natives)
6. Answer should include five of the following subcultural grouping: religion, occupation, age, sexual orientation, geographic location, gender, and disability.
7. Two underlying goals are to provide culture-specific, and culture-universal care.
8. *Culturally competent or congruent nursing c*are refers to the delivery of interventions within the cultural context of the patient. It involves the integration of attitudes, knowledge, and skills to enable nurses to deliver care in a culturally sensitive manner.
9. Four strategies include changing the subject, nonquestioning, inappropriate laughter, and nonverbal cues.
10. The Catholics, Mormons, Buddhists, Jews, and Muslims routinely abstain from eating as part of their religious practice.
11. The yin and yang theory of illness proposes that the seat of energy in the body is within the autonomic nervous system, where balance is maintained between the key opposing forces. Yin represents the female and negative forces, whereas yang represents the male positive energy.
12. The biomedical or scientific view, the naturalistic or holistic perspective, and the magico-religious view represent three major paradigms used to explain the cause of disease and illness.

MATCHING

1. e		6. a
2. c		7. c
3. a		8. a
4. d		9. e
5. b		10. c

II. Critical Thinking Questions and Exercises

DISCUSSION AND ANALYSIS

1. The goal of Leininger's research-based theory is to provide culturally congruent nursing care to improve care to people of different or similar cultures. Her theory provides care through culture care accommodation and culture care restructuring.
2. *Culture care accommodation* refers to professional nursing actions and decisions to help patients of a designated culture achieve a beneficial outcome. *Culture care restructuring* refers to the professional actions that help patients reorder, change, or modify their lifestyles toward more beneficial health care.
3. *Acculturation* is the process by which members of a cultural group adapt to or learn how to take on the behaviors of another group. *Cultural imposition* is the tendency to impose one's cultural beliefs, values, and patterns of behavior on others from a different culture.
4. *Cultural blindness* is the inability of people to recognize their own beliefs, values, and practices and those of others because of strong ethnocentric tendencies (viewing one's own culture as superior to others).
5. Refer to Chart 8-1 in the text.
6. General polymorphism is the biologic variation in an individual's response to medications that is the result of differences in age, gender, size, and body composition.
7. Differences in the five categories of alternative medicine can be found under chapter heading "Complementary and Alternative Therapies" in the text.

Chapter 9

I. Interpretation, Completion, and Comparison

MULTIPLE CHOICE

1. b	5. c	9. c
2. b	6. a	10. a
3 d	7. b	11. d
4. a	8. b	12. a

SHORT ANSWER

1. Genomic medicine encompasses the recognition that multiple genes work in concert with environmental influences resulting in the appearance and expression of disease.
2. To integrate genetics into nursing practice, the nurse (a) uses family history and the results of genetic tests, (b) informs patients about genetic concepts, (c) is aware of the personal and societal impact of genetic information, and (d) values privacy and confidentiality.
3. genotype; phenotype
4. chromosomes; autosomes; sex chromosomes; X chromosomes; one X and one Y chromosome; one sex chromosome of each pair

5. 80%; 50%
6. Answer may include five of the following: heart disease, high blood pressure, cancer, osteoarthritis, neural tube defects, spina bifida, and anencephaly.
7. Down syndrome
8. 1 in every 160, 50%
9. heart disease, diabetes, and arthritis
10. hemochromatosis (iron overload)
11. Pharmacogenetics involves the use of genetic testing to identify genetic variations that relate to the safety and efficacy of medications and gene-based treatments.
12. The nursing activities are collect and help interpret relevant family and medical histories, identify patients and families who need genetic evaluation and counseling, offer genetics information and resources, collaborate with the genetic specialist, and participate in management of patient care.

MATCHING: GENETIC TERMS

1. e		5. g	
2. h		6. d	
3. f		7. b	
4. a		8. a	

MATCHING: ADULT-ONSET DISORDERS

1. b		5. a	
2. c		6. a	
3. e		7. d	
4. d		8. f	

II. Critical Thinking Questions and Exercises

DISCUSSION AND ANALYSIS

1. Refer to Table 9-1 in the text.
2. Refer to Chart 9-1 in the text.
3. Chapter 9 readings plus personal assessments.
4. Refer to chapter heading "Inheritance Patterns" and Table 9-2 in the text.
5. Refer to chapter heading "Personalized Genomic Treatments" in the text.

Chapter 10

I. Interpretation, Completion, and Comparison

MULTIPLE CHOICE

1. d	6. a	11. b
2. d	7. b	12. a
3. b	8. a	13. b
4. d	9. b	
5. d	10. b	

SHORT ANSWER

1. use of tobacco, use of alcohol, improper diet, and physical inactivity
2. the presence of a prolonged course, the inability of a condition to resolve spontaneously, and the unlikely or rare possibility of a cure are all characteristics of chronic illness
3. 43% (about 125 million of 288 million people), 50%
4. obesity, hypertension, and diabetes
5. Refer to chapter heading "Implications of Managing Chronic Conditions" in the text.
6. Answers may include six common management problems: preventing the occurrence of other chronic conditions; alleviating and managing symptoms; preventing, adapting, and managing disabilities; preventing and managing crises and complications; adapting to repeated threats and progressive functional loss; living with isolation and loneliness.
7. The Trajectory Model refers to the path or course of action taken by the ill person, his family, health professionals, and others to manage the course of the illness.
8. Developmental, acquired and age-associated are the categories used to classify disabilities.

II. Critical Thinking Questions and Exercises

DISCUSSION AND ANALYSIS

1. A decrease in mortality from infectious diseases, lifestyle factors, longer lifespans, and improved screening and diagnostic procedures are four major causes of chronic conditions.
2. Refer to Table 10-1 in the text.
3. Refer to chapter heading "Characteristics of Chronic Conditions" in the text.
4. A *disability* is an umbrella term for impairments, activity limitations, participation restrictions, and environmental factors. An *impairment* is a loss or abnormality in body structure or physiologic function.
5. Refer to chapter heading "Overview of Chronicity" in the text.
6. Refer to chapter heading "Federal Legislation" in the text.
7. Senate bill (S. 1050-2007) would amend the Rehabilitation Act of 1973 and require that standards be set for medical diagnostic equipment to ensure accessibility and usability by those with disabilities.

EXAMINING ASSOCIATIONS

1. Explain that medical conditions are associated with psychological and social problems that can affect body image and alter lifestyles.
2. Explain that chronic conditions have acute, stable, and unstable periods, flare-ups, and remissions. Each phase requires different types of management.

3. Explain that complying with a therapeutic treatment plan requires time, knowledge, and a long-term commitment to prevent the incidence of complications.
4. Explain that the whole family experiences stress and caretaker fatigue. Social changes that can occur include loss of income, role reversals, and altered socialization activities.

CLINICAL SITUATIONS

CASE STUDY: APPLYING THE NURSING PROCESS TO THE TRAJECTORY MODEL OF CHRONIC ILLNESS

Refer to Table 10-2 in the text.

1. *Step 1.* The nurse uses assessment to determine specific problems and the trajectory phase of the chronic illness. For example, the nurse determines whether any musculoskeletal deficiencies are evident, whether fatigue is interfering with activities of daily living, and whether the patient is emotionally capable of coping with the diagnosis.
2. *Step 2.* The nurse interacts with the family and the medical team to establish and prioritize specific collaborative goals of management and support. For example, the nurse, working with the physician and physical therapist, designs an exercise program that will maximize current musculoskeletal strength while preventing excessive stress on major joints.
3. *Step 3.* The nurse can help the patient and family define a plan of action; i.e., draft a list of activities, exercises, and rest periods that can support established goals. The nurse can also identify specific criteria to be used to measure progress toward goal attainment. For example, the patient can keep a daily record of pain and joint stiffness, participation in work activities, and time allocated for recreation. The nurse can review the plan periodically with the patient.
4. *Step 4.* The nurse plans specific interventions to provide care. The nurse can help with direct care (i.e., range of motion exercises, applications of warm compresses, adjustments to the environment). The nurse can recommend referrals to counseling or agencies that can help provide services. The nurse can help the family work together to determine a lifelong approach to treatment and support.
5. *Step 5.* The nurse follows up to determine if the problem, along with treatment and management interventions, is being resolved and whether or not there is adherence to the plan. The nurse identifies environmental, social, and psychological factors that may facilitate or hinder goal achievement. For example, the nurse could explore the time commitment and types of activities required for child care and how they affect the patient. Does the patient have support from extended family members? Can the patient adjust his or her work schedule if necessary? Are there any associated systemic conditions that may compromise a plan of care, such as renal problems or swollen joints?

Chapter 11

I. Interpretation, Completion, and Comparison

MULTIPLE CHOICE

1. d	7. c	12. a
2. b	8. d	13. b
3. b	9. d	14. d
4. a	10. c	15. d
5. a	11. a	16. d
6. b		

SHORT ANSWER

1. The three goals of rehabilitation are restore the patient's ability to function independently or at a pre-illness or pre-injury level, maximize independence and prevent secondary disability.
2. Stroke recovery and traumatic brain injury, spinal cord injury, orthopedic, cardiac, pulmonary, pediatric, comprehensive pain management, and rehabilitation are specialty rehabilitation programs accredited by CARF.
3. Refer to chapter heading "The Patient With Self-Care Deficits in Activities of Daily Living" in the text.
4. Answer should include *five of the following eight diagnoses*: impaired physical mobility, activity intolerance, risk for injury, risk for disuse syndrome, impaired walking, impaired wheelchair mobility, and impaired bed mobility. Answer should also include *four of the following five goals*: absence of contracture and deformity, maintenance of muscle strength and joint mobility, independent mobility, increased activity tolerance, and prevention of further disability.
5. Answer should include four of the following: impaired physical mobility, activity intolerance, risk for injury, risk for disuse syndrome, impaired walking, impaired wheelchair mobility, and impaired bed mobility.
6. Weakened muscles, joint contractures, and deformity are common complications associated with prolonged immobility.
7. External rotation of the hip and plantar flexion of the foot (foot drop) are common complications.
8. Prolonged bed rest, lack of exercise, incorrect positioning in bed, and the weight of the bedding are four factors that contribute to foot drop.
9. Exercises are passive, active-assistive, active, resistive and isometric or muscle setting. Nursing activities are described in Table 11-1 in the text.
10. three
11. Refer to Chart 11-10 in the text.
12. Refer to Figure 11-5 in the text.
13. osteomyelitis
14. eschar does not permit free drainage of the tissue
15. carbonated soft drinks, milkshakes, alcohol, tomato juice, and citrus fruit juices

MATCHING

1. e		4. d
2. a		5. f
3. b		6. c

II. Critical Thinking Questions and Exercises

DISCUSSION AND ANALYSIS

1. Refer to Chart 11-4 in the text.
2. Refer to Chart 11-2 in the text.
3. Refer to Charts 11-3 and 11-4 and chapter heading "Patients' Reactions to Disability" in the text.
4. Refer to chapter heading "Assessment of Functional Ability" in the text.
5. Refer to Chart 11-5 in the text.
6. Refer to Table 11-2 in the text.
7. Pressure ulcers occur when pressure on the skin is greater than normal capillary closure pressure (32 mm Hg). The initial sign of pressure is *erythema* caused by *reactive hyperemia* that, if unrelieved after one hour, results in *tissue ischemia* or *anoxia*.
8. Refer to chapter heading "Promoting Pressure Ulcer Healing" in the text.
9. Refer to chapter heading "The Patient With Altered Elimination Patterns" in the text.

CLINICAL SITUATIONS

IMPAIRED SKIN INTEGRITY

1. Pressure ulcers are localized areas of infarcted soft tissue that occur when pressure applied to the skin over time is greater than normal capillary closure pressure, approximately 32 mm Hg.
2. erythema, reactive hyperemia; tissue ischemia, and anoxia
3. sacrum and heels
4. streptococci, staphylococci, *Pseudomonas aeruginosa*, and *Escherichia coli*
5. 3 g/mL; 1.25 to 1.5 g/kg/day
6. Braden and Norton scales
7. Pascal's law: As the body sinks into the fluid, more surface area becomes available for weight bearing, thus decreasing body weight per unit area.
8. Increased elevation increases the downward-pulling force of body weight, which increases pressure on the skin, which results in localized blood flow reduction.

CASE STUDY: ASSISTED AMBULATION: CRUTCHES

1. b		3. c
2. b		4. b

Chapter 12

I. Interpretation, Completion, and Comparison

MULTIPLE CHOICE

1. d	7. b
2. a	8. d
3. a	9. d
4. c	10. b
5. c	11. a
6. a	12. b

SHORT ANSWER

1. Geriatric syndromes refer to common conditions found in the elderly that tend to be multifactorial and do not fall under discrete disease categories, such as falls, delirium, frailty, dizziness, and urinary incontinence.
2. heart disease, cancer, stroke, and chronic obstructive pulmonary diseases
3. myocardial hypertrophy, fibrosis, valvular stenosis, and decreased pacemaker cells which result in reduced stroke volume
4. macular degeneration
5. thinking,and problem solving; verbal skills
6. decreased cardiac output, and decreased perfusion of the liver
7. depression
8. pneumonia, urinary tract infections, tuberculosis, gastrointestinal infections, and skin infections
9. falls

II. Critical Thinking Questions and Exercises

INTERPRETING DATA

1. 4.7%
2. 13.8%; double
3. 16.2%
4. 54; 70; 30%.

RECOGNIZING CONTRADICTIONS

1. Osteoporosis can be arrested or prevented, but not reversed.
2. If the symptoms of delirium go untreated and the underlying cause is not treated, permanent, irreversible brain damage or death can occur.
3. It is a myth that older people should avoid vigorous activity. Activity is a desired state in older adults.
4. In the older person, the baseline body temperature is usually one degree Fahrenheit lower than in a younger person. Therefore, a temperature elevation should be considered serious.

DISCUSSION AND ANALYSIS

1. Refer to Table 12-2 in the text.
2. Refer to chapter heading "Continuing Care Retirement Communities" in the text.
3. Refer to chapter heading "Cognitive Aspects of Aging" in the text.
4. Refer to chapter heading "Pharmacologic Aspects of Aging" in the text.
5. Refer to Table 12-4 in the text.
6. Refer to chapter heading "Alzheimer's Disease" in the text.
7. Refer to chapter heading "Other Aspects of Health Care of the Older Adult" in the text.
8. Refer to chapter heading "Health Care Costs of Aging" in the text.
9. Refer to chapter heading "Ethical and Legal Issues Affecting the Older Adult" in the text.
10. Refer to chapter heading "Ethical and Legal Issues Affecting the Older Adult" in the text.

CLINICAL SITUATIONS

CASE STUDY: LONELINESS

1. d	4. d
2. d	5. d
3. a	

CASE STUDY: ALZHEIMER'S DISEASE

1. a
2. acetylcholine, cerebral cortex, brain size
3. Anicept, Exelon, Razadyne, Cognex, and Namenda
4. c
5. d
6. d
7. pneumonia, malnutrition, and dehydration

CASE STUDY: DEHYDRATION

1. d	3. d
2. c	4. d

Chapter 13

I. Interpretation, Completion, and Comparison

MULTIPLE CHOICE

1. d	8. a	15. b
2. b	9. a	16. b
3. d	10. a	17. d
4. b	11. d	18. d
5. c	12. d	19. d
6. c	13. c	20. c
7. b	14. c	21. d

SHORT ANSWER

1. duration, location, and etiology
2. acute, chronic (nonmalignant), and cancer-related
3. Refer to Chart 13-2 in the text.
4. the suppression of immune function that promotes tumor growth
5. histamine, bradykinin, acetylcholine, serotonin, and substance P
6. past experiences with pain, anxiety, culture, age, gender, genetics, and expectations about pain relief
7. pain threshold; pain tolerance
8. Factors include intensity, timing, location, quality personal meaning of pain, aggravating and alleviating factors, and pain behaviors.
9. Physiologic response are tachycardia, hypertension, tachypnea, pallor, diaphoresis, mydriasis, hypervigilance, and increased muscle tone.
10. Celebrex
11. Balanced analgesia refers to the use of more than one form of analgesia concurrently to obtain more pain relief with fewer side effects.
12. respiratory depression; 24; 6 and 12
13. A placebo effect occurs when a person responds to a medication or treatment because of an expectation that the treatment will work rather than the treatment's actually effectiveness.
14. Answer may include massage, thermal therapies, transcutaneous electrical, distraction, relaxation techniques, guided imagery, and music therapy.

MATCHING

1. f
2. j
3. a
4. h
5. b
6. g
7. c
8. i
9. e
10. d

II. Critical Thinking Questions and Exercises

DISCUSSION AND ANALYSIS

1. Refer to Chart 13-1 in the text.
2. Acute pain lasts from seconds to 3 to 6 weeks (e.g., appendectomy, ankle sprain). Chronic, persistent, nonmalignant pain lasts 6 months or longer (e.g., rheumatoid arthritis, fibromyalgia). Cancer-related pain can be directly associated with the cancer and/or the result of cancer treatment (e.g., ovarian and lung cancer).
3. Refer to Figure 13-1 in the text.
4. The classic Gate Control Theory proposes that stimulation of the skin evokes nervous impulses that are then transmitted by three systems located in the spinal cord. The noxious impulses are influenced by a "gating mechanism." The concept proposed is that stimulation of the large-diameter fibers inhibits the transmission of pain, thus "closing the gate." Conversely, when smaller fibers are stimulated, the gate is opened. This mechanism is influenced by nerve impulses that descend from the brain. This theory also proposes a specialized system of large-diameter fibers that activate selective cognitive processes via the modulating properties of the spinal gate. Refer to Figure 13-2 in the text.
5. Refer to chapter heading "Factors Influencing Pain Response" in the text.
6. Refer to Figure 13-5 in the text.
7. Refer to Chart 13-4 in the text.
8. Refer to Table 13-2 in the text.
9. Refer to chapter heading "Patient-Controlled Analgesia" in the text.
10. Distraction, which involves focusing the patient's attention on something other than the pain, reduces the perception of pain by stimulating the descending control system. This results in the transmission of fewer painful stimuli to the brain.

CLINICAL SITUATIONS

CASE STUDY: PAIN EXPERIENCE

1. a
2. c
3. d
4. d

Chapter 14

I. Interpretation, Completion, and Comparison

MULTIPLE CHOICE

1. c
2. b
3. b
4. c
5. d
6. a
7. b
8. a
9. d
10. b
11. c
12. b
13. b
14. a
15. c
16. a
17. b
18. c
19. c
20. a
21. b
22. d
23. d
24. c
25. b
26. d
27. b
28. c
29. d
30. d
31. c
32. a
33. c
34. b
35. a
36. d

SHORT ANSWER

1. 66%, potassium; intravascular, interstitial, and transcultural; sodium; 50%, 6 L; plasma. (Refer to Table 14-1 in the text.)
2. Osmotic pressure is the amount of hydrostatic pressure needed to stop the flow of water by osmosis. It is primarily determined by the concentration of solutes.
3. Urine specific gravity measures the kidney's ability to excrete or conserve water. BUN, made up of urea, is an end product of protein (muscle and dietary) metabolism by the liver. Creatinine, as the end product of muscle metabolism, is a better indicator of renal function than BUN.

4. Baroreceptors, which are responsible for monitoring the circulating volume, are small nerve receptors that detect changes in pressure within blood vessels. Osmoreceptors sense changes in sodium concentration.
5. the combined actions of parathyroid hormone and vitamin D
6. bones; soft tissue
7. metastatic calcification of soft tissue, joints, and arteries
8. 7.35 to 7.45
9. 6.8 on the lower range, and 7.8 on the upper range
10. a. Low   g. High
    b. Low   h. Low
    c. High   i. Low
    d. High   j. High
    e. High   k. High
    f. Low   l. Low
11. a. Low   g. Low
    b. High   h. Low
    c. Low   i. Low
    d. Low   j. High
    e. High   k. Low
    f. Low   l. High
12. a. High   e. Low
    b. Low   f. High
    c. High   g. Low
    d. High   h. Low
13. a. Low   d. Low
    b. High   e. Low
    c. Low
14. a. Low   d. Low
    b. High   e. High
    c. Low
15. a. R-ACID   f. R-ACID
    b. M-ACID   g. M-ACID
    c. M-ACID   h. M-ALKA
    d. R-ACID   i. M-ALKA
    e. R-ALKA   j. R-ALKA
16. Na × 2 = Glucose divided by 18 + BUN divided by 3 = approximate value of serum osmolality
17. Intense supervision is required, because only small volumes are needed to elevate the serum sodium from dangerously low levels.
18. Answer may include dyspnea, cyanosis, a weak pulse, hypotension, unresponsiveness, and pain (chest, shoulder, low back).

II. Critical Thinking Questions and Exercises

DISCUSSION AND ANALYSIS

1. An early indicator of a third space fluid shift is a decrease in urinary output despite adequate fluid intake. This occurs because fluid shifts out of the intravascular space. The kidneys, receiving less blood, attempt to compensate by decreasing urine output.

2. Hydrostatic pressure (pressure exerted by fluid on the walls of the blood vessels) affects the movement of fluids through the capillary walls of the blood vessels. Osmotic pressure is pressure exerted by proteins in the plasma. Both pressures help maintain a high extracellular concentration of sodium and a high intracellular concentration of potassium.
3. The usual daily urine output is 1.0 L/kg of body weight/h. The per hour output would be: 110 lb (50 mL), 132 lb (60 mL), and 176 lb (80 mL).
4. Osmolality refers to the concentration of fluid that affects the movement of water between the fluid compartments by osmosis. It measures the solute concentration per kilogram in the blood and urine. Osmolarity describes the concentration of solutions and is measured in milliosmoles per liter (mOsm/L).
5. Refer to chapter heading "Fluid Volume Disturbances" and Table 14-3 in the text.
6. Refer to chapter heading "Electrolyte Imbalances" in the text.
7. Refer to chapter heading "Calcium Imbalances" in the text.
8. Refer to chapter heading "Chloride Imbalances" in the text.
9. Refer to chapter heading "Acid–Base Disturbances" in the text.
10. Refer to chapter heading "Acid–Base Disturbances" in the text.
11. Refer to chapter heading "Types of Intravenous Solutions" and Table 14-3 in the text.
12. Refer to chapter heading "Nursing Management of the Patient Receiving Intravenous Therapy" in the text.
13. Refer to chapter heading "Managing Local Complications" in the text.

APPLYING CONCEPTS

1. Osmosis is the movement of fluid, through a semipermeable membrane, from an area of low solute concentration to an area of high solute concentration until the solutions are of equal concentration. Diffusion is the movement of a substance from an area of higher concentration to one of lower concentration. The concentration of dissolved substances (fluid concentration gradient) draws fluid in that direction.
2. The number of dissolved particles, within a unit of fluid, determines the osmolality of a solution. It is the *osmolality* that influences the movement of fluid between compartments.
3. Tonicity is the osmotic driving force of all the solutes. Tonicity determines cellular size and hydration.
4. Osmotic pressure, determined by the concentration of solutes, is the amount of hydrostatic pressure needed to stop the flow of water by osmosis. Oncotic pressure is the osmotic pressure exerted by proteins. Osmotic diuresis is urine output caused by the excretion of substances such as glucose and mannitol.
5. Diffusion is the movement of a substance from an area of higher concentration to one of lower concentration. Filtration is the movement of water and solutes from an area of high hydrostatic pressure to

an area of low hydrostatic pressure, for example, the filtration of water and electrolytes by the kidneys.
6. Osmosis: the oncotic pressure of plasma proteins (albumin); diffusion: the filtration of water and electrolytes by the kidneys; and filtration: the exchange of oxygen and carbon dioxide between the pulmonary capillaries and the alveoli.

EXAMINING ASSOCIATIONS

1. Refer to chapter heading "Sodium–Potassium Pump" in the text.
2. Refer to Figure 14-2 in the text for an illustration of the fluid regulation cycle.
3. Three-column matching: Body fluid compartments

1. d	a. V
2. e	b. IV
3. f	c. III
4. a	d. II
5. b	e. VI
6. c	f. I

EXTRACTING INFERENCES

1. osmolality, affects the movement of water between fluid compartments
2. thirst, antidiuretic hormone (ADH), and the rennin–angiotensin aldosterone system
3. muscle contraction and the transmission of nerve impulses
4. a
5. c
6. b
7. b
8. c

CLINICAL SITUATIONS

CASE STUDY: EXTRACELLULAR FLUID VOLUME DEFICIT

1. b	3. a
2. b	4. b

CASE STUDY: CONGESTIVE HEART FAILURE

1. b	3. d
2. d	4. b

CASE STUDY: DIABETES MELLITUS

1. a	3. a
2. a	4. c

CASE STUDY: INTRAVENOUS THERAPY

1. metacarpal, cephalic, basilica, and median veins
2. subclavian or internal jugular
3. larger cannula
4. total volume (mL) divided by total time (hours) = mL/h.
5. increased tubing length and the low height of the intravenous container
6. circulatory overload, air embolism, febrile reaction, and infection
7. infiltration and extravasation, phlebitis, thrombophlebitis, hematoma, and clotting of the needle

Chapter 15

I. Interpretation, Completion, and Comparison

MULTIPLE CHOICE

1. d	10. a	19. a
2. c	11. d	20. d
3. d	12. d	21. a
4. b	13. b	22. d
5. a	14. b	23. d
6. d	15. c	24. a
7. a	16. c	25. d
8. d	17. c	
9. b	18. d	

SHORT ANSWER

1. inadequate tissue perfusion; poor oxygen and nutrient delivery, cellular starvation, cell death, organ dysfunction leading to organ failure, and eventual death
2. glucose; adenosine triphosphate (ATP)
3. blood volume, cardiac pump, and vasculature
4. stroke volume, heart rate, diameter of the arterioles
5. Mean arterial pressure (MAP) is the average pressure at which blood flows through the vasculature. MAP must exceed 65 mm Hg.
6. carotid sinus, and aortic arch; aortic arch, and carotid arteries
7. cellular, and tissue
8. lactated Ringer's solution, and 0.9% sodium chloride solution (normal saline solution)
9. limit additional myocardial damage, increase cardiac contractility, and decrease ventricular afterload
10. B-type natriuretic peptide (BNP)
11. loss of sympathetic tone, and release of biochemical mediators from cells
12. spinal cord injury, spinal anesthesia, or the depressant action of medications and glucose deficiency

MATCHING

1. c		6. d
2. a		7. c
3. a		8. b
4. e		9. b
5. f		10. e

II. Critical Thinking Questions and Exercises

DISCUSSION AND ANALYSIS

1. Refer to Figure 15-1 in the text.
2. Refer to Table 15-1 in the text.
3. Refer to Chart 15-1 in the text.

4. Refer to chapter heading "Fluid Replacement" and Table 15-3 in the text.
5. Refer to chapter heading "Complications of Fluid Administration" in the text.
6. Refer to Table 15-2 in the text.
7. Refer to Chart 15-3 in the text.

ILLUSTRATING PATTERNS

FLOW CHART: BLOOD PRESSURE REGULATION: SHOCK

A drop in blood pressure (baroreceptor response)

↓

release of epinephrine and norepinephrine from the adrenal medulla

↓

↑ heart rate and vasoconstriction=restored blood pressure

↓

A drop in blood pressure (response by kidneys)

↓

release of the enzyme renin

↓

conversion of angiotensin I to angiotensin II

↓

vasoconstriction

↓

release of aldosterone from the adrenal cortex

↓

promotes retention of sodium and water

↓

Stimulates the release of ADH by the pituitary gland

↓

causes the kidneys to raise blood volume and blood pressure

FLOW CHART: HYPOVOLEMIC SHOCK

↓ intravascular volume from hemorrhage or severe dehydration

results in

↓ venous blood return and ↓ ventricular filling

which causes

↓ stroke volume and ↓ cardiac output

which leads to

↓ blood pressure and inadequate tissue perfusion

CLINICAL SITUATIONS

CASE STUDY: HYPOVOLEMIC SHOCK

1. d
2. 20 mm Hg
3. rise, decline
4. 90
5. 30
6. colloids, Ringer's lactate, and normal saline

CASE STUDY: SEPTIC SHOCK

1. *Escherichia coli*
2. severe clinical insult that causes an overwhelming inflammatory response
3. lactic acidosis, oliguria, altered level of consciousness, thrombocytopenia, and altered hepatic function
4. 40%, and 90%
5. urine, blood, sputum, and wound drainage
6. 8 to 12 mm Hg; >65 mm Hg; >0.5 mL/kg/h; >70%
7. cardiovascular overload, and pulmonary edema

Chapter 16

I. Interpretation, Completion, and Comparison

MULTIPLE CHOICE

1. b	9. b	17. a
2. a	10. c	18. a
3. d	11. b	19. d
4. d	12. c	20. d
5. d	13. b	21. a
6. c	14. a	22. a
7. a	15. d	23. d
8. d	16. b	24. d

SHORT ANSWER

1. Men: lung, prostate, and colorectal area; women: breast, lung, and colorectal area.
2. Cancer begins when an abnormal cell, after being transformed by the genetic mutation of DNA, forms a clone and begins to proliferate abnormally ignoring growth-regulating signals.

3. carcinoembryonic antigen (CEA) and prostate-specific antigen (PSA)
4. lymph and blood
5. 75%
6. tobacco smoke
7. breast and ovarian cancer syndrome (BRCA1 and BRCA2), and multiple endocrine neoplasia syndrome (MEN1 and MEN2).
8. Answer should include four of the following: mouth, pharynx, larynx, esophagus, liver, colorectum, and breast.
9. cabbage, broccoli, and cauliflower; fats, alcohol, salt-cured and smoked meats (ham), and nitrite/nitrate-containing foods (bacon and red and processed meats) tend to increase the risk of cancer.
10. antibodies produced by B-lymphocytes, lymphokines, macrophages, natural killer (NK) cells, and T-lymphocytes
11. Answer should include three from each of the following choices:
    a. *Skin*: alopecia, erythema, desquamation
    b. *Oral mucosal membrane*: xerostomia, stomatitis, decreased salivation, loss of taste
    c. *Stomach or colon*: anorexia, nausea, vomiting, diarrhea
    d. *Bone marrow producing sites*: anemia, leukopenia, and thrombocytopenia
12. Answer should include five of the following: redness, pain, swelling, a mottled appearance, phlebitis, loss of blood return, resistance to flow, tissue necrosis, or damage to underlying tendons, nerves, and blood vessels.
13. nausea and vomiting
14. leucopenia, neutropenia, anemia, and thrombocytopenia; infection and bleeding
15. cisplatin, methotrexate, and mitramycin

MATCHING

1. a	5. d
2. b	6. g
3. f	7. h
4. e	8. c

MATCHING

1. b	4. b
2. a	5. b
3. a	

MATCHING

Refer to Table 16-6 in the text.
1. a; bone marrow suppression
2. c; nausea, vomiting, and diarrhea
3. a; stomatitis and alopecia
4. f; masculinization and feminization
5. a; bone marrow suppression
6. b; delayed and cumulative myelosuppression
7. d; bone marrow suppression
8. a; nausea, vomiting, and cystitis
9. c; proctitis, stomatitis, and renal toxicity
10. e; neuropathies
11. h; bone marrow suppression
12. g; hepatotoxicity

II. Critical Thinking Questions and Exercises

DISCUSSION AND ANALYSIS

1. Invasion is the growth of the primary tumor into surrounding host tissues in a variety of ways. Metastasis is the dissemination or direct spread of malignant cells to body cavities or through lymphatic and blood circulation.
2. Primary prevention is concerned with reducing the risk or preventing the development of cancer in healthy people through health promotion strategies. An example is teaching people the importance of stopping smoking to decrease the incidence of lung cancer. Secondary prevention involves early detection and screening efforts to achieve early diagnosis and prompt intervention to halt the cancerous process. An example is teaching principles of breast self-examination to facilitate the early detection of breast cancer. Refer to Chart 16-2 and Table 16-2 in the text.
3. Refer to Table 16-3 in the text.
4. Cell cycle-specific agents destroy cells that are actively reproducing in specific phases of the cell cycle by interfering with DNA and RNA synthesis or by halting mitosis. Cell cycle-nonspecific agents exert prolonged effects on cells, independent of cell cycle phases, which leads to cell damage or death.
5. Refer to chapter heading "Hypersensitivity Reactions" in the text.
6. Refer to chapter heading "Nursing Management in Bone Marrow Transplantation" in the text.
7. Interferons are cytokines, with antiviral and antitumor properties that stimulate the immune system to eradicate the malignant growth.
8. Refer to chapter heading "Cancer vaccines" in the text.
9. Refer to chapter heading "Administration of Chemotherapeutic Agents" in the text.
10. Refer to Chart 16-7 in the text.
11. Refer to Table 16-8 in the text.

EXAMINING ASSOCIATIONS

1. detection and screening for an early diagnosis and treatment
2. tumor cell classification
3. Incisional
4. palliative
5. a donor from an identical twin
6. interleukins
7. the thinning or complete loss of hair
8. appetite failure resulting in a wasting syndrome
9. *Pseudomonas aeruginosa*
10. acute leukemia

CLINICAL SITUATIONS

CASE STUDY: CANCER OF THE BREAST

1. b   4. d   7. a
2. d   5. d   8. d
3. a   6. c   9. b

CASE STUDY: CANCER OF THE LUNG

1. d
2. disease progression, immune competence, increased incidence of infection, delayed tissue repair, and diminished functional ability
3. fear, apprehension, fatigue, anger, and social isolation
4. c
5. answer questions and concerns, identify resources and support persons, communicate and share concerns, and help frame questions for the physician
6. infection
7. *Pseudomonas aeruginosa* and *Escherichia coli*
8. b

Chapter 17

I. Interpretation, Completion, and Comparison

MULTIPLE CHOICE

1. b   4. c   7. d
2. c   5. a   8. d
3. c   6. d   9. d

SHORT ANSWER

1. Kubler-Ross, "*On Death and Dying*"
2. Assisted suicide refers to providing another person the means to end his or her own life. Physician-assisted suicide involves a prescription by a physician of a lethal dose of medication to end life.
3. Palliative care and hospice care involve coordinated programs of interdisciplinary services provided by professional caregivers and trained volunteers to patients with serious, progressive illnesses who are not responsive to curative treatments. However, palliative care does not focus primarily on preparation for death as does hospice care.
4. Connecticut, 1974
5. neurodegenerative diseases (dementia and Parkinson's), and cardiovascular diseases
6. bronchodilators and corticosteroids
7. Decadron (dexamethasone), Megace (megestrol acetate), and Marinol (dronabinol)

II. Critical Thinking Questions and Exercises

DISCUSSION AND ANALYSIS

1. Refer to chapter heading "Death and Dying in America" in the text.
2. Refer to chapter heading "Technology and End-Of-Life Care" in the text.
3. Refer to chapter heading "Clinicians' Attitudes Toward Death" in the text.
4. Refer to chapter heading "Assisted Suicide" and the ANA's Position Statement (ANA, 1994) in the text.
5. Refer to Table 17-1 in the text.
6. Refer to Chart 17-4 in the text.
7. Refer to Chart 17-5 in the text.
8. Refer to Chart 17-6 in the text as an outline for discussion and analysis.
9. Refer to chapter heading "Goal Setting in Palliative Care at the End of Life" and Chart 17-7 in the text.
10. Refer to Charts 17-8 and 17-9 in the text.
11. Refer to Chart 17-10 in the text.
12. Refer to chapter heading "Palliative Sedation at the End of Life" in the text.
13. Refer to Chart 17-11 in the text.
14. Refer to Chart 17-13 and chapter heading "Coping With Death and Dying: Professional Caregiver Issues" in the text.

Chapter 18

I. Interpretation. Completion, and Comparison

MULTIPLE CHOICE

1. c   10. a   19. a
2. b   11. d   20. a
3. a   12. b   21. d
4. d   13. a   22. d
5. c   14. d   23. a
6. a   15. d   24. a
7. a   16. d   25. c
8. a   17. d
9. c   18. a

SHORT ANSWER

1. when the decision to do surgery is made, is transferred onto the operating room table
2. is transferred to the operating room table, the patient is admitted to the PACU
3. the number and severity of coexisting health problems and the nature and duration of the operative procedure
4. respiratory and cardiac
5. it is invasive, it requires sedation or anesthesia, it involves radiation, and/or has more than a slight risk of potential harm
6. hypoglycemia, hyperglycemia, acidosis, and glucosuria
7. 7 to 10 days; inhibiting platelet aggregation
8. dehydration, hypovolemia, and electrolyte imbalances
9. improve circulation, prevent venous stasis, and promote optimal respiratory function

MATCHING

Refer to Table 18-2 in the text.

1. d   4. c

2. a   5. b

3. e

II. Critical Thinking Questions and Exercises

DISCUSSION AND ANALYSIS

1. Refer to Chart 18-1 in the text.
2. Refer to Chart 18-2 in the text.
3. Refer to Chart 18-3 in the text.
4. Refer to Chart 18-8 in the text.

EXAMINING ASSOCIATIONS

1. Medication Administration. Refer to Table 18-3 in the text.
2. Preoperative Nursing. Refer to chapter heading "General Preoperative Nursing Interventions" in the text.

CLINICAL SITUATIONS

APPLYING CONCEPTS

Health Teaching to Prevent Postoperative Complications. Refer to Chart 18-5 in the text.

Chapter 19

I. Interpretation, Completion, and Comparison

MULTIPLE CHOICE

1. b	6. b	11. d
2. d	7. c	12. b
3. c	8. c	13. c
4. d	9. a	14. d
5. d	10. d	15. b

SHORT ANSWER

1. Refer to Glossary in the text.
2. Anesthesia is reduced with age because the percentage of fatty tissue increases as one gets older. Fatty tissue has an affinity for anesthetic agents.
3. Handling tissue, providing exposure at the operative field, suturing, and maintaining hemostasis.
4. exposure to blood and body fluids, hazards associated with laser beams, exposure to latex and adhesive substances, radiation and toxic agents
5. moderate sedation; Versed and Valium
6. thiopental sodium (Pentothal), respiratory depression
7. the subarachnoid space at the lumbar level (usually between L4 and L5)
8. epidural

9. Complete return of sensation in the patient's toes, in response to a pinprick, indicates recovery.
10. nausea and vomiting, anaphylaxis, hypoxia, hypothermia, and malignant hypothermia
11. 104°F or 42°C

MATCHING: INHALATION ANESTHETIC AGENTS

Refer to Table 19-1 in the text.

1. d   4. c

2. b   5. e

3. a

MATCHING: COMMON INTRAVENOUS MEDICATIONS

Refer to Table 19-2 in the text.

1. d   4. c

2. b   5. e

3. a

II. Critical Thinking Questions and Exercises

DISCUSSION AND ANALYSIS

1. Refer to chapter heading "Types of Anesthesia and Sedation" in the text.
2. Refer to Chart 19-1 in the text.
3. The elderly have a variety of age-related cardiovascular and pulmonary changes as well as changes in the liver and kidneys. Refer to chapter heading "Gerontologic Considerations" in the text.
4. Refer to chapter heading "The Circulating Nurse" in the text.
5. Refer to chapter heading "Basic Guidelines for Maintaining Surgical Asepsis" in the text.
6. Refer to chapter heading "Health Hazards Associated With the Surgical Environment" in the text.
7. Anesthesia awareness is a condition whereby patients are partially awake while under general anesthesia. Cardiac, obstetric, and major trauma patients are most at risk.
8. Refer to chapter heading "The Patient During Surgery" in the text.

RECOGNIZING CONTRADICTIONS

1. Older patients require <u>less anesthesia</u> and <u>take longer to eliminate</u> anesthetic drugs.
2. The <u>circulating nurse</u> controls the environment, coordinates the activities of other personnel, and monitors aseptic techniques.
3. Whenever sterility is in question, an item is considered <u>unsterile</u>.
4. Only the top of a table that is draped is considered sterile. Drapes hanging over the edge are <u>clean but not sterile</u>.
5. The unsterile arm of the circulating nurse <u>should never extend</u> over a sterile area.

CLINICAL SITUATIONS
CASE STUDY: GENERAL ANESTHESIA
1. b
2. b
3. c.

CASE STUDY: INTRAVENOUS ANESTHESIA
1. d
2. a
3. b

Chapter 20

I. Interpretation, Completion, and Comparison

MULTIPLE CHOICE
1. c
2. d
3. d
4. a
5. d
6. d
7. a
8. d
9. a
10. c
11. b
12. c
13. d
14. d
15. a
16. c
17. d
18. a
19. d
20. b
21. c
22. d

SHORT ANSWER
1. The answer should include five of the following: medical diagnosis, type of surgery performed, patient's general condition: age, airway patency, vital signs; anesthetic and other medications used; any intraoperative problems that might influence postoperative care (shock, hemorrhage, cardiac arrest); any pathology encountered; fluid administered, blood loss and replacement; tubing, drains, catheters, or other supportive aids; and specific information about which surgeon or anesthesiologist wishes to be notified.
2. respiratory function (ventilation); hypoxemia and hypercapnia
3. Hypovolemic, cardiogenic, neurogenic, anaphylactic, and septic
4. *Primary* hemorrhage occurs at the time of the operation. *Intermediary* hemorrhage occurs within the first few hours after surgery when a return of blood pressure to its normal level dislodges insecure clots. *Secondary* hemorrhage occurs some time after the operation as a result of the slipping of a ligature, which may happen because of infection, insecure tying, or erosion of a vessel by a drainage tube.
5. respiratory
6. Patient-controlled analgesia refers to self-administration of pain medication by way of intravenous or epidural routes within prescribed time/dosage limits.
7. Atelectasis and hypostatic pneumonia are reduced with early ambulation because ventilation is increased and the stasis of bronchial secretions in the lungs is reduced.
8. paralytic ileus and intestinal obstruction
9. bowel sounds, and the passage of flatus
10. Wound dehiscence refers to the disruption of the wound or surgical incision. Wound evisceration refers to the protrusion of wound contents.

II. Critical Thinking Questions and Exercises

DISCUSSION AND ANALYSIS
1. Refer to Chart 20-1 in the text.
2. Refer to Figure 20-1 in the text.
3. Pallor; cool, moist skin; tachypnea, cyanosis (lips, gums, tongue); rapid, weak, and thready pulse; narrowing pulse pressure; hypotension and concentrated urine.
4. Refer to Figure 20-3 and chapter heading "Determining Readiness for Discharge From the PACU" in the text.
5. Refer to chapter heading "The Hospitalized Patient Recovering From Surgery" in the text.
6. The respiratory depressive effects of opioids, decreased lung expansion secondary to pain, and decreased mobility are three conditions that put patients at risk for atelectasis, pneumonia, and hypoxemia.
7. Refer to Table 20-3 in the text.
8. Refer to chapter heading "Managing Potential Complications" in the text.

IDENTIFYING PATTERNS
FLOW CHART: POSTOPERATIVE CARE

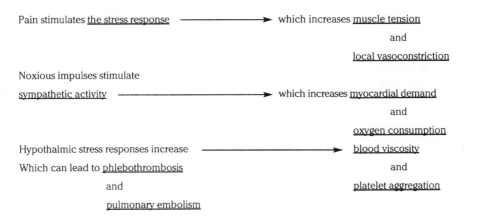

Pain stimulates the stress response ⟶ which increases muscle tension
and
local vasoconstriction

Noxious impulses stimulate sympathetic activity ⟶ which increases myocardial demand
and
oxygen consumption

Hypothalmic stress responses increase ⟶ blood viscosity
and
platelet aggregation

Which can lead to phlebothrombosis
and
pulmonary embolism

CLINICAL SITUATIONS

CASE STUDY: HYPOVOLEMIC SHOCK

1. b   4. a
2. b   5. b
3. a

CASE STUDY: HYPOPHARYNGEAL OBSTRUCTION

1. d   3. d
2. b   4. c

CASE STUDY: WOUND HEALING

1. b   3. d
2. a   4. b

Chapter 21

I. Interpretation, Completion, and Comparison

MULTIPLE CHOICE

1. d	12. a	23. a
2. b	13. a	24. d
3. c	14. a	25. a
4. a	15. b	26. a
5. c	16. d	27. c
6. a	17. c	28. b
7. b	18. a	29. b
8. b	19. d	30. b
9. b	20. c	31. c
10. d	21. d	32. d
11. b	22. d	33. d

SHORT ANSWER

1. Ventilation refers to the movement of air in and out of the airways, whereas respiration refers to gas exchange between atmospheric air and blood and between the blood and the cells of the body.
2. The epiglottis is a flap of cartilage that covers the opening of the larynx during swallowing.
3. Low or decreased compliance occurs with certain pathology. Answer should include four of the following: morbid obesity, atelectasis, pneumothorax, hemothorax, pulmonary fibrosis or edema, pleural effusion, and ARDS.
4. Partial pressure is the pressure exerted by each type of gas (e.g., oxygen, carbon dioxide) in a mixture of gases.
5. The *apneustic center* in the lower pons, and the *pneumotaxic center* in the upper pons.
6. 50
7. dyspnea, cough, sputum production, chest pain, wheezing and hemoptysis
8. asthma, COPD, cystic fibrosis, and alpha-1 antitrypsin deficiency

9. Cheyne–Stokes respirations are characterized by alternating episodes of apnea (cessation of breathing) and periods of deep breathing. It is usually associated with heart failure and damage to the respiratory center.

II. Critical Thinking Questions and Exercises

DISCUSSION AND ANALYSIS

1. Refer to chapter heading "Function of the Respiratory System" in the text.
2. Refer to Chart 21-1 in the text.
3. Refer to Table 21-1 in the text.
4. Diffusion is the exchange of oxygen and carbon dioxide at the air–blood interface. Pulmonary perfusion is the actual flow of blood through the pulmonary circulation.
5. Refer to Table 21-2 in the text.
6. Oxygen is carried in the blood dissolved in plasma or combined with hemoglobin. The higher the PaO_2, the greater the amount of dissolved oxygen.
7. Refer to chapter heading "Dyspnea" in the text.
8. Refer to Table 21-6 in the text.
9. Refer to chapter heading "Voice Sounds" in the text.

CLINICAL SITUATIONS

CASE STUDY: BRONCHOSCOPY

1. c   4. d
2. d   5. a
3. b

CASE STUDY: THORACENTESIS

1. d   4. d
2. b   5. c
3. b

INTERPRETING DATA

For an explanation of the oxyhemoglobin dissociation curve, see Chart 21-4 and chapter heading "Oxyhemoglobin Dissociation Curve" in the text.

Chapter 22

I. Interpretation, Completion, and Comparison

MULTIPLE CHOICE

1. a	8. d	15. b
2. d	9. a	16. b
3. a	10. c	17. b
4. b	11. d	18. a
5. d	12. a	19. d
6. a	13. a	20. d
7. d	14. d	

SHORT ANSWER

1. Rhinitis causes the nasal passages to become inflamed, congested, and edematous. The swollen conchae block the sinus openings and cause sinusitis.
2. *Streptococcus pneumoniae*, *Haemophilus influenzae*, *Staphylococcus aureus*, and *Moraxella catarrhalis*
3. Answer should include four of the following: severe orbital cellulitis, subperiosteal abscess, cavernous sinus thrombosis, meningitis, encephalitis, and ischemic infarction.
4. hemorrhage
5. viral; symptoms include hoarseness, aphonia, and severe cough
6. Refer to chapter heading "The Patient With Upper Airway Infection" in the text.
7. Complications may include sepsis, a peritonsillar abscess, otitis media, sinusitis, and meningitis.
8. Obstructive sleep apnea is defined as frequent loud snoring and breathing cessation for 10 seconds or longer with five or more episodes per hour. This is followed by awakening abruptly with a loud snort when the blood oxygen level drops.
9. esophageal speech, an artificial larynx, and tracheoesophageal puncture

II. Critical Thinking Questions and Exercises

DISCUSSION AND ANALYSIS

1. Refer to Chart 22-1 in the text.
2. Refer to chapter heading "Pharyngitis" in the text.
3. Refer to chapter heading "Epistaxis (Nosebleed)" in the text.

CLINICAL SITUATIONS

CASE STUDY: TONSILLECTOMY AND ADENOIDECTOMY

1. d   3. a
2. c   4. c

CASE STUDY: EPITAXIES

1. Gilberta should sit upright with her head tilted forward to prevent swallowing and aspiration of blood. She should also pinch the soft outer portion of the nose against the midline spectrum for 5 to 10 continuous minutes.
2. d
3. b
4. d

CASE STUDY: CANCER OF THE LARYNX

1. Refer to Chart 22-7 in the text.
2. squamous cell carcinoma
3. b
4. 60%, 75% to 95%
5. radiation therapy or surgery
6. 2 to 3 years

CASE STUDY: LARYNGECTOMY

1. b
2. d
3. d
4. respiratory distress, hypoxia, hemorrhage, infection, wound breakdown, and aspiration
5. d
6. Answer should include increase in temperature, tachycardia, purulent drainage, odor, redness or tenderness at the surgical site, and increased WBCs.
7. d
8. carotid artery rupture

APPLYING CONCEPTS

Refer to Chart 22-6 in the text.

Chapter 23

I. Interpretation, Completion, and Comparison

MULTIPLE CHOICE

1. d	12. d	23. c
2. a	13. a	24. a
3. c	14. a	25. a
4. d	15. d	26. a
5. d	16. c	27. a
6. c	17. a	28. b
7. a	18. d	29. a
8. a	19. b	30. b
9. c	20. b	31. c
10. d	21. d	
11. d	22. c	

SHORT ANSWER

1. Refer to Figure 23-1 and chapter heading "Atelectasis" in the text.
2. dyspnea, cough, sputum production, tachycardia, tachypnea, pleural pain, and central cyanosis
3. frequent turning, early mobilization, deep breathing maneuvers, assistance with the use of spirometry, suctioning, postural drainage, aerosol nebulizer treatments, and chest percussion
4. impaired host defenses, an inoculum of organisms that reach the lower respiratory tract, and the presence of a highly virulent organism
5. *Streptococcus pneumoniae*, *Haemophilus influenzae*, and *Staphylococcus aureus*
6. alcoholism, COPD, AIDS, diabetes, and heart failure
7. hypotension, shock, and respiratory failure
8. Superinfection is suspected when a subsequent infection occurs with another bacteria during antibiotic therapy.
9. impaired CNS function, neuromuscular, musculoskeletal, and pulmonary dysfunction
10. 60%; nonpulmonary, multiple-system organ failure

11. hypoxemia that does not respond to supplemental oxygen
12. enlargement of the right ventricle of the heart because of diseases affecting the structure or functions of the lung
13. 16%

II. Critical Thinking Questions and Exercises

DISCUSSION AND ANALYSIS

1. Refer to chapter heading "Atelectasis" in the text.
2. Refer to Table 23-2 in the text.
3. The clinical picture is characterized by tachycardia, dyspnea, central cyanosis, hypertension, hypotension, and ultimately death

4. Refer to chapter heading "Severe Acute Respiratory Syndrome" in the text.
5. Refer to chapter heading "Empyema" in the text.
6. Inadequate left ventricular function leads to a backup of blood into the pulmonary vasculature, which causes increased microvascular pressure. Fluid leaks into the interstitial space and alveoli.
7. Refer to Chart 23-6 in the text.
8. Refer to Chart 23-8 in the text.
9. Refer to chapter headings "Sarcoidosis" and "Occupational Lung Diseases: Pneumoconioses" in the text.
10. Refer to chapter heading "Types of Pneumothorax" in the text.

INTERPRETING PATTERNS

FLOW CHART: THE PATHOPHYSIOLOGY OF PNEUMONIA

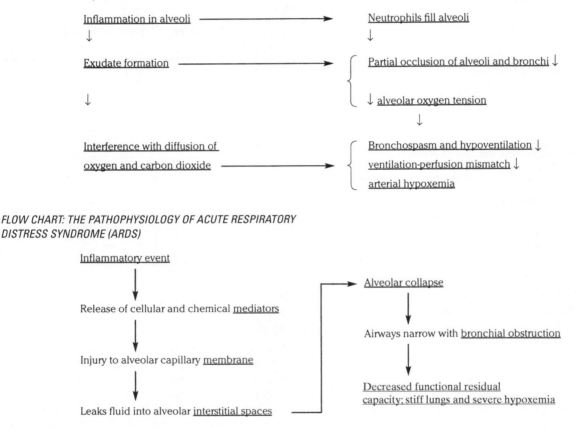

FLOW CHART: THE PATHOPHYSIOLOGY OF ACUTE RESPIRATORY DISTRESS SYNDROME (ARDS)

CLINICAL SITUATIONS

CASE STUDY: COMMUNITY-ACQUIRED PNEUMONIA

1. d	4. d
2. b	5. b
3. d	6. d

CASE STUDY: TUBERCULOSIS

1. b	4. b
2. b	5. c
3. d	

CASE STUDY: ADULT RESPIRATORY DISTRESS SYNDROME (ARDS)

1. d	4. d
2. d	5. d
3. c	

CASE STUDY: PULMONARY EMBOLISM

1. c	5. b
2. a	6. c
3. b	7. d
4. a	

APPLYING CONCEPTS

Refer to Figure 23-2 in the text.

Chapter 24

I. Interpretation, Completion, and Comparison

MULTIPLE CHOICE

1. c	7. d	13. b
2. d	8. d	14. a
3. d	9. b	15. c
4. d	10. b	16. c
5. b	11. d	17. c
6. b	12. c	18. d

SHORT ANSWER

1. chronic inflammation that results in the following: increased goblet cells and enlarged submucosal glands (proximal airways), inflammation and airway narrowing (peripheral airways), and narrowing of the airway lumen.
2. Emphysema is an abnormal distention of the air spaces, beyond the terminal bronchioles, that results in destruction of the walls of the alveoli.
3. a deficiency in alpha-antitrypsin, an enzyme inhibitor that protects the lungs
4. chronic cough, sputum production, and dyspnea on exertion
5. Answer should include five of the following: history of cigarette smoking, passive smoking exposure, age, rate

of decline of FEV_1, hypoxemia, weight loss, reversibility of airflow obstruction, pulmonary artery pressure, and resting heart rate.
6. cessation of smoking
7. alter smooth muscle tone, reduce airway obstruction, and improve alveolar ventilation
8. tracheobronchial infection, and air pollution
9. *Streptococcus pneumoniae* and *Haemophilus influenzae*
10. allergy; cough, wheezing, and dyspnea
11. status asthmaticus, respiratory failure, pneumonia, and atelectasis
12. 37 years

II. Critical Thinking Questions and Exercises

DISCUSSION AND ANALYSIS

1. Refer to Charts 24-1 and 24-2 and chapter heading "Chronic Obstructive Pulmonary Disease" in the text.
2. Refer to Table 24-1 in the text.
3. Refer to chapter heading "Oxygen Therapy" in the text.
4. Refer to chapter heading "Asthma" in the text.
5. Refer to Table 24-4 in the text.
6. The person exhibits labored breathing, prolonged exhalation, engorged neck veins, and wheezing. As obstruction worsens and wheezing may disappear, respiratory failure may occur.

IDENTIFYING PATTERNS

The Pathophysiology of Chronic Bronchitis

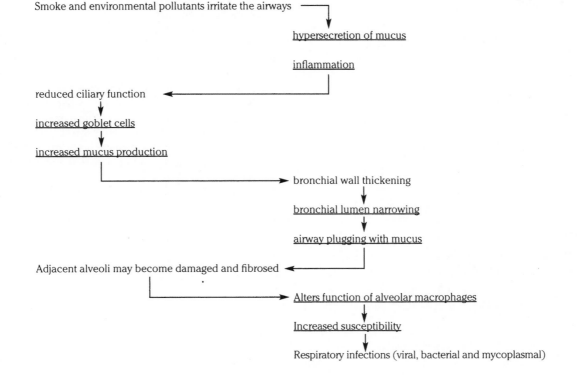

The Pathophysiology of Emphysema

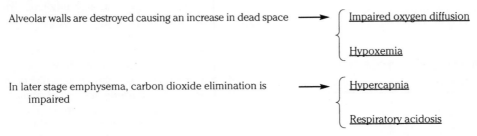

Alveolar walls are destroyed causing an increase in dead space ⟶ { <u>Impaired oxygen diffusion</u>

<u>Hypoxemia</u> }

In later stage emphysema, carbon dioxide elimination is impaired ⟶ { <u>Hypercapnia</u>

<u>Respiratory acidosis</u> }

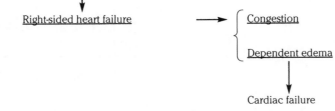

As the alveolar walls breakdown, the pulmonary capillary bed is reduced, causing increased pulmonary blood flow

↓

<u>Right-sided heart failure</u> ⟶ { <u>Congestion</u>

<u>Dependent edema</u> }

↓

Cardiac failure

CLINICAL SITUATIONS

CASE STUDY: EMPHYSEMA

1. c   4. d
2. b   5. b
3. a   6. d

Chapter 25

I. Interpretation, Completion, and Comparison

MULTIPLE CHOICE

1. a	11. c	21. c
2. b	12. d	22. a
3. a	13. d	23. c
4. b	14. d	24. d
5. d	15. a	25. c
6. d	16. c	26. c
7. b	17. a	27. b
8. c	18. d	28. d
9. d	19. b	29. d
10. a	20. d	

SHORT ANSWER

1. cardiac output, arterial oxygen content, hemoglobin concentration, and metabolic requirements
2. >50%, >48 hours
3. Answer should include five of the following: substernal discomfort, paresthesias, dyspnea, restlessness, fatigue, malaise, progressive respiratory difficulty, refractory hypoxemia, alveolar atelectasis, and alveolar infiltrates on x-ray.
4. decreased blood oxygen rather than elevated carbon dioxide levels
5. nasal cannula, oropharyngeal catheter, simple mask, partial-rebreather, and nonrebreather
6. 6 L/min
7. dislodge mucus and remove bronchial secretions, improve ventilation, and increase the efficiency of the respiratory muscles
8. 15 and 20 mm Hg, 6 to 8 hours
9. iron lung, body wrap, and chest cuirass
10. Positive pressure ventilators inflate the lungs by exerting pressure on the airway, pushing air in, forcing the alveoli to expand during inspiration.
11. A patient "bucks the ventilator" when his or her breathing is out of phase with the machine. This occurs when the patient attempts to breathe out during the ventilator's mechanical inspiratory phase or when there is jerky and increased abdominal muscle effort.
12. Refer to chapter heading "The Patient Receiving Mechanical Ventilation" in the text.
13. 10 to15 mL/K, 6 L/min, 7 to 9 mL/kg
14. Refer to Chart 25-18 in the text.

COMPLETE THE CHART

Refer to the figure in Chart 25-19 and chapter heading "Chest Drainage" in the text.

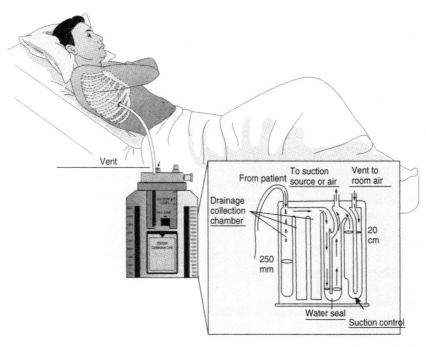

II. Critical Thinking Questions and Exercises

EXAMINING ASSOCIATIONS

1. decreased arterial oxygen tension in the blood
2. 80% to 98%
3. 12 L/min, 80% to 100%
4. inadequate capillary circulation
5. 12 to 16 per minute

DISCUSSION AND ANALYSIS

1. Refer to chapter heading "Oxygen Therapy" in the text.
2. Refer to chapter heading "Suppression of Ventilation" in the text.
3. Refer to Figure 25-4 and chapter heading "Breathing Retraining" in the text.
4. Refer to chapter heading "Breathing Retraining" in the text.
5. Refer to Chart 25-6 in the text.
6. Refer to Chart 25-10 in the text.
7. Refer to Chart 25-16 in the text.
8. Refer to Chart 25-17 in the text.
9. Refer to Chart 25-19 in the text.

APPLYING CONCEPTS: CARE OF A PATIENT WITH AN ENDOTRACHEAL TUBE

Refer to Charts 25-7 and 25-8 in the text.

CLINICAL SITUATIONS

CASE STUDY: PNEUMONECTOMY: PREOPERATIVE CONCERNS

1. d	3. d
2. a	4. a

CASE STUDY: PNEUMONECTOMY: POSTOPERATIVE CONCERNS

1. a	3. d
2. b	4. a

CASE STUDY: VENTILATOR PATIENT

1. d	3. d
2. a	4. d

CASE STUDY: WEANING FROM THE VENTILATOR

1. d	3. d
2. d	

Chapter 26

I. Interpretation, Completion, and Comparison

MULTIPLE CHOICE

1. a	7. d	13. a
2. a	8. d	14. b
3. d	9. c	15. d
4. d	10. c	16. d
5. c	11. a	
6. c	12. c	

SHORT ANSWER

1. hypertension, coronary artery disease, heart failure, stroke, and congenital cardiovascular defects
2. The atrioventricular (AV) valves separate the atria from the ventricles. The tricuspid separates the right atrium and ventricle; the bicuspid separates the left atrium and ventricle. The AV valves permit blood to flow from the atria into the ventricles. The semilunar valves are situated between each ventricle and its corresponding artery. The pulmonic valve is between the right ventricle and the pulmonary artery; the aortic valve is between the left ventricle and the aorta. These valves permit blood to flow from the ventricles into the arteries.
3. Depolarization is said to have occurred when the electrical difference between the inside and the outside of the cell is reduced. The inside of the cell becomes less negative, membrane permeability to calcium is increased, and muscle contraction occurs.
4. Preload, afterload, and contractility
5. Cardiac output (stroke volume × heart rate) would equal 5,320 mL.
6. Starling's law of the heart refers to the relationship between increased stroke volume and increased ventricular end-diastolic volume for a given intrinsic contractility.
7. Physiologic effects of the aging process may include reduction in the size of the left ventricle, decreased elasticity and widening of the aorta, thickening and rigidity of cardiac valves, and increased connective tissue in the sinoatrial and atrioventricular nodes and bundle branches.
8. hyperlipidemia, hypertension, and diabetes mellitus
9. LDL <70 mg/dL; BP <140/90 mm Hg; serum glucose <110 mg/day; and a BMI of 18.5 to 24.9 kg/m².
10. below the fifth intercostal space and lateral to the mid-clavicular line
11. creatine kinase (CK) and isoenzyme CK-MB; Troponin T and I and myoglobin
12. Cardiac catheterization is used most frequently to assess the patency of the patient's coronary arteries and to determine readiness for coronary bypass surgery. It is also used to measure pressures in the various heart chambers and to determine oxygen saturation of the blood by sampling specimens.
13. Selective angiography refers to the technique of injecting a contrast medium into the vascular system to outline a particular heart chamber of blood vessel.
14. A lowered central venous pressure reading indicates that the patient is hypovolemic. Serial measurements are more reflective of a patient's condition and should be correlated with the patient's clinical status.
15. Answer should include any four of the following: infection, pulmonary artery rupture, pulmonary thromboembolism, pulmonary infarction, catheter kinking, dysrhythmias, and air embolism.

MATCHING

1. c	4. d
2. e	5. b
3. a	6. f

MATCHING

1. d	7. b
2. g	8. j
3. a	9. c
4. f	10. h
5. i	11. e
6. k	

II. Critical Thinking Questions and Exercises

DISCUSSION AND ANALYSIS

1. Refer to chapter heading "Coronary Artery Disease" in the text.
2. Refer to Table 26-1 in the text.
3. Refer to Table 26-2 in the text.
4. Refer to Chart 26-1 in the text.
5. Type A personalities are competitive, hard-driving, and exhibit a sense of time urgency. This type personality tends to react to frustrating events with increased blood pressure, heart rate, and neuroendocrine responses. This physiologic activation, which is believed to cause cardiovascular events, is known as "cardiac reactivity."
6. Refer to Chart 26-3 in the text.
7. Refer to chapter heading "Gallop Sounds" and Figure 26-8 in the text.
8. Refer to chapter heading "Telemetry" in the text.

EXAMINING ASSOCIATIONS

Refer to Table 26-2 in the text.
1. the remainder of the body
2. Myocardium
3. third intercostal space
4. the aortic and pulmonic valves
5. abrasion of the pericardial surfaces

INTERPRETING DATA

	Angina Pectoris	Pericarditis
Duration of pain	5 to 15 minutes	Intermittent
Precipitating events and aggravating factors	Exertion, emotional stress, a large meal, exposure to temperature extremes.	Sudden onset; pain increases with inspiration, coughing, and trunk rotation
Alleviating factors	Rest, nitroglycerin, oxygen	Sitting upright, analgesics, and anti-inflammatory agents

CLINICAL SITUATIONS

CASE STUDY: CARDIAC ASSESSMENT OF CHEST PAIN

1. c
2. d
3. c
4. d
5. b

Chapter 27

I. Interpretation, Completion, and Comparison

MULTIPLE CHOICE

1. d	7. b	13. c
2. b	8. d	14. d
3. c	9. c	15. c
4. b	10. b	16. d
5. d	11. a	17. d
6. a	12. d	18. d

SHORT ANSWER

1. atria, atrioventricular node or junction, sinus node, and ventricles
2. Electrical conduction through the heart begins in the sinoatrial node (SA), travels across the atria to the atrioventricular node (AV), and then travels down the right and left bundle branches and Purkinje fibers to the ventricular muscle.
3. Answer should include five of the following: fever, hypovolemia, anemia, exercise, pain, congestive heart failure, anxiety, and sympathomimetic or parasympatholytic drugs.
4. 100 bpm
5. Ventricular tachycardia occurs when there is more than three PVCs in a row and the rate exceeds 100 bpm
6. a thromboembolic event, heart failure, and cardiac arrest
7. The difference is in the timing of the electrical current. With cardioversion, the current is synchronized with the patient's electrical events; with defibrillation, the current is unsynchronized and immediate.
8. The standard procedure is to place one paddle to the right of the upper sternum below the right clavicle and the other paddle just to the left of the cardiac apex.
9. An on-demand pacemaker is set for a specific rate and stimulates the heart when normal ventricular depolarization does not occur; the fixed rate pacemaker stimulates the ventricle at a preset constant rate, independently of the patient's rhythm.
10. Small incisions are made throughout the atria so that scar tissue forms and prevents reentry conduction of the electrical impulse.

SCRAMBLEGRAM

1. dysrhythmic
2. automaticity
3. conductivity
4. depolarization
5. diastole
6. ablation

II. Critical Thinking Questions and Exercises

EXAMINING ASSOCIATIONS

1. ventricular muscle
2. repolarization
3. U wave
4. sinus bradycardia
5. Pronestyl
6. 3:2 or 4:3

CLINICAL SITUATIONS

GRAPH ANALYSIS

1. a. T wave
   b. PR interval
   c. P wave
   d. QRS complex
   e. ST segment
2. a. Q wave is larger
   b. ST segment is elevated
   c. T wave is inverted

GRAPHIC RECORDINGS

1. P waves come early in cycle and close to T wave of previous heartbeat.
2. QRS complex is bizarre. P waves are hidden in QRS complexes.
3. Three or more PVCs in a row, occurring at a rate 100 bpm.

CASE STUDY: PERMANENT PACEMAKER

1. Yes. Heart rate can vary as much as 5 bpm faster or slower than the preset rate.
2. bleeding, hematoma formation, and infection
3. hemothorax, ventricular ectopy and tachycardia, dislocation of the lead and phrenic nerve, diaphragmatic or skeletal muscle stimulation
4. dislodgment of the pacing electrode
5. a. pacemaker model
   b. date and time of insertion
   c. stimulation threshold
   d. pacer rate
   e. incision appearance
   f. patient tolerance
6. GOALS
   a. absence of infection
   b. adherence to a self-care program
   c. maintenance of pacemaker function
   NURSING ACTIVITIES
   a. sterile wound care
   b. patient teaching
   c. patient teaching
   EXPECTED OUTCOMES
   a. free from infection
   b. adheres to a self-care program
   c. maintains pacemaker function
7. a. has a normal temperature, white blood cells within normal range, and no evidence of redness or swelling at insertion site.
   b. understands sign and symptoms of infection and knows when to seek medical attention.
   c. assesses pulse rate at regular intervals and experiences no abrupt changes in pulse rate or rhythm.

Chapter 28

I. Interpretation, Completion, and Comparison

MULTIPLE CHOICE

1. b	11. b	21. c
2. d	12. a	22. a
3. a	13. b	23. b
4. c	14. a	24. d
5. d	15. b	25. d
6. c	16. a	26. b
7. a	17. b	27. c
8. a	18. c	28. a
9. c	19. c	
10. a	20. d	

SHORT ANSWER

1. cardiovascular disease
2. atherosclerosis
3. chest pain referred to as *angina pectoris*
4. age; more than 50% are older than 65 years of age
5. Answer should include four of the following: hyperlipidemia, cigarette smoking, obesity, hypertension, diabetes mellitus, metabolic syndrome, and physical activity.
6. insulin resistance, central obesity, dyslipidemia, hypertension (>130/85 mm Hg), increased levels of C-reactive protein (proinflammation), and elevated fibrinogen levels (prothrombotic)
7. less than 200 mg/dL; 3.5:1.0; less than 100 mg/dL; greater than 60 mg/dL; 150 mg/dL
8. 25% to 35%
9. Answer should include three of the following: acute coronary syndrome or myocardial infarction, dysrhythmias, cardiac arrest, heart failure, and cardiogenic shock.
10. an elevated ST segment in two contiguous leads
11. greater saphenous vein
12. Answer should include four of the following: fever, pericardial pain, pleural pain, dyspnea, pericardial effusion, pericardial friction rub, and arthralgia.

II. Critical Thinking Questions and Exercises

DISCUSSION AND ANALYSIS

1. Atherosclerosis, the abnormal accumulation of lipid substances, causes a repetitive inflammatory response that alters the structure and biochemical properties of the arterial walls.
2. Cigarette smoking contributes to coronary heart disease in three ways. *Smoke inhalation* increases the level of blood carbon monoxide by causing hemoglobin to combine more readily with carbon monoxide than with oxygen. *Nicotinic acid* triggers the release of catecholamines, which raise heart rate and blood pressure and cause the coronary arteries to constrict. *Smoking* causes a detrimental vascular response and increases platelet adhesion, increasing the probability of thrombus formation.
3. Refer to Table 28-2 in the text.
4. Refer to Chart 28-2 in the text.
5. Refer to chapter heading "Angina Pectoris" in the text.
6. Refer to Chart 28-4 in the text.
7. Refer to Chart 28-6 in the text.
8. Refer to chapter heading "Emergent Percutaneous Coronary Intervention" in the text.
9. Refer to Table 28-5 in the text.

EXAMINING ASSOCIATIONS

1. The profile of those at highest risk for a cardiac event in 10 years.
2. Metabolic syndrome, a significant risk factor for coronary artery disease.
3. Factors, weighted by points, that indicate increased risk of having a cardiac event.
4. Modified risk factors for coronary artery disease.
5. Four primary factors of fat metabolism that affect the development of heart disease.

IDENTIFYING PATTERNS

1. Arterial lumen narrowing begins with the deposit of fatty streaks (lipids) on the intima (inner vessel wall) of the artery. Some develop into advanced lesions as atherosclerosis advances. An inflammatory response occurs and macrophages infiltrate the area, ingest and transport lipids into the arterial wall. Smooth muscle cells then proliferate and form a fibrous cap around a dead fatty core. These deposits called atheromas narrow and obstruct blood flow. A ruptured plaque can form a thrombus.
2. An atheroma, also called plaque, is a fibrous cap of smooth muscle cells that form over lipid deposits within the arterial vessels, protrude and narrow the lumen, and then obstruct blood flow.
3. The formation of a thrombus.
4. A thrombus can obstruct blood flow, cause an acute myocardial infarction, or result in sudden death.

SUPPORTING ARGUMENTS

1. (a) *Increased CO levels*: Hemoglobin combines more readily with CO than with O_2, thereby limiting the oxygen being supplied to the heart.
   (b) *Increased catecholamines*: Nicotine triggers the release of catecholamines, which cause arterial constriction and decreased oxygenation.
   (c) *Increased platelet adhesion*: Smoking increases platelet adhesion, which increases thrombus formation.
2. Calcium channel blockers are helpful adjuncts to medical management because they increase myocardial oxygen supply by (a) dilating the smooth muscle wall of the coronary arterioles, (b) decreasing myocardial oxygen demands, and (c) decreasing systemic arterial pressure.

CLINICAL SITUATIONS

CASE STUDY: ANGINA PECTORIS

1. b
2. c

3. b
4. c

CASE STUDY: DECREASED MYOCARDIAL TISSUE PERFUSION

1. a
2. b
3. b
4. thrombolytics; alteplase, and reteplase
5. a
6. b
7. a
8. d
9. the ability to walk 3 to 4 miles in an hour

Chapter 29

I. Interpretation, Completion, and Comparison

MULTIPLE CHOICE

1. d
2. b
3. c
4. c
5. a
6. a
7. d

8. c
9. c
10. a
11. c
12. b
13. a
14. a

15. d
16. b
17. a
18. b
19. a

SHORT ANSWER

1. Mitral valve prolapse is usually an inherited connective tissue disorder that causes enlargement of both mitral valve leaflets. Usually there are no symptoms. It can result in valve incompetency and regurgitation. As valve dysfunction progresses, symptoms of heart failure ensue.
2. caffeine, alcohol, and smoking
3. at the third and fourth intercostal spaces at the left sternal border, a blowing diastolic murmur
4. prophylactic antibiotics
5. Answer should include four of the following: congestive heart failure, ventricular dysrhythmias, atrial dysrhythmias, cardiac conduction defects, pulmonary or cerebral embolism, and valvular dysfunction.
6. cardiomyopathy, ischemic heart disease, valvular disease, rejection of previously transplanted hearts, and congenital heart disease
7. penicillin therapy, rheumatic fever
8. An inflamed endothelium causes a fibrin clot to form (vegetation), which converts to scar tissue that thickens, contracts, and causes deformities. The result is leakage or valvular regurgitation and stenosis.
9. streptococci, enterococci, pneumococci, and staphylococci
10. Myocarditis is an inflammatory process that usually results from an infection. The infectious process can cause heart dilation, thrombi formation, infiltration of blood cells around the coronary vessels and between the muscle fibers, and eventual degeneration of the muscle fibers themselves.
11. digitalis; digitalis toxicity
12. Listen at the left sternal edge of the thorax in the fourth intercostal space where the pericardium comes in contact with the left chest wall.

MATCHING

1. a
2. e
3. d

4. b
5. c

II. Critical Thinking Questions and Exercises

DISCUSSION AND ANALYSIS

1. On auscultation, an extra heart sound will be heard. This *mitral click* is an early sign that the valve leaflet is ballooning into the left atrium. Sometimes a murmur can be heard if the valve leaflet has stretched and regurgitation has occurred.
2. Left ventricular hypertrophy develops with mitral valve insufficiency because incomplete valve closure allows a regurgitation of blood from the left ventricle to the atrium during ventricular systole. This regurgitated blood is returned to the left ventricle, increasing the volume of blood that the left ventricle must handle. Hypertrophy of the left atrium and the left ventricle develops.
3. In aortic regurgitation, blood from the aorta returns to the left ventricle during diastole. Left ventricular dilation occurs. Left ventricular hypertrophy occurs, raising systolic blood pressure. Reflex vasodilation results as a compensatory measure. Peripheral arterioles relax, reducing peripheral resistance and diastolic blood pressure.
4. The characteristic sound is a systolic crescendo–decrescendo murmur that is low-pitched, rough, rasping, and vibrating.
5. Refer to Figure 29-3 and chapter heading "Closed Commissurotomy/Balloon Valvuloplasty" in the text.
6. Refer to Figure 29-6 and chapter heading "Valve Replacement" in the text.
7. Refer to chapter heading "Nursing Management: Valvuloplasty and Replacement" in the text.
8. All cardiomyopathies result in impaired cardiac output. The decrease in stroke volume stimulates the sympathetic nervous system and the renin–angiotensin–aldosterone response, resulting in increased systemic vascular resistance and increased sodium and fluid retention. These alterations can lead to heart failure.
9. Refer to chapter heading "The Patient With Cardiomyopathy" in the text.
10. Refer to Chart 29-4 and chapter heading "Pericarditis" in the text.

IDENTIFYING PATTERNS

FLOW CHART: MITRAL VALVE STENOSIS

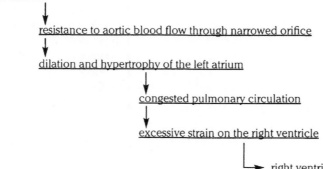

Mitral valve stenosis

↓

resistance to aortic blood flow through narrowed orifice

↓

dilation and hypertrophy of the left atrium

↓

congested pulmonary circulation

↓

excessive strain on the right ventricle

→ right ventricular failure

CLINICAL SITUATIONS

CASE STUDY: INFECTIVE ENDOCARDITIS

1. toxicity of the infection, heart valve destruction, or embolization of fragments of vegetative growth on the heart
2. a
3. headache, transient cerebral ischemia, focal neurologic lesions, and strokes
4. total eradication of the invading organism
5. c
6. congestive heart failure, strokes, valvular stenosis, and myocardial erosion
7. d

CASE STUDY: ACUTE PERICARDITIS

1. a
2. pain related to inflammation of the pericardium
3. d
4. analgesics, antibiotics, and corticosteroids
5. left sternal edge in the fourth intercostal space
6. freedom from pain and absence of complications

Chapter 30

I. Interpretation, Completion, and Comparison

MULTIPLE CHOICE

1. a	11. b	21. d
2. a	12. d	22. d
3. d	13. a	23. b
4. b	14. b	24. a
5. b	15. a	25. d
6. c	16. c	26. c
7. b	17. a	27. a
8. d	18. d	28. b
9. b	19. d	29. c
10. c	20. b	

MATCHING

1. a	6. a
2. b	7. a
3. a	8. b
4. b	9. a
5. b	10. b

SHORT ANSWER

1. Cardiac output equals the heart rate times the stroke volume (the amount of blood pumped out with each contraction).
2. Preload is the amount of myocardial stretch created by the volume of blood within the ventricle before systole. Afterload refers to the amount of resistance to the ejection of the blood from the ventricle.
3. Venous return and ventricular compliance. The diameter/distensibility of the great vessels and the opening/competence of the semilunar valves.
4. jugular venous distention; mean arterial blood pressure; a positive hepatojugular test
5. coronary artery disease, cardiomyopathy, hypertension, and valvular disorders
6. hypoxia and acidosis result from the accumulation of lactic acid
7. dilated, hypertrophic, and restrictive; dilated
8. dyspnea, cough, pulmonary crackles, low oxygen saturation, and a probable extra heart sound (ventricular gallop)
9. dependent edema, hepatomegaly, ascites, anorexia, nausea, weakness, and weight gain (fluid retention).
10. ACE inhibitors, beta-blockers, diuretics, and digitalis
11. Answer should include four of the following six: symptomatic hypotension, hyperuricemia, ototoxicity, electrolyte imbalances, dizziness, and balance problems.
12. weak pulse, faint heart sounds, hypotension, muscle flabbiness, diminished deep tendon reflexes, and generalized weakness
13. end-stage heart failure, cardiac tamponade, pulmonary embolism, cardiomyopathy, myocardial ischemia and dysrhythmias
14. pulmonary embolism
15. 100; 30:2

II. Critical Thinking Questions and Exercises

DISCUSSION AND ANALYSIS

1. The ejection factor (EF), an indication of the volume of blood ejected with each contraction, is calculated by subtracting the amount of blood at the end of systole from the amount of blood at the end of diastole and calculating the percentage of blood that is ejected. A normal EF is 55% to 65% of ventricular volume.
2. Refer to Figure 30-2 and chapter heading "Heart Failure" in the text.
3. Refer to Chart 30-1, Figure 30-2, and chapter headings "Left-Sided Heart Failure" and "Right-Sided Heart Failure" in the text.
4. Refer to chapter heading "Other Interventions" in the text.
5. Refer to Table 30-3 in the text.
6. Refer to chapter heading "The Patient With Heart Failure" in the text.
7. Refer to Figure 30-4 and chapter heading "Cardiogenic Shock" in the text.
8. Refer to Figure 30-7, Table 30-4, and chapter heading "Emergency Management: Cardiopulmonary Resuscitation" in the text.

IDENTIFYING PATTERNS

FLOW CHART: THE PATHOPHYSIOLOGY OF PULMONARY EDEMA

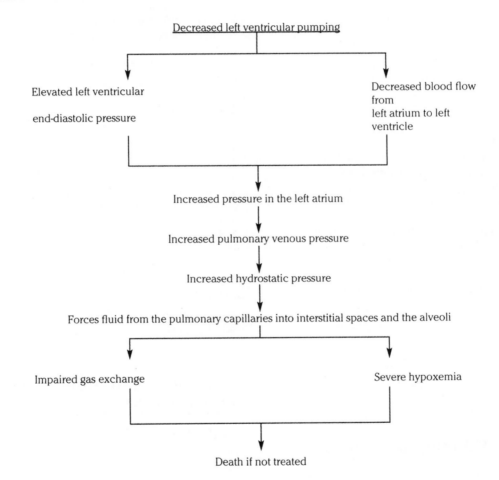

CLINICAL SITUATIONS

CASE STUDY: PULMONARY EDEMA

1. cardiac disease
2. a
3. d
4. b
5. d
6 d

Chapter 31

I. Interpretation, Completion, and Comparison

MULTIPLE CHOICE

1. d	9. b	17. d
2. b	10. d	18. d
3. b	11. d	19. c
4. a	12. b	20. d
5. a	13. b	21. d
6. b	14. d	22. b
7. b	15. d	23. a
8. c	16. a	

SHORT ANSWER

1. a driving pressure generated by the blood pressure; the pulling force created by plasma proteins
2. Intermittent claudication
3. Refer to chapter heading "Dissecting Aorta" in the text.
4. Pain, pallor, pulselessness, paresthesia, poikilothermia (coldness), and paralysis.
5. venous stasis, vessel wall injury, and altered blood coagulation
6. edema, altered pigmentation, pain, and stasis dermatitis

MATCHING

1. a	5. b
2. b	6. b
3. a	7. a
4. a	8. a

II. Critical Thinking Questions and Exercises

DISCUSSION AND ANALYSIS

1. The rate of blood flow through a vessel is determined by dividing the pressure difference (ΔP) (arterial and venous) by the resistance to flow (R).
2. The pain in intermittent claudication is caused by the inability of the arterial system to provide adequate blood flow to the tissues in the face of increased demands for oxygen and nutrients during exercise.
3. Refer to Chart 31-1 in the text.

4. Refer to chapter heading "Diagnostic Evaluation" in the text.
5. Refer to Chart 31-2 in the text.
6. Refer to Chart 31-3 in the text.
7. Refer to Chart 31-4 in the text.
8. Refer to chapter heading "Peripheral Arterial Occlusive Disease" in the text.
9. Refer to chapter headings "Thoracic Aortic Aneurysm" and "Abdominal Aortic Aneurysm" in the text.
10. Refer to Chart 31-8 in the text.
11. Refer to chapter heading "Leg Ulcers" in the text.
12. Refer to chapter heading "Varicose Veins" in the text.

EXAMINING ASSOCIATIONS

1. atherosclerosis
2. intermittent claudication
3. ratio of ankle to arm systolic pressure
4. adventitia
5. lymphatic delivery to the remainder of the body
6. lymphangitis

CLINICAL SITUATIONS

CASE STUDY: PERIPHERAL ARTERIAL OCCLUSIVE DISEASE

1. a
2. a
3. d
4. one joint level below the stenosis or occlusion
5. muscle metabolites and lactic acid
6. d
7. b
8. b
9. d

APPLYING CONCEPTS

Refer to Figure 31-1 and chapter heading "Anatomic and Physiologic Overview" in the text.

Chapter 32

I. Interpretation, Completion, and Comparison

MULTIPLE CHOICE

1. d	6. d
2. d	7. b
3. c	8. c
4. b	9. c
5. c	10. c

SHORT ANSWER

1. cardiac output; peripheral resistance
2. heart rate; stroke volume
3. 90% to 95%

4. heart, kidneys, brain, and eyes
5. myocardial infarction, heart failure, renal failure, stroke, impaired vision, and left ventricular hypertrophy
6. accumulation of atherosclerotic plaques, fragmentation of arterial elastins, increased collagen deposits, and impaired vasodilation
7. acute myocardial infarction, a dissecting aortic aneurysm, an intracranial hemorrhage, and hypertension associated with pregnancy

MATCHING

1. d	4. a
2. b	5. c
3. f	6. e

II. Critical Thinking Questions and Exercises

DISCUSSION AND ANALYSIS

1. Refer to chapter heading "Pathophysiology" and Figure 32-1 in the text.
2. Refer to chapter heading "Teaching Patients Self-Care" in the text.
3. Refer to Table 32-4 in the text.
4. Refer to Chart 32-1 in the text.
5. Refer to Tables 32-2 and 32-3 in the text.
6. Refer to chapter heading "Hypertensive Crises" in the text.

IDENTIFYING PATTERNS

FLOW CHART: THE PATHOPHYSIOLOGY OF PRIMARY ESSENTIAL HYPERTENSION

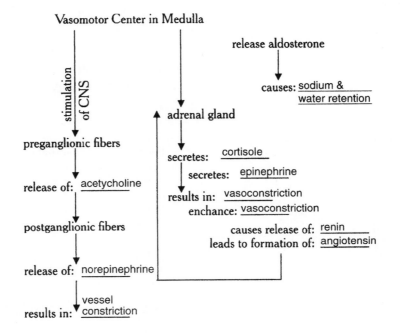

CLINICAL SITUATIONS

CASE STUDY: SECONDARY HYPERTENSION

1. b	3. c
2. d	4. d

Chapter 33

I. Interpretation, Completion, and Comparison

MULTIPLE CHOICE

1. d	13. b	25. d
2. c	14. b	26. b
3. d	15. a	27. b
4. b	16. d	28. a
5. a	17. a	29. c
6. a	18. d	30. c
7. c	19. d	31. d
8. c	20. d	32. d
9. a	21. d	33. b
10. c	22. b	34. c
11. d	23. b	
12. d	24. d	

SHORT ANSWER

1. 5 to 6
2. bone marrow
3. ribs, vertebrae, pelvis, and sternum
4. hemoglobin; transport oxygen between the lungs and the tissues
5. 15 g
6. 2 mg
7. C
8. protect the body from invasion by bacteria and other foreign entities; phagocytosis
9. albumin and globulins
10. the sternum and the iliac crest
11. 42 to 48 years
12. *Primary* polycythemia or polycythemia vera is a proliferative disorder in which all cells are nonresponsive to normal control mechanisms; *secondary* polycythemia is caused by excessive production of erythropoietin.
13. erythropoietin; reduced oxygen
14. hypochromia, microcytosis, hemolysis, and anemia

MATCHING

1. e	7. f	13. r
2. j	8. b	14. g
3. g	9. q	15. n
4. o	10. h	16. d
5. a	11. k	17. m
6. p	12. c	18. i

II. Critical Thinking Questions and Exercises

DISCUSSION AND ANALYSIS

1. Refer to Table 33-2 in the text.
2. Refer to Chart 33-1 and chapter heading "Hemolytic Anemias" in the text.
3. Refer to Table 33-3 and chapter headings "Sickle Cell Anemia" and "Sickle Cell Crisis" in the text.
4. Refer to chapter headings "Acute Lymphocytic Leukemia" and "Chronic Lymphocytic Leukemia" in the text.
5. Refer to chapter headings "Hodgkin Lymphoma" and "Non-Hodgkin Lymphomas" in the text.
6. Refer to Chart 33-8 in the text.
7. Refer to chapter heading "Disseminated Intravascular Coagulation" in the text.
8. The INR is a standard method of reporting prothrombin times. The INR is needed to regulate the dosage of Coumadin. The therapeutic range is usually between 2.0 and 3.0.

CLINICAL SITUATIONS

CASE STUDY: SICKLE CELL CRISES

1. a
2. deformed, rigid, sickle-shaped, and crystal-like formation; 7 to 10 g/dL
3. bone marrow expansion to offset anemia
4. tissue hypoxia and necrosis due to inadequate blood flow to a specific organ or tissue
5. d
6. tachycardia, heart murmurs, and cardiomegaly
7. Answer may include: stroke, infection, renal failure, heart failure, impotence, and pulmonary hypertension.
8. managing pain, preventing and managing infection, promoting coping skills, minimizing deficient knowledge, and monitoring/managing potential complications

CASE STUDY: ACUTE MYELOID LEUKEMIA

1. hematopoietic stem cell; 67; 4%
2. immature blast cells (>30%)
3. d
4. a
5. b

CASE STUDY: HODGKIN'S LYMPHOMA

1. a	3. c
2. b	4. d

CASE STUDY: BLOOD TRANSFUSION

1. d	3. b
2. b	4. b

Chapter 34

I. Interpretation, Completion, and Comparison

MULTIPLE CHOICE

1. b	11. c	21. c
2. c	12. b	22. b
3. a	13. b	23. d
4. b	14. c	24. c
5. d	15. d	25. b
6. b	16. a	26. c
7. c	17. a	27. d
8. d	18. c	28. d
9. b	19. d	29. a
10. d	20. c	

SHORT ANSWER

1. typsin, amylase, and lipase
2. mixed waves that move the intestinal contents back and forth in a churning motion; a movement that propels the contents of the small intestine toward the colon.
3. 4 hours; 12 hours
4. decreased motility and emptying, weakened gag reflex, and decreased resting pressure of lower sphincter

MATCHING

1. f	4. c
2. a	5. b
3. e	6. d

SHORT ANSWER

1. a. Low-residue diet 1 to 2 days before test
   b. Clear liquids the evening before
   c. A laxative the evening before
   d. NPO after midnight
   e. Cleansing enemas until returns are clear in the AM
2. a. NPO 8 to 12 hours before the procedure
   b. No medications affecting gastric secretions 24 to 48 hours before test
   c. No smoking in AM before test
3. a. NPO 6 to 12 hours before the procedure
   b. Spraying or gargling with a local anesthetic
   c. Administering intravenous versed before the scope is introduced
4. a. Liquids 24 to 72 hours before the examination
   b. Laxative 48 hours before procedure
   c. Laxatives until clear the AM of test, usually a polyethylene glycol electrolyte lavage solution (GoLYTELY)
   d. Clear liquids starting at noon on the day before test

II. Critical Thinking Questions and Exercises

IDENTIFYING PATTERNS

Refer to Figure 34-3 in the text.

Chapter 35

I. Interpretation, Completion, and Comparison

MULTIPLE CHOICE

1. c	9. b	17. a
2. d	10. c	18. a
3. b	11. a	19. a
4. a	12. d	20. c
5. d	13. b	21. a
6. b	14. b	22. a
7. b	15. a	
8. b	16. a	

MATCHING

Refer to Table 35-1 in the text.

1. f	5. d
2. g	6. b
3. e	7. c
4. a	8. h

II. Critical Thinking Questions and Exercises

DISCUSSION AND ANALYSIS

1. Refer to chapter heading "Mouth Care" in the text.
2. Refer to chapter heading "Dentoalveolar Abscess or Periapical Abscess" in the text.
3. Refer to chapter heading "Disorders of the Salivary Glands" in the text.
4. Refer to chapter heading "Cancer of the Oral Cavity and Pharynx" in the text.
5. Refer to Figure 35-4 and chapter heading "Neck Dissection" in the text
6. Refer to chapter heading "The Patient Undergoing a Neck Dissection" in the text.
7. Refer to chapter heading "The Patient Undergoing a Neck Dissection" in the text.
8. Refer to chapter heading "Disorders of the Esophagus" in the text.
9. Refer to chapter heading "Cancer of the Esophagus" in the text.

APPLYING CONCEPTS

Refer to Figure 35-4 in the text.
1. local-regional metastasis
2. shoulder drop and poor cosmesis (visible neck depression)
3. pectoralis major
4. altered respiratory status, wound infection, and hemorrhage
5. hemorrhage, nerve injury, and chyle fistula
6. d
7. c
8. b
9. b
10. b

CLINICAL SITUATIONS

CASE STUDY: MANDIBULAR FRACTURE

1. Rigid plate fixation (insertion of metal plates and screws into the bone to approximate and stabilize the bone) is the current treatment of choice.
2. b
3. b
4. Nasogastric suctioning is needed to remove stomach contents, thereby reducing the danger of aspiration.
5. c
6. b
7. c
8. a wire cutter

CASE STUDY: CANCER OF THE MOUTH

1. The typical lesion is a painless, indurated (hardened) ulcer with raised edges.
2. d
3. d
4. a
5. xerostomia

Chapter 36

I. Interpretation, Completion, and Comparison

MULTIPLE CHOICE

1. a
2. a
3. c (See Figure 36-2 in the text.)
4. a
5. d
6. b
7. a
8. d
9. b
10. c
11. d
12. d
13. a
14. b
15. b
16. b
17. c
18. a
19. d

MATCHING

1. e
2. b
3. d
4. a
5. c

II. Critical Thinking Questions and Exercises

DISCUSSION AND ANALYSIS

1. Refer to chapter heading "Gastrointestinal Intubation" in the text.
2. Refer to Table 36-2 in the text.
3. Refer to Table 36-3 in the text.
4. Refer to chapter heading "Monitoring and Managing Potential Complications" under chapter heading "Enteric Tubes" in the text.
5. Refer to Table 36-5 in the text.
6. Refer to chapter heading "Parenteral Nutrition" in the text.

CLINICAL SITUATIONS

CASE STUDY: THE DUMPING SYNDROME

1. Answer should include four of the following eight: caloric density, tubing size, speed of infusion, temperature and volume of feeding, zinc deficiency, contaminated formula, malnutrition, and medication therapy.
2. Answer should include three of the following six: Cleocin, Digitalis, Inderal, Lincocin, Theophylline, and quinidine.
3. a
4. d

CASE STUDY: TOTAL PARENTERAL NUTRITION

1. b
2. c
3. c
4. d
5. d

APPLYING CONCEPTS

1. a. Risk for impaired skin integrity at tube site
   b. Risk for infection related to the presence of the wound and tube
   c. Body image disturbance related to the presence of a tube
2. a. Wound infection
   b. Gastrointestinal bleeding
   c. Premature removal of tube
3. leakage of fluid
4. seepage of gastric acid, and spillage of feeding
5. 30 to 60 seconds
6. gently apply pressure with the bulb top of the syringe or elevate the syringe so that the tubing is less curved.
7. Increasing the height increases the pressure of gravity, which could result in too much force on the incisional area and the outlet.
8. An upright position facilitates digestion and decreases the risk for aspiration.

Chapter 37

I. Interpretation, Completion, and Comparison

MULTIPLE CHOICE

1. d	8. d	15. b
2. b	9. c	16. d
3. a	10. a	17. c
4. b	11. a	18. c
5. c	12. d	19. b
6. a	13. d	
7. b	14. d	

SHORT ANSWER

1. Dilute and neutralize the offending agent. To neutralize a corrosive acid, use common antacids such as milk and aluminum hydroxide. To neutralize an alkali, use diluted lemon juice or diluted vinegar.
2. Patients with gastritis due to a vitamin deficiency exhibit antibodies against intrinsic factor, which interferes with vitamin B_{12} absorption.
3. Hypersecretion of acid pepsin and a weakened gastric mucosal barrier predispose to peptic ulcer development.
4. *Helicobacter pylori* is the bacillus commonly associated with ulcer formation.
5. Hypersecretion of gastric juice, multiple duodenal ulcers, hypertrophied duodenal glands, and gastrinomas (islet cell tumors) in the pancreas.
6. A stress ulcer refers to acute mucosal ulceration of the duodenal or gastric area that occurs after a stressful event.
7. Cushing's ulcers, which are common in patients with brain trauma, usually occur in the esophagus, stomach, or duodenum. Curling's ulcers occur most frequently after extensive burns and usually involve the antrum of the stomach and duodenum.
8. The objective of the ulcer diet is to avoid oversecretion and hypermotility in the gastrointestinal tract. Extremes of temperature should be avoided, as well as overstimulation by meat extractives, coffee (including decaffeinated), alcohol, and diets rich in milk and cream. Current therapy recommends three regular meals per day if an antacid or histamine blocker is taken.
9. Hemorrhage, perforation, penetration, and pyloric obstruction
10. When peptic ulcer perforation occurs, the patient experiences severe upper abdominal pain, vomiting, fainting, and an extremely tender abdomen that can be board like in rigidity; signs of shock will be present (hypotension and tachycardia).
11. restricting a patient's ability to eat; restricting ingested nutrient absorption
12. 30 mL
13. adenocarcinoma; second and third portions of the duodenum

SCRAMBLEGRAM

1. Achlorhydria	4. Melena
2. Gastritis	5. Pylorus
3. Hematemesis	6. Pyrosis

II. Critical Thinking Questions and Exercises

DISCUSSION AND ANALYSIS

1. Refer to chapter heading "Gastritis" in the text.
2. Gastritis occurs because the gastric mucous membrane becomes edematous and hyperemic. Superficial erosion occurs. Excess mucus is produced along with a scanty amount of gastric juice. Superficial ulceration can lead to hemorrhage.
3. *Helicobacter pylori* can be diagnosed by biopsy, serologic testing for antibodies, a 1-minute ultrarapid urease test, and a breath test.
4. Refer to Table 37-1 in the text.
5. Refer to Table 37-2 in the text.
6. Refer to Table 37-4 in the text.
7. Refer to Chart 37-3 in the text.
8. Refer to Chart 37-4 in the text.
9. Refer to chapter heading "Dumping Syndrome" under chapter heading "Gastric Surgery" in the text.

EXTRACTING INFERENCES

Refer to chapter heading "Peptic Ulcer Disease" in the text.

CLINICAL SITUATIONS

CASE STUDY: GASTRIC CANCER

1. liver, pancreas, esophagus, and duodenum
2. ascites and hepatomegaly
3. esophagogastroduodenoscopy and barium x-ray of the upper gastrointestinal tract; endoscopic ultrasound; computed tomography
4. b
5. 5-fluorouracil (5-FU)

Chapter 38

I. Interpretation, Completion, and Comparison

MULTIPLE CHOICE

1. d	9. b	17. a
2. b	10. d	18. c
3. c	11. c	19. c
4. c	12. d	20. d
5. c	13. a	21. d
6. a	14. d	22. b
7. d	15. d	23. c
8. b	16. d	24. b

MATCHING

1. e	7. k	13. d
2. m	8. b	14. l
3. i	9. p	15. h
4. o	10. j	16. f
5. a	11. c	
6. g	12. n	

MATCHING

1. b-5	4. a-1
2. d-3	5. c-2
3. e-6	6. f-4

SHORT ANSWER

1. constipation, diarrhea, and fecal incontinence
2. irritable bowel syndrome (IBS) and diverticular disease
3. mucosal transport, myoelectric activity, and the actual process of defecation
4. 25 to 30 g/day; 3
5. *Clostridium difficile*
6. Peritonitis, abscess formation, fistulas, and bleeding
7. *Escherichia coli*, *Klebsiella*, *Proteus*, and *Pseudomonas*
8. adhesions; hernias, and neoplasms
9. adenocarcinoid tumors
10. Refer to Chart 38-9 in the text.

II. Critical Thinking Questions and Exercises

DISCUSSION AND ANALYSIS

1. A series of neuromuscular actions are necessary for defecation. Rectal distention stimulates the inhibitory rectoanal reflex. This causes the internal and external sphincter, as well as the muscles in the pelvic region, to relax. Intra-abdominal pressure increases to propel the colon contents.
2. Straining at stool can cause the Valsalva maneuver (forcibly exhaling with the nose, mouth, and glottis closed), which results in increased intrathoracic pressure. This pressure tends to collapse the large veins in the chest. Cardiac output is decreased and arterial pressure decreases. Almost immediately a rebound rise in arterial and venous pressure occurs. This can be dangerous for those with hypertension.
3. Refer to Table 38-1 in the text.

4. Refer to chapter heading "Irritable Bowel Syndrome" in the text.
5. *Pancreatic insufficiency* causes reduced intraluminal pancreatic enzyme activity with maldigestion of lipids and proteins. *Zollinger–Ellison syndrome* causes hyperacidity in the duodenum that inactivates pancreatic enzymes. *Celiac disease* results in the destruction of the absorbing surface of intestine as a toxic response to gluten fraction (Gliadin) (See Table 38-2 in the text.)
6. Refer to chapter heading "Management of the Patient With Chronic Inflammatory Bowel Disease" in the text.
7. Refer to Chart 38-4 in the text.
8. Refer to Chart 38-5 in the text.
9. Refer to Figures 38-7 and 38-8 in the text.
10. Refer to Table 38-5 in the text.
11. Refer to Table 38-6 in the text.
12. Refer to Chart 38-11 in the text.
13. Refer to chapter heading "Diseases of the Anorectum" in the text.

RECOGNIZING CONTRADICTIONS

1. Diarrhea refers to <u>more than three</u> bowel movements per day, increased amount of stool (>200 g/day) and increased liquidity.
2. <u>Perforation,</u> the major complication of appendicitis, occurs in <u>10% to 32%</u> of cases.
3. <u>Appendicitis,</u> the most common cause of emergency abdominal surgery, occurs in about 7% of the population.
4. <u>Sepsis</u> is the major cause of death from peritonitis.
5. The <u>distal ileum and colon</u> are the most common areas affected by Crohn's disease.
6. <u>About 75%</u> of patients with regional enteritis require surgery within 10 years of diagnosis.
7. <u>Change in bowel habits</u> is the most common symptom of colon cancer.

CLINICAL SITUATIONS

CASE STUDY: APPENDICITIS

1. c	3. d
2. c	4. d

CASE STUDY: PERITONITIS

1. d	3. a
2. a	4. a

IDENTIFYING PATTERNS

Refer to chapter heading "Irritable Bowel Syndrome" and Figure 38-2 in the text.

Chapter 39

I. Interpretation, Completion, and Comparison

MULTIPLE CHOICE

1. d	11. a	21. c
2. c	12. d	22. d
3. d	13. c	23. d
4. c	14. b	24. d
5. b	15. c	25. b
6. d	16. d	26. d
7. d	17. a	27. d
8. d	18. b	28. d
9. b	19. a	29. d
10. b	20. d	30. d

SHORT ANSWER

1. 70%
2. bleeding and bile peritonitis
3. 10%
4. hepatitis C
5. chronic liver disease, hepatitis B, hepatitis C, and cirrhosis
6. infection

MATCHING

1. c	5. d
2. e	6. g
3. b	7. f
4. a	

II. Critical Thinking Questions and Exercises

DISCUSSION AND ANALYSIS

1. Refer to Chart 39-1 in the text.
2. Refer to chapter heading "Physical Assessment" under chapter heading "Assessment" in the text.
3. *Hemolytic jaundice* is the result of an increased destruction of red blood cells that overload the plasma with bilirubin so quickly that the liver cannot excrete the bilirubin as fast as it is formed. *Hepatocellular jaundice* is caused by the inability of damaged liver cells to clear normal amounts of bilirubin from the blood. *Obstructive jaundice* is usually caused by occlusion of the bile duct by a gallstone, an inflammatory process, a tumor, or pressure from an enlarged organ.
4. Refer to Figure 39-4 and chapter heading "Ascites" in the text.
5. Refer to Chart 39-3 in the text.
6. Refer to chapter heading "Balloon Tamponade" and Figure 39-8 in the text.

7. Refer to Figure 39-11 and chapter heading "Surgical Bypass Procedures" in the text.
8. *Hepatic encephalopathy* occurs when ammonia accumulates because damaged liver cells fail to detoxify and convert ammonia to urea. Elevated ammonia levels cause brain damage. Refer to chapter heading "Hepatic Encephalopathy and Coma" and Table 39-3 in the text.
9. *Alcoholic cirrhosis*. Necrotic liver cells are replaced by scar tissue, which gradually exceeds functioning liver tissue. Liver enlargement leads to obstruction of the portal circulation, which causes the shunting of blood into vessels with lower pressures. Edema results from the concentration of plasma albumin. An overproduction of aldosterone causes sodium and water retention and potassium excretion. Anemia, gastritis, and vitamin deficiency lead to overall physical and mental deterioration.
10. Refer to chapter heading "Viral Hepatitis" and Table 39-4 in the text.

CLINICAL SITUATIONS

CASE STUDY: LIVER BIOPSY

1. d	4. b
2. b	5. d
3. c	

CASE STUDY: PARACENTESIS

Refer to Chart 39-3 in the text.

1. c	3. a
2. d	

CASE STUDY: ALCOHOLIC OR NUTRITIONAL CIRRHOSIS

1. c
2. d
3. c (1 kg = 2.2 lb)
4. c (normal protein intake is 0.8 to 1 g/kg)
5. c (normal sodium intake is 3 to 6 g/24 h without ascites; sodium restriction is minimal rather than severe)

CASE STUDY: LIVER TRANSPLANTATION

1. d	3. a
2. d	4. a

Chapter 40

I. Interpretation, Completion, and Comparison

MULTIPLE CHOICE

1. c	8. a	15. b
2. c	9. a	16. d
3. c	10. d	17. c
4. a	11. d	18. d
5. a	12. d	19. d
6. b	13. a	20. a
7. d	14. a	21. b

SHORT ANSWER

1. 30 to 50 mL
2. insulin, glucagon, and somatostatin
3. amylase; trypsin; and lipase
4. calculous cholecystitis
5. bile duct injury
6. Refer to Chart 40-3 in the text.
7. pancreatic necrosis
8. 80% to 85%; 5%

II. Critical Thinking Questions and Exercises

CLINICAL SITUATIONS

CASE STUDY: CHOLECYSTECTOMY

Brenda's Preoperative Situation

1. d	3. d
2. b	

Brenda's Postoperative Situation

1. a	3. c
2. d	

CASE STUDY: CHRONIC PANCREATITIS

1. The inflammatory process causes the replacement of cells by fibrous tissues. This results in mechanical obstruction of the pancreatic and common bile ducts and the duodenum. Atrophy of the epithelium of the ducts causes destruction of the secreting cells of the pancreas.
2. long-term alcohol consumption; 37 to 40
3. severe upper abdominal and back pain accompanied by vomiting and frequently unrelieved by opioids.
4. diabetes mellitus
5. pancreaticojejunostomy that usually relieves pain in 6 months in 85% of patients.
6. avoidance of alcohol and avoidance of foods found to cause abdominal pain and discomfort

Chapter 41

I. Interpretation, Completion, and Comparison

MULTIPLE CHOICE

1. b	9. d	15. d
2. b	10. d	16. d
3. c	11. c	17. a
4. c	12. c	18. c
5. c	13. a	19. d
6. d	14. a (use 15 to	20. d
7. a	20 kcal/kg	21. d
8. d	for IBW)	22. d

23. a	29. d	35. d
24. c	30. d	36. c
25. a	31. d	37. d
26. b	32. d	38. c
27. d	33. c	
28. c	34. a	

MATCHING

1. c	4. e
2. a	5. d
3. b	

SHORT ANSWER

1. nontraumatic amputations, blindness among working-age adults, and end-stage renal disease
2. 180 to 200 mg/dL
3. 14%
4. normalize insulin activity and blood glucose levels to reduce the development of vascular and neuropathic complications
5. nutrition management, exercise, monitoring, pharmacologic therapy, and education
6. 25 to 29; >30
7. 50% to 60% carbohydrates (the majority from whole grains), 20% to 30% fat, and 10% to 20% protein
8. 25 to 30 g
9. Lispro (Humalog) and Aspart (NovoLog)
10. ketoacidosis
11. directly stimulating the beta cells of the pancreas to secrete insulin (cannot be used in patients with type 1 diabetes)
12. abdomen, posterior surface of the upper arms, anterior surface of the thighs, and the hips
13. hypoglycemia, diabetic ketoacidosis (DKA), and hyperglycemic hyperosmolar nonketotic syndrome
14. hypotension, profound dehydration, tachycardia, and variable neurologic signs (seizures, hemiparesis, alteration of sensorium)
15. cerebral edema, hyperglycemia and ketoacidosis, hypokalemia, hypoglycemia, and fluid overload (pulmonary edema, congestive heart failure)
16. diabetic retinopathy

II. Critical Thinking Questions and Exercises

DISCUSSION AND ANALYSIS

1. Refer to Chart 41-1 in the text.
2. Refer to Table 41-1 in the text.
3. Refer to chapter heading "Insulin Therapy" in the text.
4. Insulin regulates the production and storage of glucose. In diabetes, either the pancreas stops producing insulin or the cells stop responding to insulin. Hyperglycemia results and can lead to acute metabolic complications such as diabetic ketoacidosis and hyperglycemic

hyperosmolar nonketotic syndrome. Long-term complications can contribute to macrovascular or microvascular complications.

5. *Type 1 diabetes* is characterized by an absence of insulin production and secretion due to the autoimmune destruction of the beta cells of the islets of Langerhans. *Type 2 diabetes* is characterized by deficiency of insulin production and a decreased insulin action as well as increased insulin resistance.

6. Hyperglycemia develops during pregnancy because the secretion of placental hormones causes insulin resistance.

7. "Glycemic index" is used to describe how much a given food increases the blood glucose level compared with an equivalent amount of glucose.

8. Refer to chapter heading "Complications of Insulin Therapy" in the text.

9. Refer to chapter heading "Mixing Insulins" in the text.

10. Refer to Chart 41-7 in the text.

11. Refer to Table 41-5 in the text.

12. Refer to Chart 41-9 in the text.

EXAMINING ASSOCIATIONS

1. 2	6. 2
2. 2	7. 1
3. 1	8. 2
4. 1	9. 2
5. 1	10. 1

IDENTIFYING PATTERNS

FLOW CHART: THE PATHOPHYSIOLOGIC SEQUENCE OF CHANGES THAT OCCUR WITH TYPE 1 DIABETES

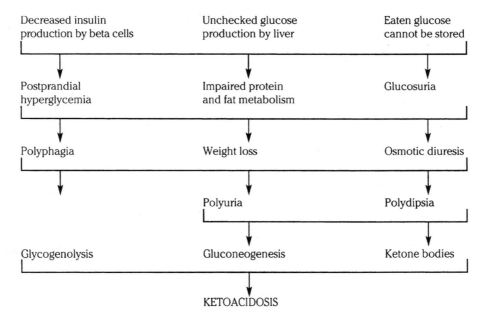

APPLYING CONCEPTS

1. Sensory neuropathy causes loss of sensation to pain and pressure; autonomic neuropathy causes an increase in skin dryness and the formation of skin fissures; motor neuropathy results in muscular atrophy.

2. 50%

3. Inadequate and compromised lower-extremity circulation interferes with the ability to get nutrients to the wound to promote healing and prevent the development of gangrene.

4. Hyperglycemia impairs the ability of specialized leukocytes to destroy bacteria, thus lowering the resistance to infection.

5. soft-tissue injury, formation of a fissure, and formation of a callus

6. bathe, dry, and lubricate the feet; inspect both feet; look for fissures on dry skin or between the toes; report any redness, swelling, or drainage; wear well-fitting, closed-toe shoes

7. Peripheral vascular disease may prevent oxygen, nutrients, and antibiotics from reaching the injured tissue.

CLINICAL SITUATIONS

Refer to Table 41-3 in the text.

CASE STUDY: TYPE I DIABETES

1. b	3. b
2. c	

CASE STUDY: HYPOGLYCEMIA

1. a	3. d
2. d	4. d

CASE STUDY: DIABETIC KETOACIDOSIS

1. d	4. a
2. a	5. b
3. d	6. d

Chapter 42

I. Interpretation, Completion, and Comparison

MULTIPLE CHOICE

1. d	11. a	21. d
2. b	12. d	22. a
3. a	13. d	23. d
4. d	14. b	24. c
5. a	15. d	25. d
6. d	16. a	26. d
7. a	17. d	27. c
8. d	18. a	28. a
9. b	19. c	29. a
10. b	20. d	

MATCHING

1. h	6. c
2. g	7. f
3. i	8. e
4. d	9. j
5. a	10. b

SHORT ANSWER

1. negative feedback
2. Answer should include four of the following: steroids, proteins or peptides, polypeptides and glycoproteins, amines and amino acids, and fatty acid derivatives.
3. vasopressin, which controls the excretion of water by the kidneys and oxytocin, which controls milk ejection during lactation
4. Cushing's syndrome or acromegaly
5. diabetes insipidus; excessive thirst (polydipsia), and large volumes of dilute urine
6. thyroxine, triiodothyronine, and calcitonin
7. autoimmune thyroiditis (Hashimoto's disease)
8. diabetes mellitus
9. Graves' disease
10. methimazole (Tapazole) and propylthiouracil (PTU)
11. Trousseau's or Chvostek's
12. glucocorticoids, mineralocorticoids, and androgens

UNSCRAMBLED WORDS

1. Pituitary
2. Hypothalamus
3. Somatotropin
4. SIADH (syndrome of inappropriate antidiuretic hormone)

5. Iodine
6. Exophthalmos
7. Tetany

II. Critical Thinking Questions and Exercises

DISCUSSION AND ANALYSIS

1. Refer to chapter heading "Diabetes Insipidus" in the text.
2. Refer to chapter heading "Thyroid Tests" in the text.
3. Refer to Chart 42-4 in the text.
4. Refer to Chart 42-7 in the text.
5. Refer to chapter headings "Adrenocortical Insufficiency (Addison's Disease)" and "Cushing's Syndrome" in the text.

CLINICAL SITUATIONS

CASE STUDY: PRIMARY HYPOTHYROIDISM

1. d	4. d
2. d	5. b
3. b	

CASE STUDY: HYPERPARATHYROIDISM

1. a
2. a
3. apathy, fatigue, muscular weakness, nausea, vomiting, constipation, hypertension, and cardiac dysrhythmias
4. kidney stones
5. d
6. b
7. c

CASE STUDY: SUBTOTAL THYROIDECTOMY

1. d	4. a
2. d	5. b
3. d	6. a

Chapter 43

I. Interpretation, Completion, and Comparison

MULTIPLE CHOICE

1. b	6. c	11. d
2. b	7. d	12. d
3. c	8. a	13. d
4. a	9. a	
5. b	10. b	

SHORT ANSWER

1. nephron; cortex
2. 400 to 500 mL

3. 300 mOsm/kg
4. aldosterone
5. increased
6. the antidiuretic hormone (ADH)
7. 7.35 to7.45; 4.5
8. urea; 20 to 30 g
9. creatine clearance

II. Critical Thinking Questions and Exercises

DISCUSSION AND ANALYSIS

1. Refer to chapter heading "Blood Supply to the Kidneys" in the text.

2. Refer to chapter heading "Nephrons" in the text.
3. Refer to Figure 43-3 in the text.
4. Refer to chapter heading "Urine Formation" in the text.
5. Refer to chapter heading "Antidiuretic Hormone" in the text.
6. Refer to chapter heading "Regulation of Acid–Base Balance" in the text.
7. Refer to Table 43-3 in the text.
8. Refer to chapter heading "Physical Assessment" in the text.

IDENTIFYING PATTERNS

FLOW CHART: PATHOPHYSIOLOGIC RESPONSES TO HYPOTENSION

Refer to Figure 43-4 in the text.

Renal perfusion decreases

and

blood pressure decreases

↓

Kidneys release <u>renin</u>

↓

Liver manufactures <u>angiotensin I</u>

which converts to

↓

<u>angiotensin II</u> (a powerful vasoconstrictor)

↓

Adrenals release <u>aldosterone</u>

↓

<u>Increases sodium retention</u>

↓

Pituitary releases <u>ACTH</u>

↓

<u>Blood pressure increases</u>

<u>Renal autoregulation occurs</u>   <u>Circulating blood volume increases</u>

Chapter 44

I. Interpretation, Completion, and Comparison

MULTIPLE CHOICE

1. d	11. c	21. d
2. d	12. a	22. d
3. a	13. d	23. d
4. d	14. b	24. b
5. b	15. a	25. b
6. b	16. a	26. b
7. a	17. b	27. d
8. c	18. d	28. d
9. c	19. a	
10. b	20. a	

MATCHING

1. a	6. j
2. b	7. h
3. c	8. f
4. e	9. g
5. d	10. I

SHORT ANSWER

1. diabetes mellitus
2. prolonged hypertension and diabetes
3. proteinuria, hematuria, decreased GFR, edema, hypertension, and decreased sodium excretion
4. The urine in the early stages of acute glomerulonephritis is characteristically cola-colored.
5. creatinine and BUN
6. proteinuria, hypoalbuminemia, diffuse edema, hypercholesterolemia, and hyperlipidemia
7. Refer to Chart 44-3 in the text.
8. (a) Prerenal conditions are hemorrhage and sepsis; (b) intrarenal conditions are crush injuries and infections, and (c) postrenal conditionsare obstruction distal to kidney(s)
9. potassium levels >5.5 mEq/L and T-wave elevations
10. Answer should include six of the following: lethargy, headache, muscle twitching, seizures, nausea, vomiting, and diarrhea. There is also dehydration and the odor of urine on the breath.
11. Answer should include six of the following: hypotension, air embolism, chest pain, dysrhythmias, pruritus, dialysis disequilibrium, painful muscle cramping, nausea, vomiting, and exsanguination.
12. arteriosclerotic cardiovascular disease
13. peritonitis
14. abdominal distention, and paralytic ileus

II. Critical Thinking Questions and Exercises

DISCUSSION AND ANALYSIS

1. Refer to Table 44-1 in the text.
2. Refer to chapter heading "Primary Glomerular Diseases" in the text.
3. Refer to chapter heading "Polycystic Kidney Disease" in the text.
4. Refer to Chart 44-5 in the text.
5. Refer to Chart 44-4 in the text.
6. Refer to chapter heading "Dialysis" in the text.
7. Refer to chapter heading "Hemodialysis" in the text.
8. Refer to chapter heading "Peritoneal Dialysis" in the text.
9. Refer to chapter heading "Renal Trauma" in the text.

APPLYING CONCEPTS

1. to support arterial flow to the dialyzer
2. to support reinfusion of the dialyzed blood
3. 2 to 3; time is needed for the venous segment of the fistula to dilate to accommodate two large-bore needles
4. squeeze a rubber ball for forearm fistulas
5. polytetrafluoroethylene; 10 days

CLINICAL SITUATIONS

CASE STUDY: CAPD

1. d	4. d
2. a	5. c
3. a	

CASE STUDY: ACUTE RENAL FAILURE

1. c	4. b
2. d	5. b
3. b	6. d

Chapter 45

I. Interpretation, Completion, and Comparison

MULTIPLE CHOICE

1. a	10. b	19. d
2. c	11. a	20. a
3. a	12. c	21. d
4. d	13. b	22. c
5. b	14. b	23. b
6. b	15. d	24. a
7. c	16. d	25. d
8. d	17. d	
9. d	18. c	

SHORT ANSWER

1. glycosaminoglycan (GAG); urinary immunoglobulin (IgA); normal bacterial flora of the vagina and urethral area
2. *Escherichia coli, pseudomonas,* and *enterococcus*
3. Urgency, burning, and pain on urination; frequency (voiding more than every 3 hours); nocturia; incontinence; suprapubic and pelvic pain; and sometimes hematuria and back pain.
4. chronic bacterial prostatitis
5. *Proteus, Klebsiella, Pseudomonas,* and *Staphylococcus*
6. Refer to chapter heading "Catheterization" in the text.
7. cloudy and malodorous urine, hematuria, fever, chills, and anorexia
8. calcium oxalate, calcium phosphate, and uric acid

II. Critical Thinking Questions and Exercises

RECOGNIZING CONTRADICTIONS

1. The majority of nosocomial infections in the hospital are caused by <u>instrumentation of the urinary tract or catheterization</u>.
2. Urethrovesical reflux refers to the backward flow of urine <u>from the urethra into the bladder</u>. (See Figure 45-1 in the text.)
3. <u>Anticholinergics</u> inhibit bladder contractions and are recommended for urge incontinence.
4. Shellfish and organ meats should be avoided for <u>uric-acid-based renal stones</u>.

DISCUSSION AND ANALYSIS

1. Refer to Chart 45-2 in the text.
2. Refer to Chart 45-3 in the text.
3. Refer to chapter headings "Acute Pyelonephritis" and "Chronic Pyelonephritis" in the text.
4. Refer to Chart 45-5 in the text.
5. Refer to Chart 45-7 in the text.
6. Refer to Chart 45-9 in the text.
7. Refer to Chart 45-10 in the text.
8. Refer to Chart 45-13 in the text.

Chapter 46

I. Interpretation, Completion, and Comparison

MULTIPLE CHOICE

1. d	8. b	15. c
2. a	9. b	16. b
3. b	10. c	17. c
4. c	11. a	18. c
5. a	12. b	19. c
6. a	13. a	20. b
7. d	14. a	

SHORT ANSWER

1. 12 to 14 years; 10 years
2. follicle-stimulating; luteinizing
3. 45 to 52 years, with a median age of 51 years; age 35 years
4. irregular or excessive vaginal bleeding, abnormal discharge, bleeding after menopause, painful intercourse (dyspareunia), bleeding after intercourse, urinary disturbances, and painful menstruation
5. six million
6. 20%
7. endometrial biopsy
8. Answer should include four of the following: headache, fatigue, low back pain, engorged or painful breasts, abdominal fullness, mood swings, general irritability, fear of loss of control, binge eating, and crying spells.
9. atherosclerosis, angina, coronary artery disease, and osteoporosis
10. Lack of body fat and low caloric intake decreases hormonal function.
11. The pill blocks the stimulation of the ovary by preventing the release of follicle-stimulating hormone (FSH) from the anterior pituitary.
12. Answer should include six of the following: a history of thromboembolic disorders, migraine headaches with visual auras, cerebrovascular disease, breast cancer, pregnancy, liver tumors, post estrogen-dependent neoplasia, congenital hyperlipidemia, and abnormal vaginal bleeding.
13. Depo-Provera, a long-acting progestin that is injected intramuscularly, effectively inhibits ovulation for 3 months.
14. An emergency dose of estrogen or estrogen and progesterone, properly timed within 5 days, can prevent pregnancy by inhibiting or delaying ovulation.
15. For in vitro fertilization, at an appropriate time, the egg is recovered by transvaginal ultrasound retrieval. Sperm and egg are coincubated for up to 36 hours so that fertilization can occur. Forty-eight hours after retrieval, the embryo is transferred to the uterine cavity by means of a transcervical catheter. Implantation should occur in 3 to 4 days.

MATCHING

1. f		5. e
2. d		6. g
3. h		7. c
4. a		8. b

II. Critical Thinking Questions and Exercises

DISCUSSION AND ANALYSIS

1. Refer to chapter heading "Health History" and Chart 46-1 in the text.
2. Refer to chapter heading "Female Genital Mutilation or Cutting" in the text.
3. Refer to chapter heading "Menopause" in the text.
4. Refer to Chart 46-5 in the text.
5. Refer to Chart 46-13 in the text.
6. Refer to chapter heading "Emergency Contraception" in the text.

RECOGNIZING CONTRADICTIONS

1. The WHI study was halted early because the results found an <u>increased risk of breast cancer, heart attack, stroke, and blood clots</u>.
2. Women born to mothers who took DES during their pregnancy have a higher than average chance of developing <u>cancer of the cervix</u>.
3. A biopsy excision of an inverted cone of tissue is performed when a Pap smear is "suspicious." The patient <u>must be anesthetized</u> for this procedure.
4. Magnetic resonance imaging uses a magnetized field to produce an image. <u>Radiation is not necessary</u>.
5. <u>Progesterone</u> is the most important hormone for preparing the endometrium for the fertilized ovum.
6. Painful cramps result from an excessive production of <u>prostaglandins</u>.
7. <u>Ectopic pregnancy</u> is the leading cause of pregnancy-related death in the first trimester.

EXTRACTING INFERENCES

1. A fertilized ovum implants in tissue other than the uterine area, usually the fallopian tube.
2. Possible causes are salpingitis, peritubal adhesions, structural abnormalities of the fallopian tube, previous ectopic pregnancy or tubal surgery, the presence of an IUD, and multiple previous abortions.
3. abdominal tenderness; sharp, colicky pain; some bleeding; gastrointestinal symptoms; and abnormal bleeding
4. the tube can be resected (salpingostomy) or removed (salpingectomy) along with an ovary (salpingo-oophorectomy)
5. determine whether any tissue remained
6. hemorrhage and shock

CASE STUDY: TOXIC SHOCK SYNDROME

1. c
2. a
3. b
4. d
5. c

Chapter 47

I. Interpretation, Completion, and Comparison

MULTIPLE CHOICE

1. d	12. a	23. d
2. d	13. a	24. c
3. d	14. c	25. d
4. d	15. b	26. d
5. b	16. c	27. d
6. a	17 d	28. a
7. c	18 d	29. d
8. b	19. c	30. b
9. d	20. d	31. c
10. a	21. b	
11. c	22. b	

MATCHING

1. f	7. n	13. k
2. d	8. o	14. b
3. p	9. i	15. l
4. e	10. a	16. g
5. h	11. j	
6. c	12 m	

II. Critical Thinking Questions and Exercises

DISCUSSION AND ANALYSIS

1. Refer to Chart 47-1 in the text.
2. Estrogen breaks down glycogen into lactic acid, which is responsible for producing a low vaginal pH. A pH level of 3.5 to 4.5 suppresses bacterial growth.
3. Refer to chapter heading "Human Papillomavirus" in the text.
4. Pelvic inflammatory disease (PID) is a condition of the pelvic cavity that may involve the uterus, fallopian tubes, ovaries, pelvic peritoneum, or pelvic vascular system.
5. Refer to chapter heading "Pelvic Organ Prolapse: Cystocele, Rectocele, Enterocele" in the text.
6. Refer to Charts 47-5 and 47-7 in the text.

CLINICAL SITUATIONS

CASE STUDY: BACTERIAL VAGINOSIS

1. a
2. b
3. c
4. a
5. a

CASE STUDY: HERPES GENITALIS

1. d
2. a
3. c
4. 50 million
5. mouth, oropharynx, mucosal surface, vagina, and cervix
6. acyclovir (Zovirax), valacyclovir, (Valtrex), and famciclovir (Famvir)
7. pain related to the presence of genital lesions, risk for recurrence of infections or spread of infection, anxiety and distress related to embarrassment, and insufficient knowledge about the disease and methods of avoiding spread and recurrences

CASE STUDY: PELVIC INFLAMMATORY DISEASE

1. uterus, fallopian tubes, ovaries, pelvic peritoneum, and pelvic vascular system
2. acute, subacute, recurrent, chronic, localized, and widespread
3. gonorrhea and chlamydia
4. ectopic pregnancy, infertility, recurrent pelvic pain, tubo-ovarian abscess, and recurrent disease
5. *Localized*: vaginal discharge, lower abdominal pain, dyspareunia, and tenderness after menses. *Generalized*: fever, general malaise, anorexia, nausea, headache, and vomiting.

Chapter 48

I. Interpretation, Completion, and Comparison

MULTIPLE CHOICE

1. b	10. d	19. b
2. b	11. d	20. c
3. a	12. c	21. b
4. a	13. d	22. c
5. d	14. c	23. a
6. d	15. d	24. d
7. a	16. b	25. d
8. b	17. b	26. c
9. d	18. b	27. c

MATCHING

1. e	5. b
2. g	6. d
3. a	7. f
4. c	

II. Critical Thinking Questions and Exercises

DISCUSSION AND ANALYSIS

1. Refer to Chart 48-1 in the text.
2. Refer to Figure 48-1 and chapter heading "Physical Assessment: Female Breast" in the text.
3. Refer to Table 48-1 in the text.
4. Refer to chapter heading "Conditions Affecting the Nipple" in the text.
5. Refer to chapter heading "Total Mastectomy" in the text.
6. Refer to Chart 48-7 in the text.
7. Refer to chapter heading "Radiation Therapy" in the text.

CLINICAL SITUATIONS

CASE STUDY: SIMPLE MASTECTOMY

1. c
2. d
3. b
4. c
5. b
6. c
7. a
8. cyclophosphamide (Cytoxan), methotrexate, and fluorouracil (CMF)

IDENTIFYING PATTERNS

Refer to Chart 48-2 in the text.

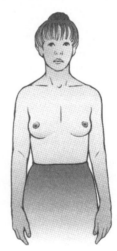

FIGURE 1/Step 1: Stand in front of a mirror. Check both breasts for anything unusual. Look for a discharge from the nipples, puckering, dimpling, or scaling of the skin.

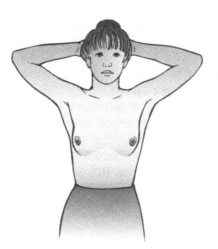

FIGURE 2/Step 2: Watch closely in the mirror as you clasp your hands behind your head and press your hands forward. Note any change in the contour of your breasts.

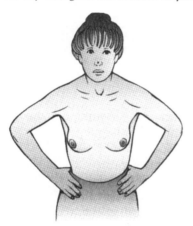

FIGURE 3/Step 3: Next, press your hands firmly on your hips and bow slightly toward the mirror as you pull your shoulders and elbows forward. Note any change in the contour of your breasts.

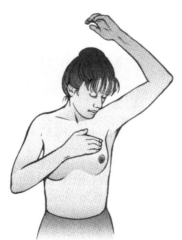

FIGURE 4/Step 4: Raise your left arm. Use three or four fingers of your right hand to feel your left breast firmly, carefully, and thoroughly. Beginning at the outer edge, press the flat part of your fingers in small circles, moving the circles slowly around the breast. Gradually work

toward the nipple. Be sure to cover the whole breast. Pay special attention to the area between the breast and the underarm, including the underarm area itself. Feel for any unusual lump or mass under the skin. If you have any spontaneous discharge during the month—whether or not it is during your BSE—see your doctor. Repeat the examination on your right breast.

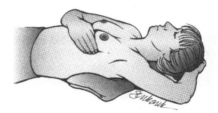

FIGURE 5/Step 5: Step 4 should be repeated lying down. Lie flat on your back, with your left arm over your head and a pillow or folded towel under your left shoulder. This position flattens the breast and makes it easier to check. Use the same circular motion described above. Repeat on your right breast.

Chapter 49

I. Interpretation, Completion, and Comparison

MULTIPLE CHOICE

1. b	8. d	15. a
2. d	9. d	16. c
3. b	10. a	17. b
4. b	11. c	18. a
5. a	12. b	19. c
6. a	13. a	
7. c	14. d	

SHORT ANSWER

1. prostrate-specific antigen (PSA) and digital rectal examination (DRE)
2. Answer should include 4 of 15 medications found in Chart 49-1 in the text.
3. *Escherichia coli*
4. Answer should include four of the following: fever, perineal prostatic pain, dysuria, urinary tract symptoms (frequency, urgency, hesitancy, and nocturia).
5. Answer should include five of the following: frequency of urination, nocturia, urgency and a sensation that the bladder has not emptied completely, hesitancy in starting urination, abdominal straining, a decrease in the volume and force of the urinary stream, recurring urinary tract infections, interruption of the urinary stream, and dribbling.
6. androgen deprivation therapy (ADT); Lupron, Zoladex, Eulexin, Casodex and Nilandron
7. hemorrhage, infection, DVT, catheter obstruction and sexual dysfunction
8. urinary incontinence

9. Heparin is given prophylactically because there is a high incidence of deep vein thrombosis and pulmonary embolism after prostatectomy.
10. Epididymitis is an infection of the epididymis that usually descends from an infected prostate or urinary tract. It passes upward through the urethra and ejaculatory duct and along the vans deferens to the epididymis.
11. human chorionic gonadotropin and alpha-fetoprotein

MATCHING

1. c	5. d
2. f	6. h
3. e	7. g
4. a	8. b

II. Critical Thinking Questions and Exercises

DISCUSSION AND ANALYSIS

1. Refer to Table 49-1 in the text.
2. Refer to chapter heading "Erectile Dysfunction" in the text.
3. Refer to Chart 49-3 in the text.
4. Refer to chapter heading "Benign Prostatic Hyperplasia (Enlarge Prostate)" in the text.
5. Refer to chapter heading "Transurethral Resection of the Prostate" in the text.
6. Refer to Chart 49-3 in the text.
7. Refer to Table 49-1 in the text.

CLINICAL SITUATIONS

CASE STUDY: THE PATIENT UNDERGOING PROSTATECTOMY

1. assessment of general health status and establishment of optimum renal function
2. acute urinary retention develops and damages the urinary tract and collecting system, or before cancer develops
3. d
4. stricture formation and retrograde ejaculation
5. Damage to the pudendal nerves may causes impotence.
6. anxiety related to the surgical procedure and its outcome, pain related to bladder distention, and knowledge deficit about factors related to the problem and the treatment protocol
7. warm compresses to the pubis and sitz baths can help relieve spasm
8. Prolonged sitting increases intra-abdominal pressure and increases the possibility of bleeding.
9. Teach the patient to tense the perineal muscles by pressing the buttocks together, holding the position for 15 to 20 seconds and then relaxing.

Chapter 50

I. Interpretation, Completion, and Comparison

MULTIPLE CHOICE

1. c	8. d	15. b
2. d	9. c	16. d
3. a	10. b	17. a
4. c	11. b	18. c
5. c	12. d	19. d
6. d	13. c	20. a
7. c	14. a	

MATCHING

Immunoglobulins

1. c	5. a
2. e	6. b
3. c	7. a
4. d	

Medications

1. d	5. b
2. b	6. a
3. a	7. e
4. c	

UNSCRAMBLED WORDS

1. Antibody
2. Complement
3. Antigen
4. Helper T cells
5. Phagocytes
6. Interferons

II. Critical Thinking Questions and Exercises

DISCUSSION AND ANALYSIS

1. Disorders arise from excesses or deficiencies of immunocompetent cells, alterations in cellular functioning, immunologic attack on self-antigens, and inappropriate or exaggerated responses to specific antigens.
2. Natural immunity, which is nonspecific, is present at birth. Acquired immunity is more specific and develops throughout life. Active acquired immunity refers to defenses developed by the person's own body. Passive acquired immunity is a temporary immunity transmitted from another source that has developed immunity through previous disease or immunization.
3. Complement is a term used to describe circulating plasma proteins that are made in the liver and activated

when an antibody couples with an antigen. Complement defends the body against bacterial infection, bridges natural and acquired immunity, and disposes of immune complexes and byproducts associated with inflammation.
4. Biologic response modifiers (BMRs) suppress antibody production and cellular immunity.
5. Stem cells continually replenish the body's supply of red and white cells. Once the immune system has been destroyed, stem cells can completely restore it with just a few cells.
6. Refer to Table 50-4 in the text.
7. Refer to Table 50-5 in the text.
8. Refer to Chart 50-3 in the text.

Chapter 51

I. Interpretation, Completion, and Comparison

MULTIPLE CHOICE

1. d
2. d
3. d
4. b
5. b
6. d
7. a
8. b (Refer to Chart 51-1 in the text.)
9. b (Refer to Chart 51-1 in the text.)
10. d (Refer to Chart 51-1 in the text.)

SHORT ANSWER

1. severe infections, autoimmunity, and cancer
2. humoral immunity, T-cell defects, combined B- and T-cell defects, phagocytic disorders, and complement production
3. mature B cells, and plasma cells
4. Pernicious anemia
5. Primary T-cell
6. severe malnutrition

II. Critical Thinking Questions and Exercises

INTERPRETING PATTERNS

1. phagocytic dysfunction
2. B-cell deficiency, probably CVID
3. T-cell deficiency
4. ataxia–telangiectasia
5. a secondary immunodeficiency

EXAMINING ASSOCIATIONS

1. B-lymphocyte
2. CVID
3. progressive neurological deterioration
4. excess occurrences of lysis of erythrocytes

Chapter 52

I. Interpretation, Completion, and Comparison

MULTIPLE CHOICE

1. c	7. c	13. a
2. c	8. c	14. c
3. a	9. c	15. b
4. c	10. c	16. b
5. c	11. d	17. c
6. c	12. b	

SHORT ANSWER

1. 33; 50%; Sub-Saharan Africa; 67%
2. unprotected sex, and the sharing of injection drug use equipment (Refer to Chart 52-1 in the text.)
3. blood, seminal fluid, vaginal secretions, amniotic fluid, and breast milk
4. retroviruses that carry their genetic material in the form of RNA rather than DNA
5. Ora Quick test
6. the ability of pathogens to withstand the effects of medications that are intended to produce toxicity
7. candidiasis
8. alpha-interferon
9. B-cell lymphomas

MATCHING

1. c	5. c
2. b	6. b
3. c	7. a
4. a	8. c

II. Critical Thinking Questions and Exercises

DISCUSSION AND ANALYSIS

1. Refer to Chart 52-2 in the text.
2. Refer to Chart 52-4 in the text.
3. Refer to Chart 52-5 in the text.
4. Primary infection is that period from infection with HIV to the development of HIV-specific antibodies. It is the time during which the viral burden set point is achieved and includes the acute symptoms and early infection phases. During primary infection, a window period occurs in which the person is infected but tests negative on the HIV antibody blood test.
5. Refer to chapter heading "Primary Infection (Acute/Recent HIV Infection, Acute HIV Syndrome)" in the text.
6. Refer to Table 52-3 in the text.
7. Refer to chapter heading "Immune Reconstitution Inflammatory Syndrome" in the text.

8. The lesions are usually brownish pink to deep purple. They may be flat or raised and surrounded by hemorrhagic patches and edema.
9. Refer to chapter heading "HIV Encephalopathy" in the text.
10. Refer to chapter heading "Treatment of Opportunistic Infections" in the text.
11. Refer to chapter heading "The Patient With HIV/AIDS" in the text.

CLINICAL SITUATION

CASE STUDY: ACQUIRED IMMUNODEFICIENCY SYNDROME

1. risky sexual practices and intravenous drug use syndrome, fluid and electrolyte imbalance, and adverse reaction to medications.
2. c
3. c
4. Refer to chapter heading "Nursing Diagnoses" and "The Patient With HIV/AIDS" in the text.
5. Answer may include opportunistic infections, impaired breathing or respiratory failure, wasting syndrome, fluid and electrolyte imbalance, and adverse reaction to medications.
6. Wasting syndrome and electrolyte imbalances and disturbances, especially dehydration
7. d
8. d
9. Refer to Table 52-3 in the text.

Chapter 53

I. Interpretation, Completion, and Comparison

MULTIPLE CHOICE

1. d	12. a
2. c	13. a
3. c	14. a
4. d	15. b
5. a	16. d
6. d	17. d
7. a	18. b
8. b	19. c (a minimum of 0.1 mg/kg)
9. b	20. c
10. d	21. c
11. d	

SHORT ANSWER

1. neutralizing toxic antigens, precipitating the antigens out of solution, coating the surface of the antigens
2. an inappropriate or exaggerated antigen and antibody interaction or response causes tissue injury
3. immunoglobulins
4. the pain and fever seen with inflammatory responses
5. Answer should include two of the following: systemic lupus erythematosus, rheumatoid arthritis, serum

sickness, certain types of nephritis, and some types of bacterial endocarditis.
6. contact dermatitis and latex allergy
7. The RAST measures allergen-specific IgE. It detects the allergen and indicates the quantity necessary to evoke an allergic reaction. Values over 2.0 are significant.
8. penicillin
9. epinephrine in a 1:1,000 dilution given subcutaneously
10. 4 to 10 hours

II. Critical Thinking Questions and Exercises

DISCUSSION AND ANALYSIS

1. An allergic reaction occurs when the body is invaded by an *antigen*, usually a protein that the body recognizes as foreign. The body responds in an effort to destroy the invading antigen. *Antibodies* (protein substances) are produced. When an interaction between the antigen and antibody results in tissue injury, an allergic reaction occurs and chemical mediators are released into the body.
2. Immunoglobulins are a group of serum proteins (antibodies formed by lymphocytes and plasma cells) that bind specifically with certain antigens to neutralize, agglutinate, and destroy various bacteria and foreign cellular material.
3. Refer to chapter heading "Histamine" in the text.
4. Refer to Figure 53-2 in the text.
5. Refer to chapter heading "Skin Tests," "Provocative Testing," and "Radioallergosorbent Test" in the text.
6. Refer to chapter heading "Allergic Disorders" in the text.
7. The systemic reactions of flushing, warmth, and itching rapidly progress to bronchospasm, laryngeal edema, severe dyspnea, cyanosis, and hypotension. Cardiac arrest and coma can occur. Onset can begin within 2 hours postexposure.
8. Refer to chapter heading "Anaphylaxis" and Chart 53-2 in the text.
9. Refer to Table 53-2 in the text.
10. Refer to Table 53-4 in the text.
11. Refer to chapter heading "Latex Allergy" in the text.

CLINICAL SITUATIONS

CASE STUDY: ALLERGIC RHINITIS

1. potential ineffective breathing patterns, related to an allergic reaction; knowledge deficit about allergy and recommended modifications in lifestyle; and impaired adjustment, related to chronicity of condition and need for environmental modifications
2. restoration of a normal breathing pattern, knowledge about the causes and control of allergic symptoms, adjustment to alternations and modifications, absence of complications

3. d
4. d
5. d
6. c

Chapter 54

I. Interpretation, Completion, and Comparison

MULTIPLE CHOICE

1. d	9. c	17. d
2. d	10. d	18. b
3. c	11. b	19. d
4. d	12. c	20. b
5. b	13. b	21. d
6. b	14. d	22. b
7. d	15. a	23. b
8. a	16. a	24. a

MATCHING

1. c	5. f
2. d	6. b
3. e	7. h
4. a	8. g

II. Critical Thinking Questions and Exercises

DISCUSSION AND ANALYSIS

1. Refer to chapter heading "Rheumatic Diseases" in the text.
2. *Exacerbation* is a period of time when the symptoms of a disorder occur or increase in intensity and frequency. *Remission* is a period of time when symptoms are reduced or absent.
3. In *inflammatory* rheumatic disease, the inflammation occurs as the result of an immune response. Newly formed synovial tissue is infiltrated with inflammatory cells (pannus formation), and joint degeneration occurs as a secondary process. In *degenerative* rheumatic disease, synovitis results from mechanical irritation. A secondary inflammation occurs.
4. Refer to Table 54-2 in the text and pages throughout the chapter for your answers.
5. Refer to Table 54-4 in the text.
6. Refer to chapter heading "Persistent, Erosive Rheumatoid Arthritis" in the text.
7. Refer to chapter heading "Polymyalgia Rheumatica" in the text.
8. Refer to chapter heading "Degenerative Joint Disease (Osteoarthritis)" in the text.
9. Refer to chapter heading "Metabolic and Endocrine Diseases Associated With Rheumatic Disorders" in the text.
10. Refer to chapter heading "Fibromyalgia" in the text.

CLINICAL SITUATIONS

CASE STUDY: DIFFUSE CONNECTIVE TISSUE DISEASE

1. b
2. b
3. Answer may include weight loss, fever, anemia, fatigue, lymph node enlargement, and Raynaud's phenomenon.
4. d
5. c
6. COX-2 inhibitors
7. d

CASE STUDY: SYSTEMIC LUPUS ERYTHEMATOSUS (SLE)

1. chemical, hormonal, environmental, and genetic
2. an increase in autoantibody production results from abnormal suppressor T-cell function, leading to immune complex deposition and tissue damage
3. pericardial friction rub, myocarditis, and pericarditis
4. severe anemia, thrombocytopenia, leukocytosis, leukopenia, and positive antinuclear antibodies
5. antimalarial
6. hypertension and atherosclerotic heart disease

INTERPRETING PATTERNS

Refer to Figure 54-1 in the text as a framework for the outline.

Chapter 55

I. Interpretation, Completion, and Comparison

MULTIPLE CHOICE

1. b	5. b
2. a	6. c
3. b	7. c
4. a	

SHORT ANSWER

1. keratinocytes, Merkel cells, Langerhans cells
2. 2 to 3 weeks
3. adipose; temperature
4. alopecia
5. sebaceous and sweat
6. vitamin D
7. Refer to Chart 55-1 in the text.
8. sclera and mucous membrane
9. hypoxia

II. Critical Thinking Questions and Exercises

ANALYZING COMPARISONS

1. skin coloring
2. jaundice

3. immune system
4. Alopecia
5. scurvy
6. Inspection
7. scales

IDENTIFYING PATTERNS

1. Telangiectasis
2. Syphilis
3. Ecchymosis or petechia
4. Urticaria
5. Kaposi's sarcoma

IDENTIFYING PATTERNS

Primary and secondary lesions: answers to 1 to 8 should include any characteristics listed for each lesion in Chart 55-3 in the text.

APPLYING CONCEPTS

1. Thinning of dermis and epidermis at their junction
   a. Appearance of wrinkles
   b. Overlapping skin folds
   c. Appearance of sags
   d. Increased vulnerability to injury
2. Loss of subcutaneous tissue of elastin, fat, and collagen
   a. Diminished protection and cushioning of underlying organs and tissues
   b. Decreased muscle tone
   c. Decreased insulating properties
3. Decreased cellular replacement
   a. Delayed wound healing
   b. Smaller vessels decrease in number and size
4. Decrease in number and function of sweat and sebaceous glands
   a. Dry and scaly skin
5. Reduced hormonal levels of androgens
   a. Decreased sebaceous gland functioning

Chapter 56

I. Interpretation, Completion, and Comparison

MULTIPLE CHOICE

1. d	11. a	21. d
2. b	12. b	22. b
3. c	13. d	23. a
4. d	14. d	24. a
5. b	15. d	25. d
6. d	16. c	26. c
7. c	17. c	27. d
8. b	18. a	28. d
9. b	19. b	29. c
10. b	20. d	30. d

SHORT ANSWER

1. prevent additional damage, prevent secondary infection, revise the inflammatory process, and relieve symptoms
2. have a high moisture vapor transmission rate. Some dressings even have reservoirs to hold excessive exudate.
3. Cytokines are proteins with mitogenic activity that release increased amounts of growth factors into a wound. This process stimulates cell growth and granulation of skin.
4. risk for impaired skin integrity related to changes in the barrier function of the skin
5. acne vulgaris
6. impetigo and folliculitis
7. *Staphylococcus aureus*
8. sepsis and keratoconjunctivitis; infection; skin and mucosal surfaces, lungs, and blood
9. skin cancer; basal cell and squamous cell carcinoma; biopsy and histologic evaluation
10. more than 10 times/year

SCRAMBLEGRAM

TERMS USED TO DESCRIBE DERMATOLOGIC PROBLEMS

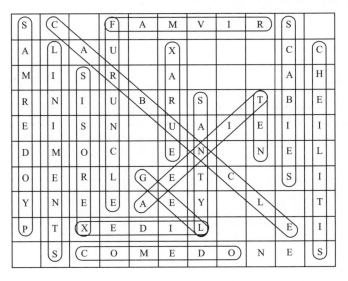

DEFINITION OF TERMS

1. Comedone
2. Cheilitis
3. Carbuncle
4. Furuncle
5. Tinea
6. Pyodermas
7. Liniments
8. Xerosis
9. Santyl
10. Gel
11. Lidex
12. Famvir
13. Scabies
14. Eurax
15. TEN

II. Critical Thinking Questions and Exercises

DISCUSSION AND ANALYSIS

1. Refer to chapter heading "Wound Care for Skin Conditions" in the text.
2. Autolytic debridement is a process whereby the body's own digestive enzymes are used to break down necrotic tissue. A foul odor occurs when cellular debris is broken down. It is normal and expected.
3. Moisture-retentive dressings result in improved fibrinolysis, accelerated epidermal resurfacing, reduced pain, fewer infections, less scar tissue, gentle autolytic debridement, and decreased frequency of dressing changes.
4. Refer to chapter heading "Folliculitis, Furuncles, and Carbuncles" in the text.
5. Refer to chapter heading "Viral Skin Infections" in the text.
6. Refer to chapter heading "Genital Herpes" in the text.
7. Refer to chapter heading "Biological Agents" under chapter heading "Psoriasis" in the text.
8. Refer to chapter heading "Photochemotherapy" in the text.
9. Refer to chapter heading "Toxic Epidermal Necrolysis and Stevens-Johnson Syndrome" in the text.
10. Refer to Chart 56-7 in the text.

CLINICAL SITUATIONS

CASE STUDY: ACNE VULGARIS

1. open comedones, closed comedones, erythematous papules, inflammatory pustules, nodules and inflammatory cysts
2. d
3. c
4. Benzoyl peroxide has an antibacterial effect because it suppresses *Propionibacterium acnes*, depresses sebum production, and helps break down and remove comedone plugs. It produces a rapid and sustained reduction of inflammatory lesions.

5. Vitamin A clears up the keratin plugs from the pilosebaceous ducts by speeding up cellular turnover and forcing the comedone out of the skin.
6. c
7. a
8. scarring and infection

CASE STUDY: MALIGNANT MELANOMA

1. c
2. Those with a melanoma gene, those with a larger number of pigmented lesions, and those with a family history of melanoma.
3. superficial spreading melanoma; trunk and lower extremities
4. d
5. c
6. c
7. d
8. 20% to 50%

Chapter 57

I. Interpretation, Completion, and Comparison

MULTIPLE CHOICE

1. b	13. a	25. c
2. b	14. a	26. b
3. d	15. a	27. b
4. c	16. d	28. c
5. c	17. b	29. c
6. d	18. c	30. b
7. b	19. d	31. c (minimum protein requirement should be 2 g/kg)
8. b	20. b	
9. c	21. c	
10. c	22. b	
11. a	23. a	32. b
12. a	24. c	

SHORT ANSWER

1. young children and the elderly (>age 60)
2. 4.9%
3. Answer should include four of the following seven: age, depth of burn, surface area, presence of inhalation injury, presence of other injuries, location of injury (face, hands), and past medical history.
4. the depth of the injury and the extent of injured body surface area
5. acute respiratory failure and acute respiratory distress syndrome (ARDS)
6. sepsis
7. 0.5 to 1.0 mL/kg/h for adults
8. *Pseudomonas*, methicillin-resistant *Staphylococcus*, and *Actinetobacter*

9. Silver sulfadiazine (Silvadene), silver nitrate, and mafenide acetate (Sulfamylon)
10. increased temperature, tachycardia, widened pulse pressure, and flushed, dry skin in nonburned areas

II. Critical Thinking Questions and Exercises

DISCUSSION AND ANALYSIS

1. Survival after large burn injury has significantly improved because of the following: research in fluid resuscitation, emergent burn treatment, inhalation injury treatment, nutritional needs, and changes in wound care practices.
2. Refer to chapter heading "Extent of Body Surface Area Injured" in the text.
3. Refer to chapter heading "Pathophysiology" under chapter heading "Overview of Burn Injury" in the text.
4. Carbon monoxide, a byproduct of the combustion of organic materials, combines with hemoglobin to form carboxyhemoglobin. Carboxyhemoglobin competes with oxygen for available hemoglobin-binding sites.
5. Refer to Chart 57-3 in the text.
6. Refer to chapter heading "Acute/Intermediate Phase" in the text.
7. Refer to chapter heading "Emergent/Resuscitative Phase" in the text.
8. Refer to chapter heading "Wound Grafting" in the text.
9. Refer to chapter heading "Hypertrophic and Keloid Scars" in the text.
10. Fluid overload may occur when fluid is mobilized from the interstitial compartment back into the intravascular compartment. If the cardiac system cannot compensate for the excess volume, congestive heart failure may result.

IDENTIFYING PATTERNS

FLOW CHART: SYSTEMIC RESPONSE TO BURN INJURY

Refer to Figure 57-3 in the text.

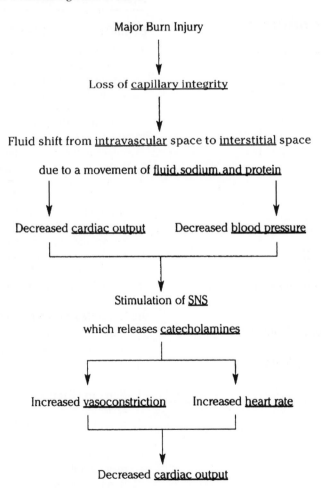

Major Burn Injury

↓

Loss of <u>capillary integrity</u>

↓

Fluid shift from <u>intravascular</u> space to <u>interstitial</u> space

due to a movement of <u>fluid, sodium, and protein</u>

↓ ↓

Decreased <u>cardiac output</u>   Decreased <u>blood pressure</u>

↓

Stimulation of <u>SNS</u>

which releases <u>catecholamines</u>

↓ ↓

Increased <u>vasoconstriction</u>   Increased <u>heart rate</u>

↓

Decreased <u>cardiac output</u>

CLINICAL SITUATIONS

See Plan of Nursing Care (Chart 57-5 in the text) for assistance with the completion of the assignment. A sample is shown below.

AIMEE'S SITUATIONS

Nursing diagnosis: Altered comfort, related to pain resulting from a burn injury

Goals: Pain relief

Nursing actions: Continue developmental growth patterns while providing for skin healing and grafting

Maintain socialization patterns consistent with Aimee's peer group

Assess Aimee's respiratory status

Rationale: Airway compromise can occur rapidly in a significant burn injury as fluid shifts occur

Expected outcome: Aimee has a patient airway and does not exhibit any respiratory distress

Chapter 58

I. Interpretation, Completion, and Comparison

MULTIPLE CHOICE

1. c	7. c	13. c
2 d	8. d	14. c
3. c	9. c	15. a
4. d	10. d	16. c
5. d	11. b	17. b
6. d	12. a	

SHORT ANSWER

1. 10 to 21 mm Hg
2. a person can see an object from 20 ft away that a person with 20/20 vision can see at 100 ft.
3. cataracts, diabetic retinopathy, glaucoma, and macular degeneration
4. glaucoma
5. pallor (lack of blood supply) and cupping of the optic nerve disc
6. laser trabeculoplasty and laser iridotomy
7. cataracts
8. irrigation with normal saline
9. *Streptococcus pneumoniae, Haemophilus influenzae,* and *Staphylococcus aureus*
10. "pink eye," dilation of the conjunctival blood vessels
11. diabetic retinopathy
12. cytomegalovirus (CMV)

MATCHING

1. b	6. e
2. c	7. g
3. f	8. d
4. j	9. h
5. a	10. i

MATCHING

1. g	7. i	13. n
2. o	8. b	14. f
3. e	9. k	15. j
4. m	10. c	16. h
5. p	11. l	
6. a	12. d	

II. Critical Thinking Questions and Exercises

EXTRACTING INFERENCES

Refer to Figure 58-1 in the text.
1. forms, stores, and secretes tears in response to reflex or emotional stimuli
2. dilates and constricts in response to light
3. the highly vascularized, pigmented part of the eye that surrounds the pupil
4. the junction of the conjunctiva
5. protects the intraocular contents from trauma and helps maintain the shape of the eyeball
6. a mucous membrane that provides a barrier to the external environment and nourishes the eye
7. the angles at either end of the slits between the eyelids; no specific function
8. covers the uppermost portion of the iris and washes the cornea and conjunctiva with tears with every blink of the eyes
9. a small, fleshy projection of the lacrimal duct

DISCUSSION AND ANALYSIS

1. Refer to chapter heading "Glaucoma" in the text.
2. Refer to chapter heading "Cataracts" in the text.
3. Refer to chapter heading "Refractive Surgeries" in the text.
4. Refer to chapter heading "Retinal Detachment" in the text.
5. Refer to chapter heading "Age-Related Macular Degeneration" in the text.
6. Refer to chapter heading "Infectious and Inflammatory Conditions" in the text.
7. Refer to chapter heading "Surgical Procedures and Enucleation" in the text.

IDENTIFYING PATTERNS

1. Blepharitis
2. stye (external hordeolum)
3. Conjunctivitis
4. Keratitis
5. Cataract

CLINICAL SITUATIONS

NURSING CARE PLAN

Elise would have several immediate, intermediate, and long-term goals. Following is an example of one with a nursing diagnosis. Page references for assistance with the completion of this care plan are in Chapter 58 of the textbook. A sample is shown below:

Nursing diagnosis:	Altered visual sensory perception related to cataract formation
Goals:	Make Elise familiar with her new environment
	Prepare the affected eye for surgery
	Encourage Elise to walk with her cane as independently as possible
Nursing action:	Assess Elise's level of knowledge about her surgery
Rationale:	Baseline information is necessary to determine teaching plan
Expected outcome:	Elise understands the purpose, process, and expected outcomes of her surgery

CASE STUDY: CATARACT SURGERY

1. smoking, diabetes mellitus, alcohol abuse, and inadequate intake of antioxidant vitamins over time
2. painless blurring of vision, sensitivity to glare, and functional impairment due to reduced visual acuity
3. a grayish pearly haze in the pupil
4. d
5. extracapsular extraction
6. one to two nights

Chapter 59

I. Interpretation, Completion, and Comparison

MULTIPLE CHOICE

1. a	9. d	17. c
2. b	10. b	18. d
3. a	11. c	19. c
4. a	12. d	20. c
5. b	13. c	21. a
6. c	14. d	22. d
7. d	15. d	
8. b	16. a	

II. Critical Thinking Questions and Exercises

DISCUSSION AND ANALYSIS

1. Refer to chapter heading "Sound Conduction and Transmission" in the text.
2. Refer to chapter heading "Evaluation of Gross Auditory Acuity" in the text.
3. Refer to chapter heading "Gerontologic Considerations" under chapter heading "Assessment" in the text.
4. Refer to chapter heading "Conditions of the Inner Ear" in the text.
5. Refer to Table 59-4 in the text.

EXAMINING ASSOCIATIONS

Answers for questions 1 to 11 are related to Figure 59-1, and can be found in Chart 59-1.

CLINICAL SITUATIONS

CASE STUDY: MASTOID SURGERY

1. infection, otalgia, otorrhea, hearing loss, vertigo, erythema, edema, and odor of discharge
2. Answer may include reduction of anxiety, freedom from pain and discomfort, prevention of infection, stabilization/improvement of learning, absence of injury from vertigo, absence of or adjustment to altered sensory perception, return of skin integrity, and knowledge about the disease process and surgical intervention.
3. a sense of aural fullness or pressure (intermittent pain may last for 2 to 3 weeks after surgery)
4. c
5. an elevated temperature and purulent drainage; serosanguineous drainage is normal
6. d
7. c
8. straining, exertion, moving or lifting heavy objects, and nose blowing

CASE STUDY: MÉNIÈRE'S DISEASE

1. Answer may include vertigo, tinnitus, fluctuating and progressive sensorineural hearing loss, a feeling of pressure or fullness in the ear, episodic and incapacitating vertigo accompanied by nausea and vomiting.
2. abnormal inner ear fluid balance caused by malabsorption in the endolymphatic sac or blockage in the endolymphatic duct
3. vertigo
4. b
5. a
6. a

Chapter 60

I. Interpretation, Completion, and Comparison

MULTIPLE CHOICE

1. d	8. d	15. a
2. b	9. d	16. a
3. a	10. a	17. c
4. d	11. b	18. b
5. a	12. c	19. b
6. a	13. a	20. c
7. b	14. c	21. c

MATCHING

1. e	4. c
2. f	5. a
3. d	6. b

II. Critical Thinking Questions and Exercises

DISCUSSION AND ANALYSIS

1. Refer to chapter heading "Blood–Brain Barrier" in the text.
2. Refer to chapter heading "Autonomic Nervous System" in the text.
3. Refer to chapter heading "Sensory System Function" in the text.
4. Refer to chapter heading "Assessment of the Nervous System" in the text.
5. Refer to chapter heading "Examining the Reflexes" in the text.
6. Refer to chapter heading "Diagnostic Evaluation" in the text.

EXAMINING ASSOCIATIONS

AUTONOMIC NERVOUS SYSTEM

Organ or Tissue	Parasympathetic Effect	Sympathetic Effect
a. Bronchi	Constriction	Dilation
b. Cerebral vessels	Dilation	Constriction
c. Coronary vessels	Constriction	Dilation
d. Heart	Inhibition	Acceleration
e. Iris of the eye	Constriction	Dilation
f. Salivary glands	Secretion	Secretion
g. Smooth muscle of		
(1) Bladder wall	Constriction	Inhibition
(2) Large intestine	Increased motility	Inhibition
(3) Small intestine	Increased motility	Inhibition

CRANIAL NERVES

Nerve No.	Column I	Column II
I	Olfactory	Smell
II	Optic	Vision
III	Oculomotor	Eye movement
IV	Trochlear	Eye movement
V	Trigeminal	Facial sensation
VI	Abducens	Eye movement
VII	Facial	Taste and expression
VIII	Vestibulocochlear	Hearing and equilibrium
IX	Glossopharyngeal	Taste
X	Vagus	Swallowing, gastric motility, and secretion
XI	Spinal accessory	Trapezius and sternomastoid muscles
XII	Hypoglossal	Tongue movement

APPLYING CONCEPTS DIAGRAM OF THE BRAIN

THALAMUS

1. Receives, synthesizes, and relays all stimuli except for olfactory stimuli. All memory, sensation, and pain impulses pass through here.
2. Relays impulses to visceral and somatic effectors

HYPOTHALAMUS

1. Maintains sugar and fat metabolism
2. Regulates water balance and metabolism
3. Regulates body temperature
4. Regulates blood pressure
5. Influences the body's response to stress
6. Maintains the sleep–wake cycle
7. Controls the autonomic nervous system
8. Regulates aggressive and sexual behavior

PITUITARY

1. Regulates growth and reproduction
2. Controls various metabolic activities

Chapter 61

I. Interpretation, Completion, and Comparison

MULTIPLE CHOICE

1. d	9. a	17. c
2. d	10. d	18. a
3. a	11. d	19. c
4. c	12. c	20. b
5. b	13. d	21. b
6. d	14. a	22. c
7. c	15. d	23. a
8. c	16. d	24. b

SHORT ANSWER

1. Answer should include five of the following: respiratory distress, pneumonia, aspiration, pressure ulcer, deep vein thrombosis, and contractures.
2. pneumonia, aspiration, and respiratory failure
3. a change in the level of consciousness (LOC)
4. brain stem herniation, diabetes insipidus, and syndrome of inappropriate antidiuretic hormone (SIADH)
5. administer osmotic diuretics and corticosteroids, restrict fluids, drain cerebrospinal fluid, maintain systemic blood pressure, control fever, reduce cellular metabolic demands
6. brain herniation resulting in death
7. cerebral edema, pain, seizures, increased ICP and neurologic status
8. cerebrovascular disease
9. status epilepticus
10. Answer should include six of the following: include bright lights, stress, depression, sleep deprivation, fatigue, foods containing tyramine, monosodium glutamate or nitrates, aged cheese, and oral contraceptives.

MATCHING

1. a and f
2. c and e
3. b
4. a
5. c

II. Critical Thinking Questions and Exercises

DISCUSSION AND ANALYSIS

1. Airway management is a vital nursing function for a patient with altered level of consciousness. The nurse should put the patient in the lateral or semiprone position with the head elevated about 30 degrees, remove secretions from the posterior pharynx and upper trachea by suctioning, perform frequent oral hygiene, auscultate the lungs every 8 hours, and initiate postural drainage and chest physiotherapy.
2. Refer to chapter heading "The Patient With an Altered Level of Consciousness" in the text.
3. Refer to chapter heading "Cerebral Response to Increased Intracranial Pressure" in the text.
4. Refer to chapter heading "Other Neurologic Monitoring Systems" in the text.
5. Refer to chapter heading "Detecting Early Indications of Increasing Intracranial Pressure" in the text.
6. Refer to chapter heading "Regulating Temperature" in the text.
7. Refer to chapter heading "During a Seizure" under chapter heading "Nursing Management" and Chart 61-3 in the text.
8. Refer to Chart 61-4 in the text.
9. Refer to chapter heading "The Epilepsies" in the text.
10. Refer to chapter heading "Migraine" in the text.

INTERPRETING PATTERNS

1. surgery involving removal of a portion of the skull
2. increased blood pressure and decreased heart rate and respirations in response to increased pressure on the medulla oblongata
3. decortication
4. unrelenting pain accompanied by nausea, vomiting, and visual disturbances
5. rhythmic waxing and waning of the rate and depth of respirations alternating with brief periods apnea

CLINICAL SITUATIONS

PLAN OF NURSING CARE: UNCONSCIOUS PATIENT

Refer to chapter heading "The Patient With an Altered Level of Consciousness" and Table 61-1 in the text.

APPLYING CONCEPTS

Refer to Table 61-1 in the text.

Chapter 62

I. Interpretation, Completion, and Comparison

MULTIPLE CHOICE

1. b
2. a
3. a
4. b
5. a
6. d
7. a
8. c
9. d
10. c
11. a
12. b
13. d
14. c
15. d

SHORT ANSWER

1. stroke; brain attack
2. 3 hours
3. age (>55 years), sex (male), race (African American), and ethnicity
4. carotid enterectomy
5. stroke, cranial nerve injuries, infection or hematoma at the incision, and carotid artery disruption
6. decreased cerebral blood flow, inadequate oxygen delivery to the brain, and pneumonia
7. brain tissue, the ventricles or the subarachnoid space
8. rebleeding or hematoma expansion, cerebral vasospasm, acute hydrocephalus, and seizures
9. hypertension

MATCHING

1. d
2. h
3. e
4. a
5. b
6. g
7. c
8. f

II. Critical Thinking Questions and Exercises

DISCUSSION AND ANALYSIS

1. Refer to Table 62-1 in the text.
2. A brain attack is a disruption of cerebral blood flow caused by either an obstruction or the rupture of a blood vessel. Blood alteration initiates a series of cellular metabolic events called an ischemic cascade. Initially, low cerebral blood flow (a penumbra region) exists. Intervention needs to occur at this time, before calcium influx and increased glutamate activate a number of damaging pathways.
3. Refer to Table 62-2 in the text.
4. On the basis of the major nursing diagnoses, the nurse would focus her care on the following interventions, which are not all-inclusive: improving mobility and preventing joint deformities, preventing shoulder pain, enhancing self-care, managing sensory–perceptual difficulties, managing dysphagia, attaining bladder and bowel control, improving communication, maintaining skin integrity, and helping with family coping.
5. Refer to chapter heading "Hemorrhagic Stroke" in the text.

CLINICAL SITUATION

Refer to chapter heading "The Patient Recovering From an Ischemic Stroke" and Charts 62-3 and 62-4 in the text.

Chapter 63

I. Interpretation, Completion, and Comparison

MULTIPLE CHOICE

1. d	8. c	15. b
2. c	9. d	16. d
3. b	10. a	17. a
4. d	11. b	18. b
5. d	12. d	19. b
6. d	13. c	
7. d	14. a	

SHORT ANSWER

1. leakage of cerebrospinal fluid from the ears and the nose
2. obstructed blood flow can decrease tissue perfusion, thus causing cellular death and brain damage
3. Answer should include five of the following: headache, dizziness, lethargy, irritability; anxiety, emotional lability, fatigue, poor concentration, decreased attention span, memory difficulties, and intellectual dysfunction.
4. difficulty in awakening, difficulty in speaking, confusion, severe headache, vomiting, and weakness on one side of the body

5. hematoma, either epidural, subdural, or intracerebral
6. coma, hypertension, bradycardia, and bradypnea
7. coma, absence of brainstem reflexes, and apnea
   Answer should include five of the following seven:
8. decreased cerebral perfusion; cerebral edema and herniation; impaired oxygenation and ventilation; impaired fluid, electrolyte, and nutritional balance; and risk of posttraumatic seizures
9. eye opening, verbal responses, and motor responses to verbal commands or painful stimuli
10. systemic infections, neurosurgical infections, and heterotrophic ossification
11. 5th cervical, 6th cervical, and 7th cervical; 12th thoracic and 1st lumbar
12. pleuritic chest pain, anxiety, and shortness of breath, and abnormal blood gas values
13. deep vein thrombosis, orthostatic hypotension, and autonomic dysreflexia
14. the urinary tract, respiratory tract, and pressure ulcers

II. Critical Thinking Questions and Exercises

DISCUSSION AND ANALYSIS

1. Head injuries, the most common cause of death from trauma in the United States, affect about 1.4 million people. Of these victims, about 50,000 die. Males between the ages of 15 and 19 years are at highest risk.
2. Refer to Chart 63-2 in the text.
3. Refer to chapter heading "Types of Brain Injury" in the text.
4. Refer to chapter heading "Intracranial Hemorrhage" in the text.
5. Brain injury can cause significant brain damage because of obstructed blood flow and decreased tissue perfusion. The brain cannot store oxygen and glucose to any significant degree. Irreversible brain damage and cell death occurs when the blood supply is interrupted for even a few minutes.
6. Acceptable medical standards for defining death, the irreversible loss of all brain function.
7. Refer to Chart 63-5 in the text for a list of activities.
8. Refer to chapter heading "Autonomic Dysreflexia" in the text.

CLINICAL SITUATIONS

PLAN OF NURSING CARE: CERVICAL SPINE INJURY

Refer to chapter heading "The Patient With Acute Spinal Cord Injury" in the text for assistance with the development of a nursing care plan for Katie.

PLAN OF NURSING CARE: PARAPLEGIA

Refer to chapter heading, "The Patient With Tetraplegia or Paraplegia" in the text for assistance with the development of a nursing care plan for Matthew.

Chapter 64

I. Interpretation, Completion, and Comparison

MULTIPLE CHOICE

1. a	7. c
2. a	8. c
3. d	9. b
4. d	10. c
5. c	11. c
6. a	

SHORT ANSWER

1. meningitis, brain abscesses, various types of encephalitis, Creutzfeldt-Jakob disease, and variant Creutzfeldt-Jacob disease
2. severe headache, high fever, a stiff neck (nuchal rigidity), photophobia, a positive Kernig sign, and positive Brudzinski sign
3. herpes simplex virus (HSV); acyclovir (Zovirax), and ganciclovir (Cytovene)
4. a protein kinase inhibitor (protein 14-3-3) in cerebrospinal fluid
5. myelin material that surrounds the nerve fibers in the brain and the spinal cord
6. relapsing–remitting, secondary progressive, and primary progressive
7. acetylcholine receptors
8. double vision, and drooping of the eyelids
9. diabetes with poor glycemic control

MATCHING

1. b	6. f
2. b	7. g
3. e	8. h
4. d	9. h
5. f	10. d

II. Critical Thinking Questions and Exercises

DISCUSSION AND ANALYSIS

1. To assess for *Kernig sign*, the nurse would ask the patient to extend one leg while the opposite thigh is flexed on the abdomen. Inability to do this is considered positive for bacterial meningitis. To assess for *Brudzinski sign*, the nurse would ask the patient to flex his neck. If flexion of the knees and hips occurs at the same time, the test is considered positive for bacterial meningitis.
2. Refer to chapter headings "Arthropod-Borne Virus Encephalitis" and "Fungal Encephalitis" in the text.
3. Demyelination refers to the destruction of myelin, the fatty and protein material that surrounds nerve fibers in the brain and spinal cord. This destruction results in impaired transmission of nerve impulses.
4. Refer to chapter heading "Myasthenic Crisis" in the text.
5. Refer to chapter heading "Guillain-Barré' Syndrome" in the text.

CLINICAL SITUATION

CASE STUDY: MULTIPLE SCLEROSIS

1. d
2. d
3. fatigue and pain
4. a
5. d
6. Rebif, Betaseron, Copaxone, Novantrone, and IV methylprednisolone

Chapter 65

I. Interpretation, Completion, and Comparison

MULTIPLE CHOICE

1. d	6. d	11. b
2. c	7. a	12. b
3. d	8. b	13. d
4. c	9. a	14. a
5. c	10. b	15. c

SHORT ANSWER

1. lung, breast, lower gastrointestinal tract, pancreas, kidney, and skin
2. headache, nausea and vomiting, and papilledema (70% to 75% occurrence)
3. hemiparesis, seizures, and mental status changes
4. intramedullary
5. Answer should include five of the following seven: Parkinson's disease, Huntington's disease, Alzheimer's disease, amyotrophic lateral sclerosis, muscular dystrophies, degenerative disc disease, and (new) postpolio syndrome.
6. tremor, rigidity, bradykinesia, and postural instability
7. fatigue, progressive muscle weakness, cramps, fasciculations (twitching), and incoordination
8. progressive muscle wasting and weakness, and abnormal elevation in blood muscle enzymes
9. C5 to C6 or C6 to C7
10. hematoma at the surgical site, causing cord compression, and neurologic deficit and recurrent or persistent pain after surgery

MATCHING

1. d	5. h
2. c	6. f
3. g	7. b
4. a	8. e

II. Critical Thinking Questions and Exercises

DISCUSSION AND ANALYSIS

1. A variety of physiologic changes can occur, such as increased ICP and cerebral edema, seizure activity and focal neurologic signs, hydrocephalus, and altered pituitary function.
2. Brain tumors are classified according to origin: those arising from the covering of the brain, those developing in or on the cranial nerves, those originating within brain tissue, and metastatic lesions originating elsewhere in the body.
3. Refer to chapter heading "The Patient With Cerebral Metastases or Incurable Brain Tumor" in the text.
4. Refer to chapter heading "Stereotactic Procedures" in the text.
5. Refer to chapter heading "Huntington's Disease" in the text.

CASE STUDY: PARKINSON'S DISEASE

1. d	3. d
2. c	4. b

PLAN OF NURSING CARE: HUNTINGTON'S DISEASE

Refer to Chart 65-5 in the text for assistance with the development of a nursing care plan for Mike.

EXTRACTING INFERENCES

Use chapter headings in the text that are relevant to tumors as a reference as well as Figure 65-1.

Chapter 66

I. Interpretation, Completion, and Comparison

MULTIPLE CHOICE

1. b	6. a
2. a	7. d
3. a	8. b
4. c	9. b
5. a	10. b

MATCHING

1. h	6. e
2. i	7. d
3. b	8. c
4. j	9. a
5. g	10. f

SHORT ANSWER

1. arthritis
2. hip fractures
3. 98%

4. 206
5. 150 mg
6. sternum, ileum, vertebrae, ribs
7. parathyroid hormone and calcitonin
8. 4 months
9. crepitus

SCRAMBLEGRAM

1. Periosteum
2. Ligaments
3. Sarcomere
4. Tendons
5. Osteoporosis
6. Scoliosis
7. Effusion
8. Arthrocentesis

DISCUSSION AND ANALYSIS

1. Protection, support, locomotion, mineral storage, hematopoiesis, and heat production.
2. Refer to chapter heading "Structure and Function of the Skeletal System" in the text.
3. Refer to chapter heading "Bone Formation" in the text.
4. Vitamin D increases calcium in the blood by promoting calcium absorption from the gastrointestinal tract and by accelerating the mobilization of calcium from the bone.
5. Refer to chapter heading "Bone Maintenance" in the text.
6. Refer to chapter heading "Bone Healing" in the text.
7. Refer to chapter heading "Skeletal Muscle Contraction" in the text.
8. Refer to Table 66-1 in the text.
9. Refer to Figure 66-4 in the text.
10. Refer to chapter heading "Diagnostic Evaluation" in the text.

EXTRACTING INFERENCES

Refer to chapter headings "Structure and Function of the Articular System" and "Structure and Function of the Skeletal System" in the text and Figure 66-2.

Chapter 67

I. Interpretation, Completion, and Comparison

MULTIPLE CHOICE

1. c	10. c	19. a
2. b	11. b	20. c
3. b	12. b	21. c
4. d	13. d	22. c
5. a	14. b	23. a
6. d	15. c	24. d
7. b	16. a	25. d
8. d	17. d	
9. b	18. a	

SHORT ANSWER

1. reduce a fracture, correct a deformity, apply uniform pressure to underlying soft tissue, and provide support and stability for weak joints
2. A fiberglass cast is light in weight and water resistant. It is more durable than plaster and water resistant.
3. necrosis, impaired tissue perfusion, pressure ulcer formation, and possible paralysis
4. The toes or fingers should be pink, warm, and easily moved (wiggled). There should be minimal swelling and discomfort. The blanch test should be carried out to determine rapid capillary refill.
5. pain, pallor, pulselessness, paresthesia, and paralysis
6. Answer should include unrelieved pain, swelling, discoloration, tingling, numbness, inability to move fingers or toes, or any temperature changes.
7. compartment syndrome, pressure ulcers, and disuse syndrome
8. to minimize muscle spasms; to reduce, align, and immobilize fractures; to lessen deformities; and to increase space between opposing surfaces within a joint
9. chlorhexidine solution
10. osteomyelitis
11. pressure ulcers, atelectasis, pneumonia, constipation, anorexia, urinary stasis and infection, and venous thromboemboli with PE or DVT
12. unilateral calf tenderness, warmth, redness and swelling (increased calf circumference)

II. Critical Thinking Questions and Exercises

DISCUSSION AND ANALYSIS

1. compartment syndrome, pressure ulcer, disuse syndrome, and delayed union or nonunion of the fracture
2. Answer should include knowledge of the treatment regimen, relief of pain, improved physical mobility, achievement of maximum level of self-care, healing of lacerations and abrasions, maintenance of adequate neurovascular function, and absence of complications.
3. Compartment syndrome occurs when the circulation and function of tissue within a confined area (casted area) is compromised. Treatment requires that the cast be bivalved; a fasciotomy may be necessary. (See Figure 67-2 in the text.)
4. Refer to Chart 67-3 in the text.
5. Volkmann's contracture is a serious complication of impaired circulation in the arm. Contracture of the fingers and wrist occurs as the result of obstructed arterial blood flow to the forearm and the hand. The patient is unable to extend the fingers, describes abnormal sensation, and exhibits signs of diminished circulation to the hand. Permanent damage develops within a few hours if action is not taken.
6. Refer to chapter heading "Nursing Management of the Patient With a Body or Spica Cast" in the text.
7. Refer to chapter heading "The Patient With an External Fixator" and Figure 67-3 in the text.

8. Refer to chapter heading "Principles of Effective Traction" in the text.
9. The major nursing goals for a patient in traction may include understanding of the treatment regimen, reduced anxiety, maximum comfort, maximum level of self-care, maximum mobility within therapeutic limits of traction, and absence of complications.
10. Refer to Chart 67-9 in the text.
11. Refer to Chart 67-10 in the text.
12. Refer to chapter heading "Total Knee Replacement" in the text.
13. Refer to chapter heading "Preoperative Care of the Patient Undergoing Orthopedic Surgery" in the text.

CLINICAL SITUATIONS

CASE STUDY: BUCK'S TRACTION

1. a
2. the patient's body weight and the bed position adjustments
3. inspect the skin for abrasions and circulatory disturbances and make certain the skin is clean and dry before any tape or foam boot is applied
4. d
5. skin color, skin temperature, capillary refill, edema, pulses, sensations, and ability to move
6. malleolus and proximal fibula
7. A positive Homans' sign indicates deep vein thrombosis.

CASE STUDY: TOTAL HIP REPLACEMENT

1. deep vein thrombosis and pulmonary embolism
2. dislocation of the hip prosthesis, excessive wound drainage, thromboembolism, infection, and heal ulcer pressure
3. c
4. d
5. leg shortening, inability to move the leg, abnormal rotation, increased pain, swelling and immobilization at the surgical site, acute groin pain in affected hip, and a reported "popping" sensation
6. b
7. b
8. 3; 24

Chapter 68

I. Interpretation, Completion, and Comparison

MULTIPLE CHOICE

1. d	7. d	13. d
2. b	8. c	14. b
3. b	9. c	15. d
4. c	10. d	16. c
5. a	11. d	17. b
6. c	12. b	

SHORT ANSWER

1. Answer should include five of these conditions: acute lumbosacral strain, unstable lumbosacral ligaments, weak lumbosacral muscles, osteoarthritis of the spine, spinal stenosis, intervertebral disk problems, and unequal leg length.
2. risk for ineffective tissue perfusion; peripheral related to swelling; acute pain related to surgery, inflammation, and swelling; impaired physical mobility related to foot-immobilizing device, and risk for infection related to the surgical procedure/surgical incision
3. reduced bone density, deterioration of bone matrix, and diminished bone architectural strength.
4. age 45 and 55, after menopause
5. Calcitonin, which inhibits bone resorption and promotes bone formation, is decreased. Estrogen, which inhibits bone breakdown, is decreased. Parathyroid hormone, which increases with age, enhances bone turnover and resorption.
6. a deficiency in activated vitamin D (calcitriol), which promotes calcium absorption from the gastrointestinal tract
7. calcitonin, bisphosphonates, and plicamycin

II. Critical Thinking Questions and Exercises

DISCUSSION AND ANALYSIS

1. Refer to Chart 68-2 in the text.
2. Refer to chapter heading "Bursitis and Tendinitis" in the text.
3. Refer to chapter heading "Impingement Syndrome" and Chart 68-4 in the text.
4. Refer to chapter headings "Carpal Tunnel Syndrome" and "Dupuytren's Disease" in the text.
5. Refer to chapter heading "Common Foot Problems" in the text.
6. Refer to Figure 68-4 in the text.
7. Refer to Figure 68-7 in the text.
8. Refer to chapter heading "Paget's Disease of the Bone" in the text.
9. Refer to chapter heading "Septic (Infectious) Arthritis" in the text.

APPLYING CONCEPTS

Refer to Figure 68-6 as a reference and chapter heading "Common Foot Problems" in the text.

CLINICAL SITUATIONS

CASE STUDY: OSTEOPOROSIS

1. the rate of bone resorption is greater than the rate of bone formation
2. women have a lower peak bone mass than men and estrogen loss affects the development of the disorder
3. c
4. a
5. c
6. d

Chapter 69

I. Interpretation, Completion, and Comparison

MULTIPLE CHOICE

1. d	9. d	17. a
2. b	10. a	18. c
3. d	11. b	19. a
4. b	12. b	20. d
5. c	13. a	21. c
6. d	14. d	22. d
7. a	15. b	
8. b	16. d	

MATCHING

PART I

1. c	3. b
2. a	4. e

PART II

1. c	3. a
2. b	4. d

SHORT ANSWER

1. tissue death due to anoxia and diminished blood supply
2. the rubbing of bone fragments against each other
3. osteomyelitis, tetanus, and gas gangrene
4. Early: Answer should include three of the following: shock, fat embolism, compartment syndrome, deep vein thrombosis, thromboembolism, DIC, and infection. Delayed: Answer should include three of the following: delayed union and nonunion, avascular necrosis of bone, reaction to internal fixation devices, complex regional pain syndrome (CRPS), and heterotrophic ossification.
5. stabilizing the fracture to prevent further hemorrhage, restoring blood volume and circulation, relieving the patient's pain, providing proper immobilization, and protecting against further injury
6. deep vein thrombosis, thromboembolism, and pulmonary embolus
7. Colles' fracture
8. deep vein thrombosis
9. atelectasis and pneumonia
10. abduction, external rotation, and flexion
11. flexion contracture of the hip

II. Critical Thinking Questions and Exercises

EXAMINING ASSOCIATIONS

1. an injury to the ligaments around a joint
2. subluxation

3. surgical repair
4. failure of the fractured bone ends to unite
5. allograft
6. trochanteric region

DISCUSSION AND ANALYSIS

1. Refer to chapter heading "Contusions, Strains, and Sprains" in the text.
2. Refer to chapter heading "Types of Fractures" in the text.
3. Refer to chapter heading "Types of Fractures" in the text.
4. Refer to Chart 69-2 in the text.
5. Refer to chapter heading "Fat Embolism Syndrome" in the text.
6. Refer to chapter heading "Compartment Syndrome" in the text.
7. Refer to chapter heading "Avascular Necrosis of Bone" in the text.
8. Refer to chapter heading "Hip" under chapter heading "Fractures of Specific Sites" in the text.

EXTRACTING INFERENCES

1. medial collateral ligament; acute onset of pain, point tenderness, and joint stability; hemarthrosis
2. anterior or posterior cruciate ligament (ACL); near-normal ROM has returned; 6 to 12
3. meniscal injury; MRI; an effusion into the knee joint; 1 to 2 days

CLINICAL SITUATIONS

CASE STUDY: ABOVE-THE-KNEE AMPUTATION

1. d	5. a
2. d	6. d
3. d	7. b
4. d	8. d

Chapter 70

I. Interpretation, Completion, and Comparison

MULTIPLE CHOICE

1. c	8. d	15. d
2. a	9. a	16. d
3. d	10. c	17. c
4. d	11. c	18. d
5. c	12. d	19. d
6. d	13. d	
7. a	14. d	

SHORT ANSWER

1. Colonization is used to describe microorganisms present without host interference or interaction.
2. Infection indicates a host interaction with an organism.
3. the smear and stain, the culture and organism identification, and the antimicrobial susceptibility
4. The World Health Organization and the Centers for Disease Control and Prevention
5. coagulase-negative staphylococci and diphtheroids; *Staphylococcus aureus*, and *Pseudomonas aeruginosa*
6. *Clostridium difficile*, methicillin-resistant *Staphylococcus aureus* (MRSA) and Vancomycin-resistant *Enterococcus* (VRE)
7. Pneumococcus and meningococcus
8. Refer to Table 70-3 in the text.
9. Tamiflu, Relenza
10. Refer to Table 70-4 in the text.
11. sexually transmitted diseases; 19; Chlamydia trachomatis and *Neisseria gonorrhoeae*
12. West Nile virus, Legionnaire's disease, pertussis, Hanta virus, and viral hemorrhagic fevers
13. pneumonia; Zithromax, Erythrocin, and Biaxin
14. Ebola and Marburg viruses

MATCHING

1. a	5. f
2. d	6. c
3. b	7. g
4. e	8. h

II. Critical Thinking Questions and Exercises

EXAMINING ASSOCIATIONS

Use Figure 70-1 to fill in each blank. Use terms on the perimeter of each link as a guide for choosing a nursing intervention.

DISCUSSION AND ANALYSIS

1. Refer to chapter heading "The Infectious Process" in the text.
2. Refer to chapter heading "Isolation Precautions" in the text.
3. Refer to Chart 70-2 in the text.
4. Refer to chapter heading "Common Vaccines" in the text.
5. Refer to chapter heading "Planning for an Influenza Pandemic" in the text.
6. Refer to Chart 70-5 in the text.
7. Refer to chapter heading "The Patient With a Sexually Transmitted Disease" in the text.

Chapter 71

I. Interpretation, Completion, and Comparison

MULTIPLE CHOICE

1. c	8. b	15. c
2. b	9. c	16. d
3. d	10. a	17. d
4. c	11. d	18. d
5. b	12. d	19. a
6. b	13. c	
7. a	14. d	

SHORT ANSWER

1. Refer to Chart 71-1 in the text.
2. hepatitis B, hepatitis C, and human immunodeficiency virus (HIV)
3. speak, breathe, or cough; 3 to 5 months
4. tachycardia, hypotension, thirst, apprehension, cool and moist skin, and delayed capillary refill
5. weakness, hypotension, tachycardia, thirst; 104°F
6. drowning
7. 1 to 9 years
8. 4 to 12 hours
9. syrup of ipecac

II. Critical Thinking Questions and Exercises

DISCUSSION AND ANALYSIS

1. Refer to chapter heading "Providing Holistic Care" in the text.
2. Refer to chapter heading "Triage" in the text.
3. Refer to chapter heading "Establishing an Airway" and Charts 71-3 and 71-4 in the text.
4. Refer to chapter heading "Control of External Hemorrhage" in the text.
5. Lactated Ringer's solution is initially useful because it approximates plasma electrolyte composition and osmolality, allows time for blood typing and screening, restores circulation, and serves as an adjunct to blood component therapy.
6. Refer to chapter heading "Crush Injuries" in the text.
7. Refer to chapter heading "Heat Stroke" and Chart 71-7 in the text.
8. Refer to Chart 71-9 in the text.
9. Refer to chapter heading "Ingested (Swallowed) Poisons" in the text.
10. Refer to chapter heading "Carbon Monoxide Poisoning" in the text.
11. Refer to chapter heading "Alcohol Withdrawal Syndrome/Delirium Tremens" in the text.
12. Refer to chapter heading "Sexual Assault" in the text.
13. Refer to chapter heading "Posttraumatic Stress Disorder" in the text.

APPLYING CONCEPTS

Refer to Chart 71-3 in the text.

CLINICAL SITUATIONS

1. Refer to chapter heading "Intra-Abdominal Injuries" in the text.
2. Refer to chapter heading "Anaphylactic Reaction" in the text.
3. Refer to Chart 71-11 in the text.
4. Refer to Table 71-1 in the text.
5. Refer to chapter heading "Psychiatric Emergencies" in the text.

Chapter 72

I. Interpretation, Completion and Comparison

MULTIPLE CHOICE

1. c	6. b	11. a
2. d	7. d	12. b
3. b	8. b	13. d
4. c	9. c	14. a
5. b	10. b	

SHORT ANSWER

1. anthrax; chlorine
2. Department of Health and Human Services; Department of Justice; Department of Defense and Department of Homeland Security
3. California, Colorado, and North Carolina
4. The Incident Command System is a management tool for organizing personnel, facilities, equipment, and communication for any emergency. Its activation during emergencies is mandated by the federal government.
5. the degree and nature of the exposure to disaster, loss of loved ones, existing coping strategies, available resources and support, and personal meaning attached to the event
6. *Defusing* is a process by which an individual receives education about recognition of stress reactions and management strategies for handling stress. *Debriefing* is a more complicated intervention; it involves 2- to 3-hour processes during which participants are asked about their emotions, symptoms, and any other psychological ramifications.
7. anthrax and smallpox
8. ciprofloxacin or doxycycline; 100%
9. 30%
10. Pulmonary chemical agents act by destroying the pulmonary membrane that separates the alveolus from the capillary bed. When this happens, the individual cannot release carbon dioxide or acquire oxygen.

II. Critical Thinking Questions and Exercises

DISCUSSION AND ANALYSIS

1. Refer to Chart 72-1 in the text.
2. Refer to chapter heading "Components of the Emergency Operations Plan" in the text.
3. A critically ill individual with a high mortality rate would be assigned a low triage priority because it would be unethical to use limited resources on those with a low chance of survival. Others who are seriously ill and have a greater chance of survival should be treated.
4. Some cultural considerations include language differences, a variety of religious preferences (hygiene, diet, medical treatment), rituals of prayer, traditions for burying the dead, and the timing of funeral services.
5. Some common behavioral responses are depression, anxiety, somatization (fatigue, malaise), posttraumatic stress disorder, substance abuse, interpersonal conflicts, and impaired performance.
6. Refer to chapter heading "Blast Injury" in the text.
7. Refer to chapter heading "Anthrax" in the text.
8. Refer to chapter heading "Smallpox" in the text.
9. Refer to chapter heading "Nerve Agents" in the text.
10. Refer to chapter heading "Types of Radiation" in the text.
11. Refer to chapter heading "Acute Radiation Syndrome" in the text.